PUBLIC HEALTH

AN UNHEALTHY CONCEIT

GARY JOHNS

AND

SAMARA MCPHEDRAN

Connor Court Publishing

Public Health: an unhealthy conceit

Gary Johns and Samara McPhedran

Published in 2026 by Connor Court Publishing Pty Ltd

Connor Court Publishing Pty Ltd
PO Box 7257
Redland Bay QLD 4165
sales@connorcourt.com
www.connorcourt.com

ISBN: 9781923568914

Cover Design by Maria Giordano

Image: Wikipedia Commons

Printed in Australia

Table of Contents

Figures

Tables and Text Boxes

Introduction

Public health. Could there be anything more benign or praiseworthy? The term evokes images of sanitation reaching the impoverished slums of Dickensian London or smiling children spared from the ravages of smallpox and polio. From mass vaccination campaigns that have nearly eradicated some of the world's most debilitating and contagious diseases, to environmental and urban engineering initiatives that have significantly lowered childhood deaths from gastrointestinal illnesses, the accomplishments of public health have improved countless lives worldwide.

Infant and child mortality rates have significantly dropped because diseases that were particularly deadly to infants and young children, such as measles, smallpox, polio, tuberculosis, and others, have been stopped through inoculation. Medical science played a vital role, as did mothers' and carers' awareness and vigilance. Adult mortality has also decreased dramatically because ischaemic heart disease and cerebrovascular disease—and, to a lesser extent, cancers—have been curtailed through improvements in treatment and in managing risk factors like smoking. Both medical science regarding cause and effect and consumer awareness of these issues have been essential, with public health playing a key role in raising awareness and understanding.

There is no doubt that widespread awareness and education campaigns on topics such as cancer, transmissible diseases, hygiene, and nutrition have had a profoundly positive impact. To give credit where it is due, there is much to thank public health for. Or, at least, to thank the brand of public health that is genuinely concerned about health. There is also little doubt that interventions can reduce harm. Tobacco consumption decreased by half in the last 20 years (Figure 4.1). Alcohol consumption per capita, which rose substantially during the 1970s and 1980s, has returned to the levels of the 1960s.[1] In allied fields of behavioural concern, it is possible to improve by changing behaviour. Campaigns about skin cancer and how to be sun-safe, for example, have made inroads into mortality from that cause.[2] Road deaths and accidents have been reduced through legislation that lowered speed limits, required seatbelt use, and tested driver competence. The campaigns were driven largely by surgeons.[3]

These success stories are undeniable. They are also where our thinking is meant to begin and end. We are not meant to contemplate, even for a moment, that public health could be in any way self-serving. We are certainly not meant to consider the possibility that public health could be used for political purposes or can actively cause harm. But it has. The focus of public health has shifted firmly towards the social and political, at the expense of health. Marking this divide, we see one brand of public health that continues to work hard at providing people with sound, scientifically based, medically supported information so that they can make good choices, while the other brand – although hiding behind the façade of science and medicine — is concerned only with using coercive, authoritarian means to remove an individual's right to make bad choices, punish them for doing so, or both.

What we see today is the culmination of a long march. As early as 1923, for example, public health was defined as:

> *The science and the art of preventing disease, prolonging life, and promoting physical health and efficiency through organized community efforts for the sanitation of the environment, the control of community infections, the education of the individual in principles of personal hygiene, the organization of medical and nursing services for the early diagnosis and preventative treatment of disease, and the development of the social machinery which will ensure to every individual in the*

1 Australian Bureau of Statistics, 2019. *Apparent Consumption of Alcohol, Australia.*

2 Australian Institute of Health and Welfare, 2016. *Skin Cancer in Australia*

3 Australian Bureau of Statistics, 2010. *Year Book Australia, 2009-10* and Bureau of Infrastructure and Transport Research Economics, 2022. *Road Trauma Australia, Statistical Summary 2021*

> *community a standard of living adequate for the maintenance of health.*[4] (Emphasis added)

Public health – unlike medicine – therefore only exists through social action. And who is best positioned to take 'social action'? That, invariably, is the government, with its extensive array of levers and coercive powers – legislation and taxation being at the top of those. Seen in this light, it is no wonder that public health has long been preoccupied with securing the state's powers to advance its own ends.[5]

The coercive leanings of public health are, of course, disguised behind a carefully manufactured guise of altruism. In Australia, for example, the Commonwealth's National Preventive Health Strategy claims that it simply wants to stop Australians from becoming ill by tackling the 'causes of the causes' of ill health.[6] The Public Health Association of Australia boldly claims, 'Our goal is to make everyone in Australia less sick.'[7] The Australian Health Promotion Association 'seeks to advance the health of all people in Australia.'[8] Their journal, Health Promotion Journal of Australia, addresses 'social and ecological determinants of health.'[9] Others, publishing in the Australian and New Zealand Journal of Public Health, extend the brief to include the 'commercial determinants of health.'[10]

---

4 Winslow C E A, 1923. *The Evolution and Significance of the Modern Public Health Campaign.* Yale University Press: New Haven, 1

5 Flanigan J, 2024. Political Ideology and Public Health. *Social Philosophy and Policy* 41(2), 508

6 Commonwealth of Australia Department of Health, 2021. *National Preventive Health Strategy, 2012-2030.* Another example is the Australian Prevention Partnership Centre https://preventioncentre.org.au/work/research-projects/. Note, all references to the Commonwealth are to the government of the Commonwealth of Australia.

7 Public Health Association Australia https://www.phaa.net.au/Web/Web/About/About.aspx

8 Australian Health Promotion Association https://www.healthpromotion.org.au

9 https://onlinelibrary.wiley.com/journal/22011617

10 Heenan M, Ralph M & Shantosh J, 2024. Why public health acts could be our best chance to stem the tide of non-communicable diseases. *Australian and New Zealand Journal of Public Health*, 2. See also, Gilmore A B, 2023. Defining and conceptualising the commercial determinants of health. *The Lancet* 2023(401), 1194

Aside from claims of just wanting everybody to be healthy, the authoritarian branch of public health turns to economic arguments – saying, for instance, that drinking, smoking, gambling, and gluttonous fat slob 'sinners' are ruining the nation and that stopping them would save billions of dollars. In truth, the public health lobby seeks to use government powers to regulate consumer choice or to tax all consumers for the consumption habits of a few, despite evidence that taxation can be punitive or ineffective, or lead to serious unanticipated consequences, such as the creation of black markets and tax evasion. The public health lobby insists that anything that even remotely touches upon health in any way, shape or form, no matter how tangentially or distantly, is fodder for public health meddling.

Social, not medical issues

What is more, public health now concerns itself chiefly with social, not medical, issues – or, as it likes to call them, 'the social determinants of health'. However, the observation that, for example, the poor may, on average, be less healthy than the rich does not suggest a remedy. Making poor people less poor through tax transfers may help, but taxation and transfers have their downsides; they punish the doers but do not make the poor any more capable. They can make everyone poorer by discouraging entrepreneurs. What about Aboriginal health? A belief in Aboriginal community control became the public health answer to 'closing the gap', but there has not been a payoff for the health of Aborigines. The advocates overlooked measuring actual health outcomes; instead, they focused on measuring ownership and control, which are political goals.

The next trend was gender dysphoria, where the belief in gender overrode the science of sex. The gender affirmation model assumes only one solution to what are frequently complex mental health problems. It is an ideology based on minority rights, not health. Then came the COVID-19 response. Which public were public health advisers thinking of when their fearmongering advice led governments to strangle entire economies, the education of children, and lives with vaccines that had barely passed standard scientific scrutiny?[11] The public health advisers suffered under the delusion that the state could stop a virus. Politicians and media editors were sometimes eager participants, other times captive to the authority borne by those who, although holding medical qualifications, were quick to decide that 'first, do no harm' meant that only certain types of harm should be considered. The actual harm their advice caused was immense.

Public health ideologues demonise commercial actors, big tobacco, big alcohol, big pharmacy, big sugar and the like, who allegedly protect their interests, 'often at the expense of public health, the environment and democracy.'[12] These ideologues cite health-harming and planet-harming industries, including tobacco, alcohol, gambling, pharmaceuticals, ultra-processed foods and beverages, firearms and weapons, automobiles, social media and technology, oil and gas, and chemicals. Indeed, almost every product that makes life in the modern world more comfortable, efficient, and enjoyable, and not a single communicable disease among them.[13]

The ideologues aim to ensure that the next generation of public health practitioners learns more than mere epidemiology, biostatistics, evaluation methods, and health economics. They want these graduates to be players in a political game that holds that the social, political, and economic determinants of health are the primary causes of poor health and health inequities, and that government regulations and progressive

11 In April 2023 a class action was filed on behalf of three lead applicants against the Australian Government, the Department of Health and Aged Care Secretary and the Deputy Secretary of Health Products Regulation Group in the Federal Court of Australia on Covid-19 vaccination injured parties to recover compensation for injuries obtained as a result of taking one or more Covid-19 vaccines. The matter is ongoing although an interlocutory matter was decided in *Rose v Secretary of the Department of Health and Aged Care* [2025] FCA 339. Leave to appeal has been sought.

12 Lacy-Nichols J et al, 2022. The public health playbook: ideas for challenging the corporate playbook. *Lancet Global Health* 10(7), e1067. See also, Backholer K et al, 2021. Australia in 2030: what is our path to health for all? *Medical Journal of Australia* May 214(Supplement 8), S5

13 Heenan M, Ralph M & Shantosh J, 2024, 2

taxation are the most effective tools for protecting public health. To them, public health is the sword and shield against the forces of evil. Evil, such as online food delivery,[14] and the vaguest of concepts, food insecurity.[15] And for good measure, a global 'syndemic' (they probably mean sindemic to reflect better what is a moral crusade), the triple whammy of malnutrition, now incorporating underfed and overfed, and climate change.[16] And, of course, there is the mere slip of pretence at rationality, return on investment, to reduce future national health expenditure.[17]

Proper public health – such as putting an end to smallpox — is based on science: the science of disease transmission, physiological reality, and cause-and-effect. Too often, however, public health is an ideological pursuit that uses medicine as a cover: medicine in the service of ideology. Some argue that this new type of social issue-focused public health emerged in the second half of the 20th century. This makes it easier to believe that the elite group of bureaucrats, academics, and NGOs who use the mantle of public health to seek power and push their own views about the world – along with a never-ending ticket to leech off the public purse – are an aberration. It makes it seem as if the most egregious examples of public health authoritarianism are recent

---

14 Miles H et al, 2022. Describing and characterising on-demand delivery of unhealthy commodities in New Zealand. *Australian and New Zealand Journal of Public Health* 46(4). See also, Pettigrew S et al, 2023. The inexorable rise of automated food deliveries and potential anticipatory policy actions. *Australian and New Zealand Journal of Public Health* 47(4)

15 Lindberg R et al, 2024. Revising a right to food road map: perspectives of Australian key informants. *Australian and New Zealand Journal of Public Health* 48(5). See also, Carrad A, 2022. Australian local government policies on creating a healthy, sustainable, and equitable food system: analysis in New South Wales and Victoria. *Australian and New Zealand Journal of Public Health* 46(3), 332

16 Swinburn B A et al, 2019. The global syndemic of obesity, undernutrition, and climate change: the Lancet Commission report. *Lancet* 393(10173), 791. See also, Weeramanthri T S et al, 2020. *Climate Health WA Inquiry: Final Report.* Department of Health, Government of Western Australia

17 Masters R et al, 2017. Return on investment of public health interventions: a systematic review. *Journal of Epidemiology Community Health* 71, 827. See also, Public Health Association of Australia, 2018. Top 10 public health successes over the last 20 years. *PHAA Monograph Series No. 2*

developments, brought about by sheer coincidence – or perhaps by an unpleasant minority who have risen to positions of influence. In fact, not much has changed since the mid-19th century. The ideologies and ambitions of an elite class have long guided public health.

From its emergence as a response to industrialisation in the mid-19th century, public health has continually sought authority in the name of the greater good. From the early 20th century, it has used statistics to find new problems with increasingly broad causes. From the 1960s, it came to focus on non-communicable conditions associated with individual behaviours like smoking. From the 1980s, overeating, overworking, drug and alcohol use, sedentary lifestyles, social and psychological stress, mental health problems, and suicide became pressing concerns. This was particularly so in countries that enjoyed good economic and hygiene standards and, therefore, may have been questioning why they really needed taxpayer-funded public health types telling them how to live, causing those public health types to panic that their influence, power, and position may evaporate if they did not come up with more problems that only they could solve.

Today, public health is invoked in the context of unemployment, social isolation, poverty, low education levels, violence, corruption, crime, civil war, war in general, genocide, the spread of weapons of mass destruction, environmental degradation, fires, hurricanes, floods, climate change, mass migration, displacement of populations, and economic decline. Can these things affect well-being? Certainly, but just because something affects well-being does not mean it requires a public health response. Public health, however, vehemently disagrees. And it is this ever-expanding gambit of the public health response that motivates this book.

Public health's ever-expanding sphere provides it with an almost endless licence to meddle, but it also raises the question: what, exactly, is public health? It has been said that:

> *What is considered part of the domain of applicability of public health*

> *is flexible to the point of near universal inclusivity: almost anything can be viewed as a public health issue....*[18]

Public health is certainly not medicine. Medicine focuses on the diagnosis and cure of individuals, based on relationships between cause and effect. Cause and effect have never really interested public health. Instead, it has long co-opted epidemiology to identify and monitor 'determinants' of 'health' in each population (which can range from members of a particular group who engage in activities such as drinking alcohol to an entire country or, indeed, the entire world). It has also long relied on the coercive powers of the state to address those determinants.

Often, public health now means trying to force individuals to change their behaviour and societies to change their structures. Public health is fundamentally about social engineering. Public health is also about defining who is, and who is not, worthy – as we saw during the COVID-19 pandemic. The health apartheid measures of that time, initially embraced with enthusiasm, have since become a source of shame for anybody with a conscience – even some of those who fiercely embraced and actively peddled them. But public health as a tool for giving power to the elite to decide who should be excluded from nice society — meaning, the society that conforms to those elites' worldview and interests — has a long tradition. It continues to be used as a tool for setting certain groups above others.

It has been the practice of governments since the beginnings of the welfare state to restrict, to some degree, individuals' choices for their own good and that of society. It is also common for governments to impose additional obligations on those receiving welfare benefits. In both instances, a degree of regulation is justified when harm is apparent, its cause is direct, its effects are irreversible, and the means to stop the damage are not too taxing. But governments, with the frantic urging of the public health industry, have begun to act as if your body belongs to them. They have become parents, telling childlike citizens how to

18 Rickles D, 2011. Public health. In F. Gifford (Ed) *Handbook of the Philosophy of Science*. Volume 16. Elsevier: Netherlands.

behave: instructing, forbidding, taxing, and berating them about their personal choices. The degree of regulation is not justified when the harm is not obvious, direct, or irreversible, and when the means to prevent it are too burdensome.

There is a significant amount of unjustified intervention, often referred to as paternalism, in the name of public health. The result of paternalism is that sinners sometimes lose more than they gain; occasional indulgers and non-sinners almost always lose. Of course, taxpayers are vitally interested in the expense imposed by sinners on others – spillover costs are a genuine concern. Beyond that, trying to save people from themselves is a moral question. It should not involve the taxpayer. But to paraphrase Australian economist Jonathan Pincus, public health lobbyists are past masters at making 'each person's decisions a matter of momentous financial consequence for others', which 'gives them an excuse to control those decisions.'[19] The public health activist's trick has been to argue that 'if it only saves one life' it is worth it and saving one life saves you money. This is not true. Trying to convince others to live better is the work of missionaries, not scientists. Public health experts should be stripped of their pseudo-scientific attire and cloaked in sackcloth and ashes.

Context

Whatever claims public health may make on improving the health of all Australians, it must do so in the context of three salient facts. Australians live longer and healthier lives. A male born in 2010 can expect to live 80 years, while a female can expect to live 84 years. A century earlier, a male could expect to live to 55 years, while a female could expect to live to 59 years (Figure I.1). The rate of improvement, however, has slowed dramatically in the last 30 years or so. Any new investments are likely to bring modest returns in terms of longevity.

19 As recalled by Henry Ergas, Sugar coating hard truths about obesity tax. *The Australian* 28 November 2016

Figure I.1 Life expectancy (years) at birth in Australia, by sex, 1881 to 2021

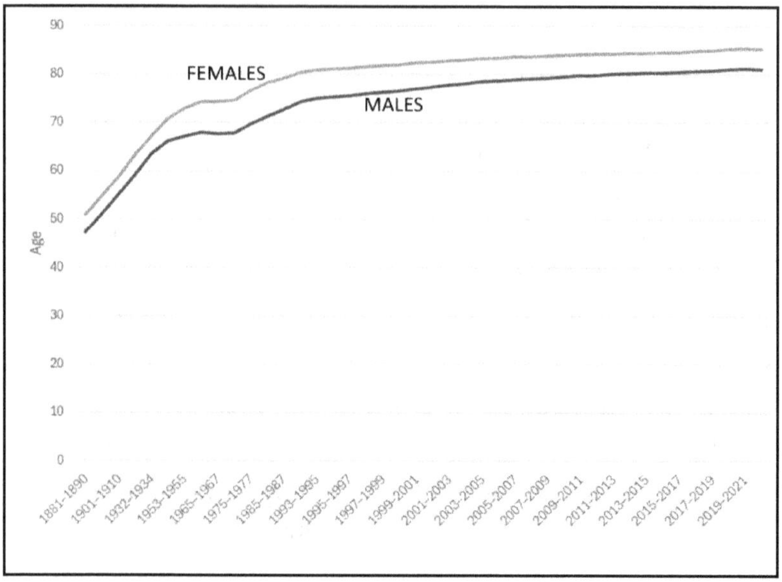

Source: Australian Institute of Health and Welfare, 2024. *Deaths in Australia*

Second, while the likelihood of living longer without disability continues to rise, so do the years of living with disability (Figure I.2).[20] Life expectancy is rising, life free from disability is rising, and years of life with disability are rising. The medical costs of longevity are rising. Third, non-medical costs of healthy ageing are also rising.[21] Any public health study that claims to demonstrate savings in harm prevention or health promotion, for example, should be treated with caution. Public health studies often focus on end-of-life health costs while overlooking the health costs of additional years of life, for example, by disregarding welfare payments or assuming that promoting healthy ageing will lower healthcare costs.[22] How much of any advances in public health, as opposed to medical science, can be made is bound to be highly scrutinised.

20 Australian Institute of Health and Welfare, 2024. *Australian Burden of Disease Study 2024*

21 Snowdon C, 2015. Death and taxes: why living longer costs money. Institute for Economic Affairs, *Discussion Paper* 67, 30

22 Snowdon C, 2015, 30

Figure I.2 Life expectancy and life-adjusted life expectancy over time by sex at age 65

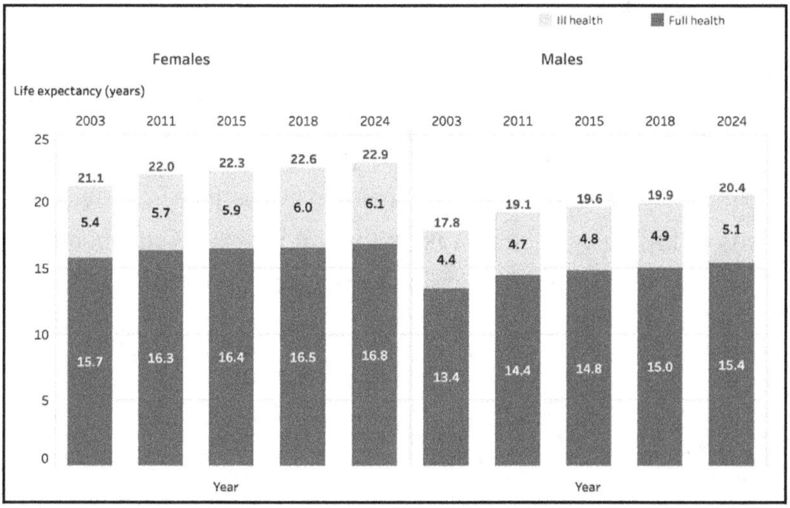

Source: Australian Institute of Health and Welfare, 2024. *Australian Burden of Disease Study 2024*

Chapter outlines

This book draws on some of the most high-profile current examples of how the noble-sounding mantle of public health has been exploited as a smokescreen for ideology, political agendas, and personal power grabs. In doing so, it shows how public health has misled the public about its actual goals, purpose, and desires. We do not delve into the details of, for example, the discovery of pathogens or the development of vaccines. Those are fascinating topics, but they rightly belong in the realm of medicine, where tangible, physical facts and direct cause-and-effect matter. This book focuses on where public health resides — the social and political. Most importantly, it opens a conversation about how to combat the insidious influence of public health actors.

1. Public Health: history repeats

Some argue that the new public health, which focuses primarily on social issues, emerged in the second half of the 20th century. This makes it easier to believe that the elite group of bureaucrats, academics, and

NGOs who use the mantle of public health to seek power and push their views about the world, along with a never-ending ticket to raid the public purse, are an aberration.

It makes it seem like the most egregious examples of public health excesses — like fat taxes, climate change and the COVID-19 response — are recent developments, brought about by sheer coincidence — or, perhaps, by an unpleasant minority who happen to have risen to positions of influence. The fact is, not much has changed since the mid-19th century. The ideologies and ambitions of an elite class have long guided public health.

The public health approach

2. Health Determinants: change society

What causes some individuals to lead less healthy and shorter lives than others? What are effective remedies? Unless the causes of illness are well understood and responses are effective, public health will not positively contribute to health outcomes. There are two competing strategies in public health: one that emphasises external causes —things that happen to people —and the other, rooted in genetic science, which asserts that DNA influences most illnesses, including behaviours that are likely to result in poor health.

The dominant group in public health focuses on the external environment (social and other determinants of health). For them, the holy grail is achieving equality in health outcomes or, even more ambitiously, equity in health, reflecting a deep concern over unfair outcomes caused by social, economic, and political processes. The minority group, guided by genetics, understand that bodies and health outcomes are inherently unequal.

3. Public Health Acts: instruments of oppression

Public health relies on the state's coercive powers. This came to the forefront during COVID-19, when emergency declarations, along with State and Territory public health legislation and subsequent directions, gave license to many travesties. Lawmakers and large sections of society tolerated it, and some watchdogs were asleep.

The Australian Human Rights Commission raised concerns about the increasing authoritarianism in response to COVID-19. Unfortunately, the Victorian Equal Opportunity and Human Rights Commission seemed indifferent to Victorians confined for an unprecedented time under the Human Rights and Victoria's *COVID-19 Omnibus (Emergency Measures) Act* of May 2020. The Commissioner prioritised workplace equality and addressed racism but paid little attention to the widespread confinement of the population and the arrests of individuals for peaceful protests.

While it is comforting to think that such measures could (or would) only ever be used during unusual events like COVID-19, the reality is that public health legislation is now so broad that it can apply to almost anything. Those powers were in place long before the declaration of the pandemic. Most importantly, they have not gone away. Public Health Acts continue to grant government officials astonishing powers.

4. Taxation: no cure-all

Most taxes result in some loss of economic efficiency as they distort 'usual' economic behaviour. The deadweight loss from taxation arises from the reduced incentive effects associated with additional taxation. This is because it drives a wedge between the prices paid and received for goods and services. This has been estimated at 27.5 cents in the dollar, on average.

Much worse is when swingeing taxes designed to stop people smoking create a black market, for example, in illegal tobacco. The costs to taxpayers are immense, and the harm caused by organised crime is immense, and the same poor sods still smoke despite years of taxing and years of health campaigns.

Case studies

5. COVID-19: society is not a hospital ward

The script for a future pandemic response has already been written: 'Lock 'em up and wait for a vaccine.' This strategy was devised by politicians who harvested votes in Queensland, Western Australia, and Victoria. It was advised by Chief Medical Officers who enjoyed the limelight, as well as by media owners and journalists who thrived on a fearful, lockdown-obsessed audience during the COVID-19 pandemic. There is little reason to believe the response to the next pandemic will differ unless the influence of such individuals changes, creating space for alternative views.

The Commonwealth's Inquiry into the COVID-19 response asserted that interventions from the Commonwealth, such as JobKeeper, and from the states and territories, like rent relief and eviction moratoriums, mitigated the pandemic's impact. For instance, the Inquiry relied on an assertion that the number of households facing housing 'affordability stress' would have surged by 74 per cent without these interventions. But had the lockdowns, school closures, and mandated vaccinations not closed businesses and caused job losses (accounting for any net increase in illness that would have occurred without these measures), would affordability stress have been as severe? Is the 74 per cent a sign of success or failure?

6. Transgender Affirmation: a profession duped

The now prominent and controversial response to gender dysphoria, the affirmation model, represents a very dark chapter of medical practice. Gender affirmation therapy begins with social validation towards the opposite sex, gonadotropin-releasing hormone analogues in children to delay puberty, followed by cross-sex hormone therapy to achieve the desired masculinisation or feminisation. Potential surgical procedures include breast reduction or augmentation, hysterectomy or orchiectomy, and vaginoplasty or phalloplasty.

Professor John Whitehall has described the result as an 'ersatz similarity with the opposite sex.' The power of the 'therapeutic ritual' between patient and doctor — a force strong enough to create a placebo effect regardless of both diagnosis and cure — has been evident in the affirmation model popular in the treatment of gender dysphoria, especially among the young. Science is the least important aspect.

7. Aboriginal Health: measuring ideology

Is socioeconomic disadvantage the determining factor in Aboriginal life expectancy? Aboriginal men living in the most socioeconomically disadvantaged areas have a life expectancy that is about five years lower than that of those living in the least disadvantaged areas. Aboriginal females in the most disadvantaged areas have a life expectancy of around three years lower than those in the least disadvantaged areas. It is part of the answer, as better-off people, not just Aborigines, tend to take better care of their health. That journey, however, is not a medical journey. It may have something to do with behaviour and culture, but not in a way that public health officials would want to hear.

One string among many of the public health lobby's bow is the claim that Aboriginal community-controlled health services are better for Aboriginal clients. Is it true, or just ideology dressed as science? The sector conflates methods for achieving better health outcomes with measuring outcomes. The measures are those of intermediaries, such as cultural safety, but not years of life. Most government programs are evaluated to determine their effectiveness and the worthiness of the investment. Most evaluations will state an explicit theory of change, that is, a specific and measurable description and illustration of how and why a program is supposed to work. What happens, though, when the theory of change for Aboriginal community-controlled organisations is based on the principles of self-determination and cultural integrity?

8. Mental Health and NDIS: diagnostic inflation

Patrick McGorrie and Ian Hickie argue that the mental health of young Australians represents a public health crisis. McGorrie argues that despite the 'scale and urgency of the crisis', the political will is yet to emerge to solve it. Is it accurate to say that a response is yet to emerge? If the bottom line is that every young Australian should receive the medical care they and clinicians desire, then McGorrie is correct. However, that is not the real world of limited resources and competing priorities, such as the crises in public hospitals and aged care, the rise in disability, and the NDIS response, which alone threaten Australia's public finances.

An ageing population may account for inadequacies in hospitals and aged care. More visits to doctors have also placed resources under pressure; since Medicare was introduced in 1984, visits to general practitioners have increased from 3.8 to 6.8 per person per year, and visits to other medical professionals have also ballooned. Given the budget deficit and the ongoing demands for service, is there room for further investment in health at the current standard of living?

Tackling the public health lobby

9. Costs and Benefits: honest evaluation

A decade ago, St Vincent's Health Australia urged political parties to commit to a target of reducing alcohol-related illness by 20 per cent by 2025. St Vincent's has been working with alcoholics and others since 1964, so, understandably, they might be frustrated that there are still alcoholics. This may explain their desire for a national policy. They pursued this goal, knowing that only 3.4 per cent of drinkers fall into the harmful category. Echoing tobacco regulation, St Vincent's calls for a ban on all alcohol advertising and sponsorship, alcohol taxation based on its content and level of harm, pictorial health warnings, and various restrictions on trading hours.

The Commonwealth Department of Health's national alcohol strategy warns that the risks associated with alcohol are often underestimated. Perhaps not. A typical statistical sleight of hand in such warnings is the distinction between relative and absolute risk. Alcohol consumption is linked to certain cancers, for example, but most drinkers consume in moderation. Relative risk describes how much something increases (or decreases) the likelihood of an outcome. For instance, consuming alcohol may raise the relative risk of breast cancer by about 10 per cent per standard drink per day. That figure sounds significant until the absolute risk is considered. Absolute risk assesses the actual likelihood of developing a disease.

10. Things to do

The public health lobby is driven by ego and ideology, harming society. Too many medical and allied professionals want to save the world from itself and will use all means necessary, particularly taxpayers' money and government fiat, to achieve population health outcomes. The overriding value in public health, according to one of its young enthusiasts, is that of equity, a highly freighted concept that drives a never-ending search for optimal outcomes for all. No stone is to be left unturned to help even those who did not ask for it.

At its centre, it is, as Professor Jessica Flanigan observed, progressive and statist.[23] Public health, in conjunction with more conventional patient point-of-entry medical interventions, is driving nations into debt. The result will be a very unappealing equity, a highly prescribed environment where health is valued above all else and health practitioners rule the polity. Public health needs to be reined in.

Public health enthusiasts are not alone in seeking influence or persuading public officials to adopt their worldview. However, they carry a medical authority that makes their perspectives less likely to be challenged. This book analyses public health's overall objectives and the tactics it uses to advance its agenda. Those objectives and tactics apply to any issue

23 Flanigan J, 2024, 508

in which public health becomes involved. However, to encourage open debate on current issues where public health is having an unhealthy influence, and to reduce the potential harms the public health lobby is likely to cause, this book has also produced a series of specific and immediate recommendations, detailed in chapter ten, and summarised here.

1. *Stop insidious ideology: let people do their job*
   Professions must reclaim the scientific realm and not play politics.
2. *Push back on the use of legislation: amend Public Health Acts*
   Chief Health Officers must never have powers applicable during the COVID-19 pandemic.
3. *Challenge coercive control: restrict mandatory vaccination*
   The law should not license an overly protective mindset.
4. *Oppose the WHO pandemic Agreement*
   One false move at the UN and the world panics.
5. *No more bureaucracy: oppose the Centre for Disease Control*
   CDC risks the single-minded pursuit of a public health approach, increasingly recommended for almost every type of social ill that touches health.
6. *Real-time evaluations of non-pharmaceutical interventions*
   All non-pharmaceutical interventions should be evaluated in real time, including risk-benefit analyses.
7. *Oppose social justice ideological contagion in AHPRA*
   The regulator should never interfere with the ethical doctor-patient relationship.
8. *Stick with matters directly related to health*
   Medical doctors are not well-equipped to assess societal risk in public policy.
9. *Enough with social determinants: challenge public health centres*
   Coercion and control are common techniques used to engage in social engineering.
10. *Remove taxation privileges from public health organisations*
    Public health organisations should demonstrate public benefit and the absence of harm.

1

Public Health: history repeats

[P]ublic health is not a science, but a form of social activism, one whose benefits appear profound enough to society that it is institutionalized and heavily subsidized by governments.[1]

Sander Greenland, Professor of Epidemiology and Statistics

To understand how public health has gotten to where it is today, we must first appreciate the circumstances surrounding its emergence. Modern public health is a product of 19th-century England, the first industrial country, beginning in earnest in 1832 when Parliament appointed a Royal Commission to inquire into the operation and administration of the Elizabethan-era Poor Laws. This provided just the opportunity that Edwin Chadwick had been seeking to create for himself. Chadwick was a lawyer of middling ability whose career had been relatively lacklustre until that point, but who nevertheless showed great skill at ingratiating himself with the influential and well-connected. Chadwick had been employed as an assistant by and remained a fervent believer in the philosophies of social reformer Jeremy Bentham. Bentham, of course, is best remembered as an early progressive thinker whose ideas about thc greatest good for the greatest number were fundamental to the creation of the modern welfare state.

Chadwick became an assistant to the Commission and then a

1 Greenland S, 1988. Probability versus Popper: an elaboration of the insufficiency of current Popperian approaches for epidemiologic analysis. In K. Rothman (Ed) *Causal Inference*. Epidemiology Resources Inc., 96

commissioner. The Royal Commission provided a vehicle for Chadwick to promote his mentor's ideology. In its first report, published in 1834, primarily written by Chadwick, the Commission recommended a series of amendments to address a newly identified problem: labour supply. The 1834 Poor Law Amendment Act, based on recommendations in Chadwick's report, had the ostensible — and wholly laudable — objective of reducing poverty, but its broader aim was to free the labour market and stimulate investment. As factories came to dominate production, an increasing number of workers were required. Labour had to be found and moved to cities where factories were located.[2] The Poor Laws, which held individual parishes responsible for providing relief and finding employment for the poor within their districts, had helped maintain a reserve of rural labour and prevented workers from migrating to towns.[3] This was unacceptable to the new industrial middle class and its advocates – many of whom sat in parliament and more than a few of whom were, themselves, factory owners. Since the system of poor relief was alleged to be the chief obstacle to a supply of factory labour, the remedy proposed was to do away with assistance to the able-bodied poor,[4] thus freeing labour for the economic self-interest of the middle classes.

This new system, of course, would require monitoring. Chadwick's report recommended the establishment of a permanent Commission to oversee the operation of the new laws.[5] The Commission would issue orders and regulations to guide local officials in administering the law. It would necessarily require paid jobs for Commissioners and a Secretary. After successfully identifying problems that could only be solved through paid government positions, Chadwick became the Secretary. Happily, at least for Chadwick's self-advancement, the Poor Law Amendment

2 Rosen G, 1958. Industrialism and the sanitary movement (1830-1875). In G. Rosen, *A History of Public Health*. MD Publications: New York

3 Rosen G, 1958

4 Fee E & Brown T M, 2005. The Public Health Act of 1848. *Bulletin of the World Health Organization*, 83(11), 866-867

5 House of Commons, 1842. *Report on the Sanitary Condition of the Labouring Population of Great Britain*. Parliament of Great Britain: London

Act's intervention into the labour market raised a larger question. How to organise life in an increasingly complex industrial, urban society?[6] The same processes that created the market economy, the factory, and the modern urban environment also contributed to the development of health problems. This had been foreshadowed not in the context of medicine, but in 18th century writings about how the unemployed poor could be used as manufacturing labourers and the difficulties that might arise from that.

As the 19th century progressed, an increasing number of people moved to towns and worked in factories. Populations grew rapidly, and the expansion of the urban population outpaced any increase in available housing. Large numbers of workers were compelled to live in densely populated urban districts close to their workplaces, as their employment was often casual and they had to be present or risk missing out on work. Alongside the influx of low-income workers and the growth of urban communities, those of higher income tended to move to suburban and rural areas, exacerbating the neglect of poorer districts. Initially, it was assumed that individuals in those areas would either decide to address their physical and social needs or that someone would do it for them out of financial interest or moral principle. Instead, shops and saloons flourished, but little else. Sanitary arrangements received negligible attention, since expenditures for such facilities were not considered lucrative. Infrequent sewage and garbage removal, and the neglected state of the courts and alleys around which houses were built, gave rise to their use as rubbish dumps for all residents of the surrounding premises.

Health conditions deteriorated, and death rates increased. Between 1831 and 1844, the mortality rates per thousand population in Birmingham rose from 15 to 27, in Bristol from 17 to 31, in Liverpool from 21 to 35, and in Manchester from 30 to 34.[7] Epidemics such as cholera were rampant, and factories and congested dwellings began to be recognised as providing conditions in which diseases could flourish. From the 1830s,

6 Rosen G, 1958

7 Rosen G, 1958, 202

urged on by the Poor Law Commission, a series of Acts were passed concerning the damaging aspects of factory labour and the conditions under which the workers lived. Impetus for growing sanitary measures rested on the fact that diseases such as cholera could affect anybody, but tended to begin in the slums and then spread. Dealing with the health of the poor thus benefited the health of the better off. More crucial, though, were the economic arguments.

In 1838, the Poor Law Commission reported that three medical inspectors employed to investigate the prevalence and causation of preventable diseases in London had offered the opinion that 'the expenditures necessary to the adoption and maintenance of measures of prevention would ultimately amount to less than the cost of the disease now constantly engendered.' Statistics began to be gathered and used to demonstrate the economic impacts of poor health, such as lost productivity and the average cost to the medical system for a patient. Discussing the impact of disease on the workers, the Select Committee on the Health of Towns — a parliamentary group consisting of various titled notables — declared in 1840:

> *The property which the country has in their useful labours will be so far lessened, and the unproductive outlay necessary to maintain and restrain them so far augmented...some such measures are urgently called for, as claims of humanity and justice to great multitudes of our fellow men, and as necessary not less for the welfare of the poor than the safety of property and the security of the rich.*[8]

In other words, when a disease or injury happens to the poor, that is one thing. However, when it affects the interests of the well-to-do by interfering with labour supply and incurring costs, then something must be done. Chadwick continued his advocacy, producing in 1842 *The Report on the Sanitary Condition of the Labouring Population*, in which he highlighted connections between unsanitary living conditions and disease:

8 House of Commons, 1840. *Report from the Select Committee on the Health of Towns*. Parliament of Great Britain: London, xiv

> *The defects which are most important...and which come most immediately within practical legislative and administrative control, are those chiefly external to the dwellings of the population and principally arise from the neglect of drainage.*[9]

Public health was, therefore, about the conditions in which people lived. And those were things that governments could change. Further Chadwickian reports were presented to Parliament in 1844 and 1845. Overcrowding and congestion, poverty, crime, ill-health, and heavy mortality were shown to be commonly found together. The reports contained several recommendations that should be incorporated into new legislation. Most important was a proposal to give the national government the power to investigate and supervise the execution of all general measures for regulating the sanitary conditions of larger urban communities. This proposal placed responsibility for public health in the hands of centralised government and — naturally — involved the creation of a new government department.

The dominoes started to fall quickly after that. In 1846, lobbying from the Liverpool municipality, where sanitary conditions were deplorable and cholera outbreaks were common, prompted Parliament to pass the *Liverpool Sanitary Act*, the first comprehensive sanitary measure in England. While primarily dealing with sewerage, it also established a Borough Engineer position to oversee sanitation projects and to allow unspecified works to improve public health. Coincidentally, Liverpool had an exceptionally high number of starving, diseased Irish fleeing the famine, and concerns about a potential proletariat uprising were spreading throughout middle-class England, all of which contributed to a sense of emergency in which disease, migration, and threats to the social order became intertwined.

In 1846 and 1848, two *Nuisances Removal and Diseases Prevention Acts* were passed. While dealing mainly with problems such as filthy dwellings, accumulations of refuse and dung, and foul or offensive privies, the term 'nuisances' was sufficiently wide as to encompass anything that could

9 House of Commons, 1842, 25

be seen as a threat to health. Then, in 1848, the *Public Health Act* was passed. Overall, it facilitated the expansion of government powers and the growth of the central bureaucracy that Chadwick and his ilk had long sought. Among other measures, such as establishing positions for a chief medical officer and health inspectors, this Act established a prestigious and powerful Board of Health, on which Chadwick sat. However, things took a turn as people started to realise just how much power public health had over their lives. The Board's strong centralising tendencies and attempts to diminish local authorities' autonomy did not go over well. Nor did the tendency of its field staff to use their new powers to tell people what to do. This rapidly alienated those individuals and groups whose lives and livelihoods were directly affected. Opposition grew, particularly in the name of property rights and individual freedoms.

Even the media — initially cheerleaders for greater government intervention in the name of public health — changed their tune, with The London Times saying: '...we prefer to take our chance of cholera and the rest than be bullied into health.'[10] When even cholera is seen as a better option, something has gone very, very wrong. Criticism was so widespread that in 1854, Parliament (in an act of bravery that would be inconceivable today) refused to renew the Public Health Act. The first National Board of Health came to an end. This was everybody's fault, except the Board itself, which maintained that they were victims of their brilliance. They were simply smarter, more efficient, and more competent than everyone else. The Seventh Earl of Shaftesbury, Anthony Ashley-Cooper, who served on the Board and had previously been heavily involved with the Select Committee on the Health of Towns,[11] bemoaned that:

---

10 London Times, 1854. *Editorial.* 1 August

11 The Earl was the child of a relatively wealthy family. He attended exclusive schools and complained about how badly he was treated there and how those experiences taught him about the horrors of oppression. He was also very interested in lunacy laws and treatment of the insane. A notable achievement was his sponsorship of two 1845 Acts, *For the Regulation of Lunatic Asylums* and *For the Better Care and Treatment of Lunatics in England and Wales*. Among other things, these Acts established a Lunacy Commission. The Earl became its chair.

> *The parliamentary agents are our sworn enemies ... because we have reduced ... their fees ... The civil engineers also, because we have selected able men ... The College of Physicians ... because ... we proved that many a Poor Law medical officer knew more than all the flash and fashionable doctors of London. ... the Boards of Guardians, for we exposed ... their reluctance to ... relieve the suffering poor ... they hated us with a perfect hatred.*[12]

Chadwick was finally relegated to the sidelines and forced to give up his grand ideological crusade. Naturally, he is still feted in public health circles as a visionary and founder of modern public health. In fairness, he certainly set an example that today's bureaucrats, toadies, and professional rent-seekers continue to emulate. Thus, even though some physicians drew community attention to ill health among the poor, medicine had little to do with the emergence of public health legislation, public health officials, and the agendas that drove their creation. Instead, the emergence of public health was driven by power, money, and ideas about morality. It was characterised by activists – or social reformers as they are euphemistically termed – co-opting the apparatus of government to advance their own views and interests.

Aside from the obvious material perks and social status afforded by the creation of various departments, Committees and Boards, those ideologies were nowhere near as altruistic as their proponents sought to portray. Public health crusaders came from the middle and upper classes, who, although largely segregating themselves from the dirty poor people, were nevertheless increasingly worried that the miasmas wafting from poor communities posed a risk to their own health and comfort (not to mention costing them money).

The economic liberalism and increased productivity of the Industrial Revolution were seen by many in the 19th century as developments that would end scarcity, improve people's lives, and reduce poverty and suffering. However, as Welsh industrialist and philanthropist Robert Owen observed in 1817, the new order:

---

12 Rosen G, 1958, 223

> *...generates a new character in its inhabitants; and as this character is formed upon a principle quite unfavourable to individual or general happiness, it will produce the most lamentable and permanent evils, unless its tendency be counteracted by legislative interference and direction.*[13]

The actual change brought about by 19th century public health was not sanitation reform. It was about positioning capitalism as a force that cared little for people and could not be trusted to 'do the right thing' on its own, while concurrently establishing state intervention as a necessary tool for righting the wrongs the system inflicted. These ideas rapidly spread from England to other industrialised countries.

The rise of public health has been described as a political and social paradox, where the introduction of economic freedom, which was meant to free markets and reduce the need for governmental intervention, control, and regulation, instead led to an enormous increase in the administrative functions of the state – all in the name of doing good. Since its inception, public health has been a sphere in which competing views on economic freedom, capitalism, social welfare, state powers, and social justice have played out. And once the activists succeeded in establishing a case for state interference in the name of health, this approach began to be seen as a distinct theory and program of social action that was inextricably linked with the emerging welfare state:

> *Disease is largely a removable evil ... it continues to afflict humanity, not only because of incomplete knowledge of its causes and lack of individual and public hygiene, but also because it is extensively fostered by harsh economic and industrial conditions and by wretched housing in congested communities. These conditions and consequently the diseases which spring from them can be removed by better social organization.*[14]

---

13 Owen R, 1817. *Observations on the effect of the manufacturing system: with hints for the improvement of those parts of it which are most injurious to health and morals: dedicated most respectfully to the British* legislature. Second Edition. Multiple publishers: London, 5

14 Biggs H, 1911. Public health is purchasable. *Monthly Bulletin of the Department of Health of the City of New York*, 1(10), 226

Endless new problems – with the numbers to prove it

> *The reduction of the death rate is the principal statistical expression and index of human and social progress.*[15]

There is no doubt that early modern public health efforts, primarily focused on practical environmental management, such as enhanced waste removal and improved sewage systems, made significant inroads into mortality rates from common communicable diseases. By the early 20th century, urban environments were less squalid, and death rates from the dread diseases, such as cholera, that had driven the rise of public health in the previous century had fallen markedly.

This was not enough for health workers (mainly female social workers and nurses) who sought to improve the lot of poor communities. An array of vice, suffering, and social ills continued to assail their senses. The measures that had brought about change so far were unable to address new problems, such as poor maternal and child welfare and inadequate nutrition, observed among the poor. Clearly, more public health, with a much broader focus, was needed to address society's ills further. The growing medical and scientific knowledge about bacteria greatly helped this. However, the discovery of germs and their relationship with illness,[16] only emphasised the difference between the political world of public health and the physical world of medicine:

> *The discovery of bacteria, which proved such a boon to public health's disease control efforts, also brought it into competition with physicians, inasmuchas control measures such as immunizations were carried out not in the environment but on individual patients, who were the purview of the private doctor.*[17] ***(emphasis added)***

New programs were funded to educate mothers about infant nutrition and

---

15 Biggs H, 1911, 226

16 Which, incidentally, showed that Chadwick's belief that miasmas caused disease were wrong – demonstrating that public health may not accurately identify cause.

17 Committee for the Study of the Future of Public Health; Division of Health Care Services, 1988. *The Future of Public Health.* National Academy Press: Washington, D.C., 5

proper care, enhance knowledge about common skin conditions such as scabies and ringworm, and develop informational posters and pamphlets on maintaining good health. Public health workers (still, mostly nurses and social workers) multiplied accordingly. This marked the start of public health's long march away from simply trying to prevent the spread of communicable diseases that could, in theory, affect anyone, to instead focusing on non-communicable conditions connected to (other) people's lifestyles. It was around the time that social workers were identifying more problems that only they could help address that Winslow's 1923 definition of public health permanently embedded social engineering as a fundamental component. He saw public health as the development of the social machinery that would ensure every individual a standard of living adequate for maintaining their health.[18]

Most definitions since then are equally couched in terms that can include almost anything.

> *Improving quality of life and promoting health for all... the wide range of individual and collective efforts to improve health, forestall disease, and protect health.*[19]
>
> *The process of mobilizing and engaging local, state, national, and international resources to assure the conditions in which people can be healthy.*[20]
>
> *...collective action for sustained population-wide health improvement.*[21]

Importantly, these definitions make it clear that public health only occurs through action, either by a community or, more typically, by government. Public health is defined by its desired outcomes, as made clear in the Constitution of the World Health Organization (WHO),

---

18 Winslow C E A, 1923, 1

19 Fielding J, 2014. Foreword. In T H Tulchinsky & E A Varavikova (Eds) *The New Public Health* Third Edition. Academic Press: Netherlands, xix

20 Detels R & Breslow L, 2005. Current scope and concerns in public health. In R Detels J R McEwen, R Beaglehole and H Tanaka (Eds) *Oxford Textbook of Public Health 4th Ed. Vol. l. The Scope of Public Health.* Oxford University Press: Oxford, 3

21 Beaglehole R, Bonita R, Horton, R Adams O & McKee M, 2004. Public health in the new era: improving health through collective action. *Lancet*, 363, 2084.

which enshrines the 1940s concept of public health as a state of complete physical, mental, and social well-being. Completing the process begun under Chadwick, the government has now taken centre stage to ensure the mission is adequately addressed.[22]

But how can governments identify who has the most pressing problems that require public health interventions? From its earliest days, the answer was invariably: the poor. However, the early 20th century also marked a change in thinking about poverty. Poverty was no longer considered the natural punishment of the poor for their shortcomings.[23] Instead, it came to be seen as a social problem or, as public health began to call it, a social disease that had to be addressed through social measures. Thus, public health, with its moral foundation of Benthamite welfarism and zeal to be a progressive counterforce against the evils of capitalism, had a problem. It had to find a way to demonstrate that specific unfortunate populations were experiencing the social ills that public health workers said they were, without appearing to pass judgement.

Fortunately, an emerging discipline had the answer. In a 1928 journal article, The Statistician's Place in Public Health Work, U.S. economist and statistician Edgar Sydenstricker – one of the earliest public health researchers, invited by the then-League of Nations to establish its health epidemiology arm — argued that public health differs from medicine because public health has a social objective. To help meet its social objectives, it had an obligation to collect, tabulate, publish and interpret vital statistics, including those that 'distinguish between endemic conditions and the occurrence of unusual or epidemic conditions,' not to mention determine 'the money cost of administrative, preventive, and control activities.'[24]

Taking inspiration from Chadwick's decision that the poor were the

---

22 Committee for the Study of the Future of Public Health; Division of Health Care Services, 1988, 7

23 Rosen G, 1958, 466

24 Sydenstricker E, 1928. The statistician's place in public health work. *Journal of the American Statistical Association* 23(162), 117

problem, and then collecting information about the poor to prompt action on that problem, public health hitched itself to the emerging discipline of epidemiology to objectively identify who was less healthy and how that might relate to their more impoverished living conditions and other circumstances. While certainly not the first to use numbers, Sydenstricker promoted their application to determine relationships among variables, such as poverty, diet, and pellagra,[25] and to act based on these correlations. Sydenstricker noted that one of the roles of a public health statistician was to observe the association of x and y and that the scope of public health to do this was limited only by the amount of data and extent of statistical sophistication available to it. The language he used was different to what it is today, but this marked the emergence of public health's reliance on statistics about risk factors– things that are so typically distant from an effect that they cannot be called causes in the scientific sense of the word — to justify itself. The trouble is that while cause and effect are persuasive in prompting people to act, correlations are generally less compelling. Public health had to find a way to discuss causes without being overly concerned with them. Often, public health actions are taken without identifying the actual causes of a phenomenon. This is because the cause is irrelevant to using epidemiological results to drive decisions.

Public health's early marriage to epidemiology gave it a probabilistic or statistical conception of causality, which works backwards from data on patterns of correlation among variables within a sample of individuals to draw inferences about causes across populations. This enabled public health to discover endless disparities between different groups of people, which it could attribute to endless causes.[26] These were not causes of health disparity in the same way that a pathogen is a cause of disease. Public health was interested in cause as a relative concept, which is now understood as having meaning only in terms of its removal, associated

25 A disease caused by a lack of the vitamin niacin (vitamin B3).

26 It did not matter whether miasmas or germs caused cholera, just that better toilets fixed the problem. Guesses that produced results one hundred years ago do not justify the hundreds of millions of dollars spent on public health programs today.

with diminished risk.[27] Public health thus began to shift its moral focus to addressing risk factors, such as low income or education, or behaviours that placed individuals at risk. However, knowing about a risk factor cannot, by itself, permit causal inferences. Nor can it tell us the direction of an association or how it would change under different background conditions.

Public health sees a causal association as one in which 'an alteration in the frequency or quality of one category is followed by a change in the other.'[28] As long as something changes, that is enough for public health to claim success, and the need to manipulate something to find out what else changes provides the ideal justification for any intervention. Of course, public health interventions have never occurred in isolation. For instance, programs to educate mothers about milk hygiene were introduced alongside advancements in pasteurisation and the provision of clean milk. This means it is almost impossible to isolate any real impact those programs may have had, over and above everything else that was going on. Public health is nearly impossible to assess scientifically. This is because the counterfactual—what would have happened in the absence of this measure—is seldom present, especially when something like an education campaign or a piece of legislation is implemented nationwide. But by concentrating on risk factors, this critical detail becomes largely irrelevant.

The breakthrough for public health's reliance on risk factors came in 1950, when associations were found between smoking and lung cancer. Subsequently, medical science established clear causal relationships. This is why public health always invokes its anti-smoking efforts whenever it is criticised on any front. Just like Chadwick's lucky guess about sanitation occurred despite him having a completely mistaken view about miasmas as a cause of disease, the direct physiological relationship

27 Maxwell Parkin D & Bray F, 2005. Descriptive studies. In W Ahrens and I Pigeot (Eds) *Handbook of Epidemiology*. Springer: London, 157–230

28 MacMahon T F & Pugh B (Eds) 1970. *Epidemiology: Principles and Methods*. Little Brown & Co: Boston, 17–18

between smoking and lung cancer is the rare exception in public health that we are meant to believe is the rule. Thus, public health, through its emphasis on risk factors for certain populations, came to focus on ways of changing individual behaviours. Unhealthy environments suddenly shifted from those that were unsanitary or where adequate resources to support good health could not be accessed, to those in which harmful or risky products such as tobacco could be advertised or readily obtained, or where restrictions were not imposed to make it harder for people to make bad choices.

Figure 1.3 When you're on a good thing, stick to it

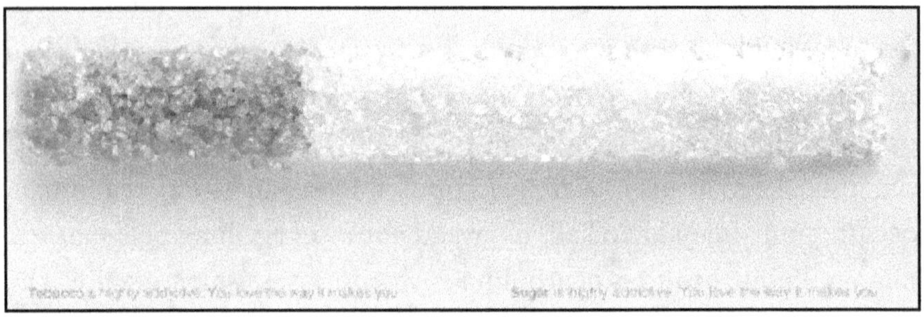

The words read ... *Tobacco is highly addictive ... Sugar is highly addictive ... Somewhere in the world, it takes a life every six seconds.*

Source: Diabetes Association of Sri Lanka, https://www.adsoftheworld.com/campaigns/1-in-every-6-seconds

An attempt to replicate the tobacco-cancer-specific link to harm was made with sugar in the brilliant advertisement from the Diabetes Association of Sri Lanka (Figure 1.3), which displays raw and white sugar in the shape of a filtered cigarette and compares the death rates associated with tobacco and sugar. There are doubts about the equivalence, for example, a study found that 'focusing public health messages on sugar may mislead on the need to reduce fat and overall energy consumption', but the intention is clear.[29] Making sugar out to be as harmful as tobacco is powerful marketing.

29 Anderson J J et al, 2017. Adiposity among 132479 UK Biobank participants; contribution of sugar intake vs other macronutrients. *International Journal of Epidemiology*, 46(2), 492–501

Statistics and 'othering': the backbone of public health

It has become an unassailable fact within public health that if we seek to reduce risks to people's wellbeing (many of which are now described as social determinants – see chapter 2), we must examine society and the social networks in which individuals find themselves. It is only there, or so the argument runs, that manipulation can lead to the elimination of the mechanisms that contribute to some ill. The idea is that social factors are ultimately responsible for health disparities. This sleight of hand greatly increases the complexity of issues related to causality, while simultaneously justifying the manipulation of populations and societies. And, of course, social conditions are not the same for everyone, so public health interventions tend to focus on targeting those individuals judged most likely to develop disease (whether an actual disease, or the social ills that public health describes as diseases). Something does not need to be common, widespread, or frequent for public health action to be required. There only needs to be inequality (or, perhaps, the increasingly preferred and hard to define, inequity) in how it is distributed in the population, or in how its risk factors manifest, for it to merit attention.

Importantly, this epidemiological approach provides the justification needed to single out not only specific groups but also individuals. The statistical scaffolding makes it seem as if this is an unbiased, value-neutral process that exists outside social influences.

> *Public health professionals rely on expert knowledge derived from such areas as epidemiology and biostatistics ... to maximize the influence of accurate data and professional judgment on decision-making—to make decisions as comprehensive and objective as possible.*[30]

Who gets to be a public health professional or expert? Just as Chadwick with his law degree styled himself as a public health expert, any qualification today suffices: epidemiology, biostatistics, nursing, midwifery, economics, social work, sociology, psychology, architecture, town planning, environmental health, engineering, gender studies,

30 Committee for the Study of the Future of Public Health; Division of Health Care Services, 1988, 4

bioethics, and veterinarians (and more besides) all get a look in. However, as postmodernists point out, measuring health, illness, and mortality within a population is a central feature of power and biopolitics in modern societies. They have highlighted how classification systems and statistics are misused by dominant groups in society to perpetuate acts of oppression. They have even suggested that classification systems and understandings of disease are developed for those purposes and used to advance the self-interest and power of the elite classes: 'each category valorizes some point of view and silences another.'[31]

There is no doubt that the ultimate goal of public health is to manipulate societies. But for whose benefit? To understand this, we need to recognise that public health has often been employed in ways that have little to do with the care or compassion that public health professionals like to profess. Public health, from the Dickensian slums to the present, has always been about othering, a discursive process by which a dominant in-group (us) constructs one or many dominated out-groups (them) by stigmatising difference (real or imagined).[32] Othering defines and secures one's own identity by distancing or dehumanising another identity. Its purpose is to reinforce notions of our own normality, and to set up the difference of others as a point of deviance. The person or group being othered experiences this as a process of marginalisation, disempowerment and social exclusion. This effectively creates a separation between us and them.[33]

Othering determines people's proper place, and when they step out of that, they are typically presented as a threat. Catchy new name for the old sociological concept of in-groups and out-groups though it is, it is nevertheless useful in describing how public health thrives from dividing society into different groups. Othering has been at the centre of public

31 Bowker G & Star S L, 2000. *Sorting Things Out: Classification and Its Consequences*. MIT Press: Cambridge, MA, 5.

32 Staszak J-F, 2020. Other/Otherness. In A Kobayashi (Ed) *International Encyclopedia of Human Geography*. Second Edition. Elsevier: New York, 25-31

33 Grove N J & Zwi A B, 2006. Our health and theirs: forced migration, othering, and public health. *Social Science & Medicine*, 62, 1931–1942

health since its early days. A prominent example lies in how tuberculosis was viewed in early 20th century Los Angeles. Los Angeles publicised itself as a grand wellness retreat where the best and most desirable of people could come to be blessed by endless sunshine and surrounded by idyllic living conditions, healthy air, fresh food, and the opportunity for a better life. Predictably, this sparked massive waves of migration from other parts of the U.S., Europe and Asia. Equally predictably, many of those immigrants were not the type that city publicists had in mind.

Statistics (of course) soon painted a picture of crisis, suggesting that tuberculosis, much like the cholera epidemics that had sparked the public health movement in the UK, was more likely to be found among poor immigrants (especially Mexicans) than nice people. Poverty (as always) was highlighted, with around two-thirds of patients dying of tuberculosis said to have family incomes of less than one thousand dollars.[34]

Health officials, with the help of anti-immigration groups, began to highlight the prevalence of tuberculosis among immigrants routinely, depicted them as agents rather than victims of disease, and produced reams of statistical information about the burdens this caused for the health care system. Calls for border control grew. Race reared its head: 'the white elite were especially ready to embrace an exclusionary strategy because they viewed themselves as a uniquely blessed people; they could sustain an illusion of invulnerability only by banishing anyone identified with weakness and danger.'[35]

The Board of Health wrote in 1906 that many people who died of tuberculosis 'contracted the disease from cases coming here without the means for proper care...infected strangers, living in dark and ill-ventilated rooms, eating at cheap restaurants and expectorating everywhere, will infect more natives than ten times the number who reside in good homes where care is exercised.'[36] While ignorance was one explanation for the

---

34 Abel E K, 2007. *Tuberculosis and the Politics of Exclusion: A History of Public Health and Migration to Los Angeles*. Rutgers University Press: New Brunswick

35 Abel E K, 2007, 2

36 California State Board of Health, 1906. *Monthly Bulletin* 2(7), 65

carelessness of the afflicted undesirables, it was not uncommon to find expressions that the poor failed to comply with public health advice because they were both vicious and stupid. Nice people did not like being confronted with sickness. Pasadena residents who signed petitions urging the Los Angeles County Board of Supervisors to close a health camp for patients in 1909 argued not only that they were a threat to the wellbeing of others but also that 'while we have every sympathy with the victims of the disease we do not think it fair or right to be compelled to hear their distressing coughing day and night continuously.'[37]

Adding to this affront, consumptives represented a high proportion of charity recipients. Charitable societies were at the forefront of anti-immigration efforts, urging an end to the practice of encouraging poor tuberculosis sufferers to travel to Southern California for their health. The New York Charity Organization Society, the city's major philanthropic society, sent a letter to 8,600 physicians stating that 'difficult as it may be for a poor man to recover from tuberculosis in this city, he is better off here among his friends and relatives, where there are more adequate hospital and dispensary facilities, than he is far from home, where he is thrown entirely upon his resources and where the great number of consumptives willing to work at the lowest wages make the finding of employment ... almost impossible.'[38] In 1909, the Los Angeles County Board of Supervisors followed the example of private charities. It enacted a rule requiring that consumptives seeking public assistance be given one-way train fares out of town.

When the Los Angeles County Board of Supervisors announced plans to construct four new buildings for the overcrowded county hospital in 1902, the Municipal League, the major Progressive organisation, protested that the proposal would involve exorbitant expense to taxpayers. In addition, the league claimed, the new buildings would serve as an 'apparent invitation to indigent invalids from all over the Union to come to this

37 Petitions to the Board of Supervisors, August 20, 1908, file OD949H, LACBS. Cited in: Abel E K, 2007, 32

38 Abel E K, 2007, 35

country and be cared for.'[39] Health authorities defined the right kind of people as white and middle-class and worked relentlessly to advance their interests. After the defeat of an early state quarantine bill, all exclusionary strategies were carefully targeted solely at the poor. Public health officials argued that illness was not a normal and inevitable part of life in Southern California. All advocates of services for tuberculosis sufferers would have to acknowledge those attitudes.

Public health workers wondered why their programs were not being greeted with open arms. Reports complained about patients who missed clinic appointments, rebuffed public health nurses, and refused to cooperate with programs designed to help them. Health authorities put this down to ignorant, vicious people overcome by inertia. Public health workers (mostly female nurses and social workers) prided themselves on demonstrating unlimited 'tact' and sympathy.[40] Some acknowledged that they scolded clients who failed to heed what, to those middle-class denizens, was entirely reasonable public health advice, such as eating fresh food and living in airy, clean apartments. It seems to have escaped their awareness that those things cost money that the poor did not have.

The well-meaning, while extolling a kinder approach to consumptives, did their utmost to further 'other' the unwell. Describing poor Mexican immigrants' overcrowded and substandard housing, for instance, they stressed the filthy walls and floors and the odours that assail the visitor, implying that Mexican tenants were dirty and smelly. Eugenics reared its head, suggesting that the high tuberculosis rate among Mexicans indicated that their bodies were innately inferior to those of whites. Alongside this, bureaucrats presented single case studies as evidence of widespread problems. Edythe Tate-Thompson, the director of the Bureau of Tuberculosis, highlighted the danger of unrestricted immigration:

> *Last year an aged Mexican in the last stages of tuberculosis came across the border ... he was sent to the already overcrowded ward of the tuberculosis hospital. He ... decided he would not stay in bed*

39 Abel E K, 2007, 36

40 Abel E K, 2007, 53

> *in spite of a fever of 104 degrees, so he left the hospital and later was picked up on the street again and returned. ... While the patient waiting to be readmitted, he died ... the hospital was blamed, yet the episode of dying people entering this country is not unusual.*[41]

Tate-Thompson ensured that her work figured prominently in the growing campaign to limit migration, promote racial segregation, and deport Mexicans. She continued to harangue politicians about how much Mexicans were costing certain sections of the state.[42] Despite public health's burgeoning love of numbers, no statistical support for her case studies was forthcoming — but her rhetoric certainly scared politicians. By 1937, Tate-Thompson was demanding funding for more social workers, who had sufficient language skills to tell Mexicans to accept deportation.

Interestingly, in the 1998 tuberculosis survey in the UK, it was found that more than half of the persons infected had been born abroad. Recently arrived immigrants showed the highest rates, and many were refugees and asylum seekers from African countries, the Middle East and former Yugoslavia. This prompted a political focus on newly arrived migrants from certain countries, who were perceived as posing a risk to the British population's health. Perhaps not coincidentally, this occurred at a time of mounting political anxiety over immigration.[43]

Public health needs to respond to the current discourse of othering or risk being co-opted into a system of heightened social control and marginalisation.[44] Recently, academics have come to the startling realisation that public health problems are not simply there waiting to be found, but are constructed at times and in particular places by people with different viewpoints. Academics have also observed

41 Edythe Tate Thompson. Cited in Abel E K, 2003. From exclusion to expulsion: Mexicans and tuberculosis control in Los Angeles, 1914-1940. *Bulletin of the History of Medicine*, 77(4), 823-849

42 Abel E K, 2003, 823-849

43 von Unger H, Scott P & Odukoya D, 2019. Constructing im/migrants and ethnic minority groups as 'carriers of disease': power effects of categorization practices in tuberculosis health reporting in the UK and Germany. *Ethnicities* 19(3), 518–534

44 Grove N J & Zwi A B, 2006, 1939

a tendency to moralise in policy and popular discourse about health. Reams of academic papers now castigate how public health is (ab)used by neo-liberal, capitalist powerbrokers to other people with disability, gay men, gender diverse people, refugees, and so on. Unsurprisingly, othering is applied only to the groups progressives purport to care about.

Traditionally, public health othering has been based on poverty or ethnic/racial minority status. However, since the emergence of discourses of human rights, social justice, and health equity in the 1990s, minorities are not only perceived as a risk (to the general population) but also as at risk, or vulnerable, and thus worthy of full moral consideration. New studies, though, have identified othering as occurring between groups of (otherwise similar) individuals with behavioural differences– specifically, compliance or non-compliance with public health recommendations. The authors suggest that:

> *... our data suggest an emergence of a new consideration of acceptance or non-acceptance of social norms as they relate to public health recommendations. The implications of this new class of Othering are troubling as Othering serves to normalize and justify different treatment for different groups, typically as a hierarchical power relationship, in western cultures archetypically based on racial or gender divides.*[45]

Yet barely a word is spoken anywhere about how public health is increasingly used to other, say, people who politically disagree with progressive preoccupations, who adopt libertarian philosophies, who challenge the orthodoxy of the health bureaucracy itself, or who want to be left alone to make their own life choices (bad for them though those may be). Those othered groups are certainly not seen by the public health establishment as vulnerable or worthy of moral consideration. Quite the opposite. Fischer and Poland, for example, show how community policing in anti-smoking campaigns stigmatises and excludes those who smoke. They note, 'Behind the calculus of risk lies the assumption of a 'perfect' life free of risk. As such, the calculus of risk reveals a profound intolerance for the unhealthy or 'deviant'

45 Van Scoy L J et al, 2022. 'Us-Versus-Them': othering in COVID-19 public health behavior compliance. *PLoS ONE* 17(1) e0261726, 11

'Other' as embodiments of risk (and of difference).'[46]

Othering serves to categorise certain segments of the population as unruly or problematic citizens and thus lacking full citizenship. As Foucault notes, stigmatisation and exclusion are 'basic dimensions of social normalization'.[47] Using health, or health attitudes, to define others as pathological, deviant, or risky to the whole, thus serves an agenda of exclusion. While some academics recognise that 'the practice of claiming the authority to define others as unruly, which in some sense denies them the status of the full citizen, should be treated with great care and the implications debated openly',[48] this has had little impact on public health discourse and practice. Indeed, the role of public health in the othering process is generally only discussed in relation to neoliberal biopolitics – a more modern version of capitalism that so affronted 19th-century activists, even as they benefited from it.

What's next?

Despite hiding behind the virtues of helping the unfortunate, the blandness of numbers, and a handful of successes driven by advances in medical and scientific knowledge, public health has always had questionable motives and objectives. While piously advocating a better society for all, public health has long been a vehicle for the use and abuse of power, self-interest, and the viciousness of segregation, denigration, and exclusion. This may be why, in a glimmer of hope for the future, medical doctors, cautioned from their earliest training to do no harm, are apparently turning their backs on public health.

> *One of the important changes in recent decades has been the way in which doctors in clinical practice have moved away from engagement*

46 Fischer B & Poland B, 1998. Exclusion, 'risk', and social control: reflections on community policing and public health. *Geoforum* 29(2), 195

47 Foucault M, Bertani M, Fontana A, Ewald F & Macey D, 1997. *'Society Must Be Defended': Lectures at the Collège de France, 1975-1976.* Macmillan: London, 62

48 Thompson L & Kumar A, 2011. Responses to health promotion campaigns: resistance, denial and othering. *Critical Public Health* 21(1), 114

> *with preventative medicine and the major public health issues of the day. This is in stark contrast to the successes of the broader medical profession during the later half of the twentieth century in relation to issues such as tobacco, seat belts, crash helmets, and car windscreens.*[49]

It is no wonder physicians are becoming wary of public health activism in which ideology, political power, and revulsion towards the unclean have long featured. Looking at the history of public health – the history that is often swept under the carpet in favour of the wonders of sanitation, vaccinations, and the like – three instruments weaponise an assault on the scientific method, perverting it and replacing it with ideology.

1. While individuals with good intentions toil, public health has always been about the ambitions and self-advancement of a few. From Chadwick onwards, the rewards have been great for those who shout the loudest about wanting to improve the well-being of the unfortunate, and find endless problems that only they have the answer to (if they are given enough government largesse, that is). The example of Chadwick, however, shows that it is possible to purge these conceited social climbers. Remove the incentives, end the gravy train, and make an example of the 'Chadwicks of today', and public health will begin to attract and promote quite different types of people.

2. Public health has always relied on getting control over and using the powers of government. It has always linked itself to Commissions, Boards, paid government positions, new government departments, and the like, which it then uses to perpetuate itself. Public health's very existence has always relied on extending the reach of government. This may be reasonable when it means digging new drains or having state-run garbage collection – in other words, tangible things in the physical world that relate directly and causally to health. It is not reasonable when intervention means the government doing little other than regulating what choices individuals should and should not make, and meting out punishment to individual citizens for the choices they do make. Take away its government levers and powers to regulate individuals, and

49 Scally G, 2014. Public health profession. *Encyclopedia of Health Economics* 3, 208

public health would rapidly shift its focus and scope back to simple persuasion through education.

3. Public health has always been political, and must be seen that way. Despite hiding behind a cloak of gentle benevolence, its actual goals and objectives have always been ideological. Public health has a long history of being used to advance bigotry, discrimination, and vicious othering. Public health has long been a political response designed to quell worries—and the prospect of civil unrest—about perennial problems like housing, immigration, and crime. Yank away the cloak, and suddenly, public health looks nowhere near as caring and compassionate as it makes itself out to be. Instead, it is revealed as just another political tool in a battle for supremacy of a preferred view of the world.

The public health approach

History teaches that public health aficionados are motivated to empire-build and are skilled at finding more problems that require more public health intervention. The problems that public health says are connected to health grow remote from health.

Public health's objective is to bring about a society that conforms to the standards that it deems to be good. To ensure that it is not subject to limits, public health has developed strategies – termed the public health approach — that allow it to justify inserting itself into many aspects of people's lives.

Public health employs numerous strategies to achieve its aims, but its three overarching approaches are 'social determinant' arguments, law, and taxation.

In the highly ideological straitjacket of socially determined health, where sociology trumps genetics and enhances the argument that only public control can solve public health problems.

The main instruments of public control are the Public Health Acts, employed to devastating effect during the COVID-19 response, along with legislative measures more generally to constrain what people can do and punish those who defy the public health lobby.

More recently is reference to WHO instruments, which although not Australian law, appear to be increasingly relied upon for 'authority'.

For other 'sins' such as smoking, drinking and over-eating, there is taxation.

2

Health Determinants: change society

What causes some individuals to lead less healthy and shorter lives than others? What are effective remedies? If public health concerned itself with understanding the causes of illness and developing effective responses to those causes, then it would make a positive contribution to health outcomes. That is what medical science does. Public health, on the other hand, has had to look further afield and brand itself as the champion of *prevention*, with great fondness for such homilies as 'prevention is always better than cure'. The problem in this view is that if public health is about prevention, then it 'will have to focus on all of the causes of public health problems ... such a conception of public health could be limitless, as almost all human activities (and many inactivities) may affect health.'[1]

Once epidemiology enabled public health to identify risk factors, it was a short step to examine broader environments that statistically correlate with them. Today, these are called social determinants, which, according to the WHO, are:

> *...the conditions in which people are born, grow, live, work and age, and people's access to power, money and resources.... These are the*

1 Dawson A & Verweij M (Eds) 2007. *Ethics, Prevention, and Public Health.* Oxford University Press: Oxford, 17

> *unfair and avoidable differences in health status seen within and between countries.*[2] *(Emphasis added)*

The *Social Determinants of Health Alliance* is a public health advocacy group that employs the slogan, 'fair, just, right, equitable'. It gathers substantial data indicating a link between poor health and poverty, suggesting that equality must be the solution.[3] Their intellectual leader is epidemiologist Professor Sir Michael Marmot, who, in the introduction to a United Nations report, stated, 'Health [inequity] … is a matter of social justice and … social injustice is killing people on a grand scale.'[4] Marmot elaborated on his theories at length during the 2016 Boyer Lectures.[5] Unfortunately, Marmot and his Australian supporters lack practical solutions beyond addressing the inequitable distribution of power, money, and resources, which essentially call for lobbying governments for increased income transfers from one group to another or advocating a socialist revolution. The *Health in All Policies Collaboration* expands upon the Marmot prescription by suggesting that medical and allied professionals utilise their skills to promote the ideology that a more equal society is healthier.[6]

In other words, public health insists that social factors are ultimately responsible for health disparities. Invoking social determinants greatly increases the complexity of causality, while simultaneously justifying the manipulation of societies. And, of course, determinants are not spread equally, so public health interventions tend to target 'those individuals who are judged most likely to develop disease.'[7]

---

2 United Nations, 2025. *Social Determinants Of Health: Key Facts*

3 Social Determinants of Health Alliance, http://socialdeterminants.org.au accessed 23 October 2016. Now called Climate and Health Alliance.

4 Commission on Social Determinants of Health, 2008. *Closing the Gap in a Generation*, i

5 Australian Broadcasting Commission, 2016. Fair Australia: social justice and the health gap. *2016 Boyer Lectures*

6 Gakh M, 2015. Law, the health in all policies approach, and cross-sector collaboration. *Public Health Reports* 130(1), 96

7 Rose G, 1992. *The Strategy of Preventive Medicine.* Oxford University Press: Oxford, 13

An example is young people who were allegedly ignored during the COVID-19 outbreak. The solution? Expand voting rights in Australia to 16-year-olds.[8] No matter how the young voted, the same advisers who advised the adults to lock down schools during COVID-19 would remain in place. The link between voting and ill health is so remote as to be incredible, but it is where public health with a social determinants frame leads.

The social determinants revolution has swept through public health institutions. The Australian Institute of Health and Welfare (AIHW), for example, presents variations in health determinants in diagrammatic form (Figure 2.1). The argument runs that the distribution of power and resources that comes with the socioeconomic gradient in a society results from various social and structural determinants. Variations in power and resources can lead to differences in these determinants. For example, having less power and fewer resources can heighten a person's exposure to health risks, making them more susceptible to illness and injury, and it can amplify the social and economic repercussions they may face due to poor health. The model also illustrates that this relationship is 'compounding', with the social and economic outcomes of poor health 'negatively impacting upstream determinants' that further limit an individual's access to power and resources.[9] From this vast array of determinants, which, if they could be changed, would make a difference to health?

---

8 Kapeke K et al, 2024. Young voices, healthy futures: the rationale for lowering the voting age to 16. *Medical Journal of Australia* 221(10), S18

9 Australian Institute of Health and Welfare, 2024. *What Are Determinants of Health?*

Figure 2.1 How differences in health determinants contribute to health

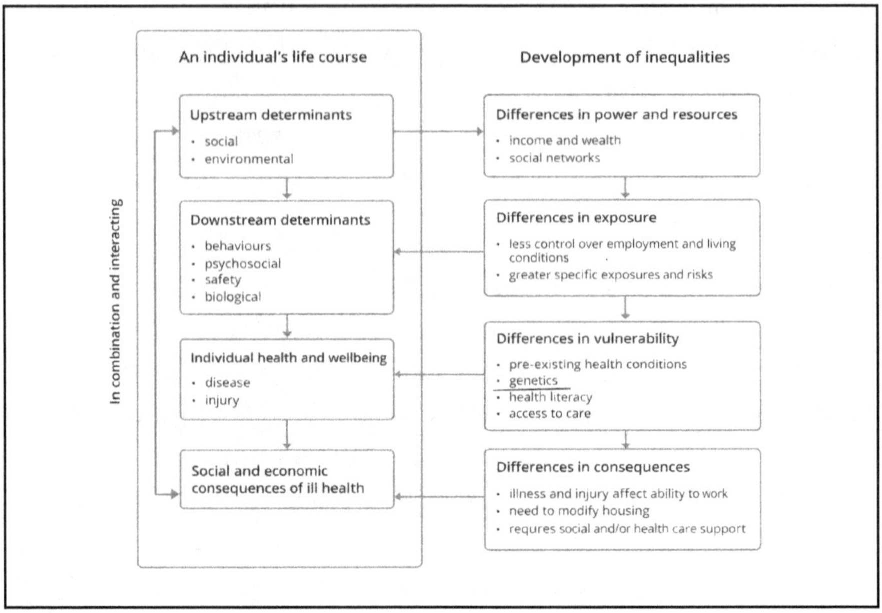

Source: Australian Institute of Health, 2024. *What Are Determinants of Health?*

While the public health lobby is busy sharpening its tools to change society, the dominant cause of differential health outcomes, genetics, remains out of reach. This may explain why it is buried in Figure 2.1. Those who focus on differential epidemiology study the impact of intelligence and personality on health.[10] They have established that there is a positive relationship between intelligence and survival.[11] They have established that cognitive ability, along with personality, consistently predict various health outcomes. Genetics accounts for approximately 50 per cent of all psychological traits, from personality to mental abilities.[12]

10 Deary I J, Weiss A & Batty G D, 2010. Intelligence and personality as predictors of illness and death: how researchers in differential psychology and chronic disease epidemiology are collaborating to understand and address health inequalities. *Psychological Science in the Public Interest* 11(2), 67

11 Sánchez-Izquierdo M et al, 2023. Intelligence and life expectancy in late adulthood: a meta-analysis. *Intelligence* 98, 7

12 Plomin R, 2018. *Blueprint: How DNA Makes Us Who We Are.* Penguin Random House, viii

The so-called mediating factors, such as socioeconomic factors,[13] and family background,[14] have a modest influence on health outcomes.[15] The likely explanation is that intelligence enhances an individual's health because it represents 'learning, reasoning, and problem-solving skills useful in preventing chronic disease and accidental injury and in adhering to complex treatment regimens.'[16]

The AIHW could also have mentioned, although this might be too controversial for a government agency, that personality traits such as conscientiousness and agreeableness influence things like employment prospects, which, in turn, affect income and health. These traits, for instance, affect how punctual individuals are, their willingness to follow instructions, their politeness towards customers, and their ability to collaborate with colleagues.[17] The AIHW and the government would need to face the uncomfortable truth that, for example, the unemployed tend to have poorer health because they generally exhibit a less conscientious and less agreeable personality profile than employed citizens.[18]

Furthermore, inadequate language skills can foster such a personality. Perkins notes that children from professional families hear an average of over 2,000 words per hour, compared to over 1,000 for working-class children and only about 600 for children of welfare claimants.[19] The cumulative vocabulary of these children is vastly different. The reality is that parents at the lower end of the socioeconomic spectrum hardly communicate with their children, which leads to detrimental

13 Deary I J, 2010, 67

14 Iveson, M H et al, 2018. Intelligence and all-cause mortality in the 6-Day Sample of the Scottish Mental Survey 1947 and their siblings: testing the contribution of family background, *International Journal of Epidemiology* 47(1), 89

15 Fries J & Pietschnig J, 2022. An intelligent mind in a healthy body? Predicting health by cognitive ability in a large European sample. *Intelligence* 93, 11

16 Gottfredson L S & Deary I J, 2004. Intelligence predicts health and longevity, but why? *Current Directions in Psychological Science*, 13(1), 1

17 Perkins A, 2016. *The Welfare Trait: How State Benefits Affect Personality*. Palgrave Macmillan

18 Perkins A, 2016, 133

19 Perkins A, 2016, 82

effects on their education. To illustrate the magnitude of the challenge in overcoming poor language skills, 60,000 children, or 20 per cent of those born in Australia, are born to mothers who are receiving welfare benefits.[20] These children are more likely to struggle with language skills than their peers. They are more likely to suffer ill health. Why is this discussion missing in government studies?

Perkins believes that a 'welfare state which increases the number of children born into disadvantaged households risks imposing a significant per capita headwind on society.' Each of those children will, on average, 'create a burden for the welfare state and the criminal justice system that is four times larger than the burden imposed by average individuals.'[21] More importantly, schooling has limited power to change upbringing and does not influence genes. Even children subjected to a very expensive program of intensive preschool tutoring are twice as likely as others to fall back on welfare or become involved in crime. A crucial finding is the willingness among welfare recipients 'to have extra children in order to increase welfare income, then to neglect those children.'[22] These statistics are supported by a study of vulnerable individuals in NSW, which found that females in the most vulnerable group are 25 times more likely to have children who eventually enter out-of-home care.[23] Women from poor backgrounds are less likely to follow contraceptive practices. Despite reported high contraceptive usage, nearly 40 per cent of women were at risk for unintended pregnancy, primarily due to inconsistent contraceptive use and reliance on ineffective contraception. Strategies may be needed to improve the consistency of effective contraceptive use or to place greater emphasis on long-acting contraceptives for specific subpopulations at higher risk for unintended pregnancy, yet the public health lobby is generally silent on naming sub-groups for fear of

20 Johns G, 2015. *No Contraception, No Dole: Tackling Intergenerational Welfare.* Connor Court, 130

21 Perkins A, 2016, 174

22 Perkins A, 2016, 159

23 New South Wales Government, 2018, 173

offence.[24]

These insights may seem somewhat fatalistic, but the evidence is robust. There is little point in wishing and hoping that everyone had the same inclination to make healthy choices or, indeed, to respond to information that would ensure they make sensible (to others) decisions. Unfortunately, this is not the case. Choices made under pressure, geared towards the immediate future, can be disastrous. Diabetics, for instance, may take their medication only 50 to 70 per cent of the time. An Australian study of elderly individuals with chronic ailments who visited a general practitioner more than 50 times in a year, 85 per cent of whom were on welfare, found that 40 per cent failed to adhere to their medication regimen.[25] Brilliant pharmacology amounts to nothing when someone forgets to take their tablet and no amount of public health nagging is likely to change this.

That DNA 'matters more than everything else' combined regarding the stable psychological traits that define who we are[26] seems not to trouble the AIHW. The fact that the connection between intelligence, personality, and illness is quite robust and has long been recognised also seems not to trouble public health institutions. While Figure 2.1 acknowledges genetics, its effects appear minimal. The upstream determinants — power, resources and exposure — are given significant weight, not because they have much impact, but because they create an extensive agenda for intervention with a misguided, and even detrimental pursuit of health equity. They articulate that health inequalities are differences in health among groups, and that health inequities are 'avoidable and unjust'.[27] The commitment to this ideology, despite the known impact of

24 Ong J et al, 2012. Contraception matters: indicators of poor usage of contraception in sexually active women attending family planning clinics in Victoria, Australia. *BMC Public Health* 23(12),1108

25 Laba T-L et al, 2018. Medication non-adherence in a cohort of chronically ill Australians: a case of missed opportunities. *Australian Journal of Medical Practice* 47(8)

26 Plomin R, 2018, x

27 Australian Institute of Health and Welfare, 2024. *What Are Determinants of Health?*

social interventions, some ineffectual, some adverse, and indeed, some unknown, all expensive, is astonishing.

Not only are individuals unique, but so are groups. Health equity is sought for priority populations, namely, the poor, Aboriginal people, and other favoured minorities. Alas, for the public health social determinants mindset, disparities do not equate to discrimination.[28] Differential outcomes do not imply unfairness; indeed, so long as they are not based on deliberate acts of repression, they may be essential for all to prosper.[29] All benefit from the best and brightest and their brilliant gifts to society. Public health officials must ask whether people are treated differently or if they behave differently. While it is possible to transfer funds and provide medical services to groups, it may not be feasible to 'prepare and orient people' to the behaviours necessary for improved health.[30] It is impossible to alter their genetic makeup, and it is difficult to change a culture that changes behaviour relevant to health.

An example of the unscientific approach by social determinants public health advocates is a paper on Aboriginal dental health from the Indigenous Oral Health Unit at the University of Adelaide. 'Oral disease is a direct reflection of societal disadvantage and is arguably a more visible representation of one's social position than any other trait. The disparities in oral health outcomes established by *colonisation* are perpetuated and widened by *neoliberalism* in Australia [and] … inadequately meet the oral health needs of Aboriginal and Torres Strait Islander Peoples.'[31] [emphasis added] These ideologues might consider that most people of Aboriginal descent are about as well off as other Australians.[32] The

28 Sowell T, 2019. *Discrimination and Disparities*. Basic Books

29 Deaton A, 2013. *The Great Escape: Health, Wealth, and the Origins of Inequality*. Princeton University Press 2015 Edition

30 Sowell T, 2019, 216

31 Poirier B et al, 2025. The causes of the causes: Aboriginal and Torres Strait Islander oral health and the neo liberalisation of Australia's dental health system. *Humanities and Social Sciences Communications* 12, 53

32 Shepherd S et al, 2020. Closing the (incarceration) gap: assessing the socio-economic and clinical indicators of indigenous males by lifetime incarceration status. *BMC Public Health* 20(1), 1

minority who are suffering reside on their lands, barely engaged in the modern economy and reliant on government support, which, while vastly superior to anything they experienced before colonisation, is insufficient to overcome a destructive culture,[33] the ravages of alcohol[34] and violence.[35] These environments are so powerful that even those who would survive and prosper under normal circumstances are less likely to lead healthy lives. Others survive because of personal characteristics. How does the social determinants approach help public health in this example? It denies that genetics, culture, or group behaviour explain ill health. When public health advocates are confronted with these facts, they either resort to the implausible concepts of colonisation, or to its alleged antidote, self-determination.

To the long list of possible social determinants has latterly been added commercial determinants.[36] The inclusion of commercial determinants shows that traditional social determinants like income and where you live are no longer enough to satisfy public health's reach, and that it is entering a bold new phase of interference with society. Commercial determinants of health refer to the activities undertaken by commercial organisations that public health perceives to affect people's health, either directly or indirectly. The argument suggests that private-sector commercial organisations (such as greengrocers and gymnasiums, or alcohol and fast food retailers) can have a positive or negative impact on health, particularly through multinational corporations.[37] What if a greengrocer or gymnasium is owned by a multinational? What do these analysts desire in a greengrocer? For example, a greengrocer in a major

---

33 Walter M, 2017. Doing Indigenous family. In M Walter, K Martin & G Bodkin-Andrews (Eds) *Indigenous Children Growing Up Strong: A Longitudinal Study of Aboriginal and Torres Strait Islander Families*. Palgrave Macmillan

34 d'Abbs P & Hewlett N, 2023. *Learning from 50 Years of Aboriginal Alcohol Programs*. Springer

35 Webb S, 1995. *Palaeopathology of Aboriginal Australians: Health and Disease Across a Hunter-gatherer Continent*. Cambridge University Press. Jarrett S, 2013. *Liberating Aboriginal People from Violence*. Connor Court. Pinker S, 2011. *The Better Angels of Our Nature: A History of Violence and Humanity* Penguin

36 https://www.aihw.gov.au/reports/australias-health/what-are-determinants-of-health

37 Gilmore A B et al, 2023,1194

outlet is likely to have far more sophisticated logistics, resulting in lower food waste and greater scrutiny of use-by dates and other quality control measures than might have been the case with a local greengrocer. There has been substantial growth in gymnasiums over the last 30 years, although a decline in some team sports may have offset this growth. Would the ownership of gymnasiums matter?

The social determinants model also claims that the 'profit motive conflicts with good health outcomes.' Are positive outcomes only achievable in a communist state? Do public officials not have their own agendas, specifically to criticise capitalism and praise public ownership? The exploration of the supposedly nefarious intentions of private enterprise has expanded beyond tobacco, alcohol, and discretionary foods, along with 'the large commercial organisations behind them,'[38] (or big tobacco, big alcohol, and big food, as public health likes to style them to make them sound extra sinister), to such things as examining 'social media's impact on mental health and the fossil fuel industry's role in pollution and climate change,[39] things that public health has latched onto to try and maintain its relevance. The consumption of tobacco and alcohol has decreased in Australia over recent decades; how is this connected to the ownership of production? Beyond the blatant ideology evident in these studies of the profit motive, there is a notable lack of contributions to effective health interventions. How does this framework assist a General Practitioner, a hospital physician, a nurse, an allied health professional, or an employer? What significance can be ascribed to any factor? How would it inform government decisions on resource allocation?

Unsubstantiated allegations like privatisation and reductions in government regulations are claimed to lead to various issues – misleading packaging, inappropriate marketing to children, harm to local communities and the environment during production, low pay

38 Lacy-Nichols J, Johnson M & Cullerton K, 2023. Commercial lobbying and political contributions: an Australian scoping review. *Australian and New Zealand Journal of Public Health* 47(4), 100073

39 Gilmore, 2023, 1194. See also MacKean C et al, 2024. *State of the Nation's Food Industry Report*. The Food Foundation

levels and hazardous work environments, greenwashing, spreading misinformation and disinformation, lobbying to block or delay regulations aimed at limiting harms, investment in health-harming products, and tax avoidance. Using Global Burden of Disease data, the ideologues estimated that four commercial products – tobacco, alcohol, ultra-processed food, and fossil fuels – were responsible for 19 million global deaths in 2019, which accounts for 34 per cent of all deaths and 41 per cent of non-communicable disease deaths.[40]

The sleight of hand lies in the phrase 'accounted for'. Were these deaths entirely attributable to these products? Would other harmful alternatives have replaced them if they hadn't existed? Would these deaths not have been premature if different factors contributed? Are those who now survive living longer, healthier lives, or are they enduring lives plagued by other ailments that diminish their satisfaction? Was the decline in consumption a result of improved harm awareness and specific behavioural interventions (such as banned advertising and better labelling) along with taxation, and if so, who carries the tax burden? These products are in demand by consumers. They are legal and widely valued. The latter, fossil fuels, underpin a healthy lifestyle, providing affordable energy and pharmaceuticals (strangely, public health seems reticent to take on 'big pharma' and has recently tended to label those who do as anti-vaxxers or other cranks). How these papers could be relied upon by the AIHW, especially one focused on public health, is beyond belief.

A bloated and ineffective empire

In the contest between nature (genes) and nurture (environment) in influencing health, individuals select, modify, and even create experiences based on their genes. Genetics accounts for about half of the correlations between what is often termed environmental measures and psychological traits. For example, the apparent environmental effects of

40 Gilmore, 2023, 1194

parenting on children's psychological development stem from parents responding to their children's genetic differences.[41] It is argued that broader environmental influences are random experiences rather than systematic forces like families. These experiences can affect people, but their impacts are often temporary; 'after these environmental bumps, we bounce back to our genetic trajectory.'[42] This is not to suggest that there is no value in trying to help; for instance, extended or enhanced education can improve knowledge and, consequently, people's ability to manage their health,[43] but the effects are limited. This is not what public health wants to hear, because for public health to maintain its relevance, it is vital that humans be viewed solely as products of society and therefore agree to whatever manipulations of society public health calls for.

The following two graphs further illustrate the influence of the social determinants of health ideology on the capture of public policy and institutions. The Australian Burden of Disease Study,[44] published by the AIHW, suggests that the years of life lost (YLL) rate due to all diseases is significantly higher in remote Australia compared to major cities (Figure 2.2). It indicates that 44 per cent of YLL could have been prevented if the rate for those living in remote Australia matched that of major cities.

41 Plomin R, 2018, ix

42 Plomin R, 2018, ix

43 Anton C J et al, 2012. Social origin, schooling and individual change in intelligence during childhood influence long-term mortality: a 68-year follow-up study. *International Journal of Epidemiology* 41, 398

44 Australian Institute of Health and Welfare, 2021. *Australian Burden of Disease Study 2018*

Figure 2.2 Years of life lost by remoteness area, 2018, persons

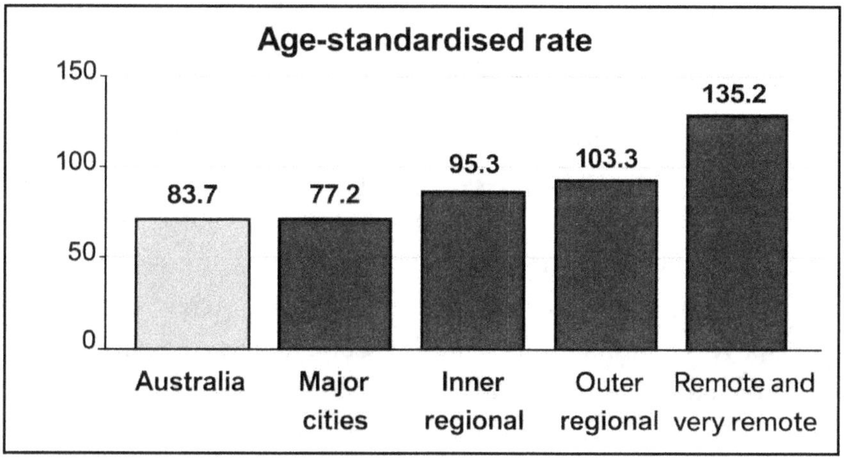

Source: Australian Institute of Health and Welfare, 2021. *Australian Burden of Disease Study 2018*

The study also indicates that the YLL rate for all disease sources is significantly higher among individuals in the lowest socioeconomic group than among those in the highest socioeconomic group (Figure 2.3). Thus, 44 per cent of the YLL in the lowest group could have been avoided if they had the same rate as the highest group.

Figure 2.3 Years of life lost by socioeconomic group, 2018, persons

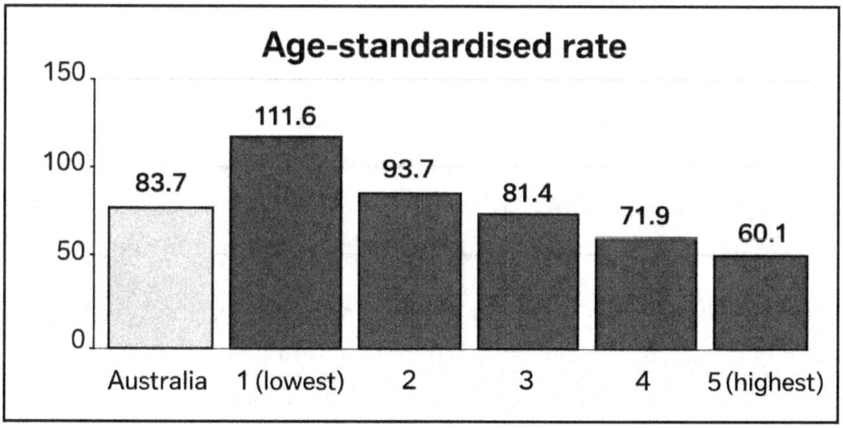

Source: Australian Institute of Health and Welfare, 2021. *Australian Burden of Disease Study 2018*

In these instances, the use of 'if' raises the question of why a gap exists between groups, whether by class or race (proxy measured by remoteness). The social and economic determinants are assumed causes, yet little else is considered. If it were possible to relocate people to cities and place them in higher social classes, would they experience improved health? The rationale for these measures is that they are available, appealing, and acceptable. These are the images that some policymakers find comfortable; for example, the oppression of the class system leads to poor health, or the lack of resources from indifferent governments and taxpayers contributes to ill health. For example, the AIHW argues that 'if the poor were as healthy as the rich, they would be 21 per cent better off.'[45] They further say that 30 per cent of the burden of disease (a measure combining the impacts of dying early and living with illness) is caused by 'modifiable risk factors' and, therefore, is preventable.

Class differences do not explain health differentials in a way that leads to effective change. The AIHW acknowledges that the concept of social determinants of health can serve as a platform for interventions in various policy fields, such as transport, housing, environment, education, and social services. However, it cautions that health determinants differ in their modifiability.[46] The more upstream (social) determinants, such as education, employment, income, and family structure, can be difficult to modify successfully. Modification for the more downstream determinants can be more specific. For instance, programs and policies aimed at influencing health behaviours—such as legislation against smoking in cars with children, restrictions on alcohol sales to young people, and enforcing seat belt usage— can help reduce the burden of illness and injury. Action must be based on the effectiveness and cost of the restrictions, including their impact on consumers.

When effectiveness is unproven or minimal, and costs are high, public health becomes merely an exercise in changing society: it is not for the faint-hearted. For example, most Australians (67 per cent of those born

45 Australian Institute of Health and Welfare, 2016. *Impact and Causes of Illness and Deaths in Australia 2011*, vii

46 Australian Institute of Health and Welfare, 2012. *Australia's Health 2012*, 13

between 1976 and 1982) earn more than their parents did at a similar age, particularly those from poorer families.[47] The returns to longevity may be relatively minor, judging from the longevity of Australians, which has risen far more slowly after the gains of the last half of the 20th century (shown in I.1). Furthermore, around 85 per cent of individuals whose parents were in the bottom income decile have moved out.[48] In terms of social determinants, surely this shift would work wonders for relative health inequities? The greater story is of a society solving its health problems by pursuing old-fashioned progress. And for the intervention-inclined, it is not as if taxpayers are not assisting those in need. While the poorest 20 per cent of the population earn three per cent of all private incomes, after receiving benefits and paying taxes, their share of income increases to 13 per cent.[49] It seems that a just society is always out of reach and, for public health aficionados, only more intervention can solve it.

Who can be blamed for obesity?

Take the example of obesity. Whose needs should be prioritised? Should a person with a shorter-than-average lifespan be considered more deserving than someone likely to live longer yet risk having their expected life cut short by a preventable disease? Are those genetically advantaged less deserving? This latter question stems from an assumption obscured by an ideology prevalent in the social sciences, which posits that every person is a blank slate and that their circumstances are determined by external forces that they can influence.[50] In the health context, this implies they should enjoy a long life like others and that those who do not are somehow deprived due to various preventable factors. (Presumably,

47 Australian Government Productivity Commission, 2024. *Fairly Equal? Economic Mobility in Australia*, Research paper, Canberra, 2

48 Australian Government Productivity Commission, 2024, 3

49 Australian Bureau of Statistics, 2018, *Government Benefits, Taxes and Household Income, Australia*

50 Pinker S, 2003. *The Blank Slate: The Modern Denial of Human Nature.* Penguin 2019 Edition

no one argues that individuals who enjoy long lives should die earlier to attain greater health equality). Unless the illness is specific and the causes are well understood, it is nearly impossible to assist every person meaningfully. More importantly, misguided policies waste valuable resources that could be better allocated to other health concerns.

In developed countries over the past thirty years, rates of obesity and morbid obesity have increased as the average adult consumes more calories, protein, fat, and sodium than those in the 1970s.[51] The reason is that calorie intake tends to rise with income. This is presumably due to a shift in food composition, such as greater consumption of fats and sugars alongside fruits and vegetables.[52] In Australia, the level of poverty has decreased, yet rates of obesity, particularly childhood obesity, have surged among the poorer population. Overall, everyone is consuming more, but the poor (who aren't as disadvantaged as before) are eating even more and often making poor food choices. The rise of processed food has played an important role, but although the public health lobby is quick to demand taxes on such goods, it has shown little genuine interest in the reasons why people choose those foods. For some, for example, a bag of corn chips and a bottle of soft drink are now the only real pleasure in life they can afford and the hit of fat and sugar means happiness in otherwise hard, empty, and unfulfilling lives. Others grew up in homes where nobody knew how to cook fresh, healthy foods, or could not be bothered. Others are too focused on just trying to put food on the table to feed hungry mouths to worry too much about what that food is. Yet as always, public health shows little interest in the lives of those others whom it seeks to help.

A McKinsey study concluded, 'Obesity is a complex, systemic issue with no single or simple solution.'[53] But that does not stop people from

51 United States figures. Kranjac A & Wagmiller R, 2016. Decomposing trends in adult body mass index, obesity, and morbid obesity, 1971-2012. *Social Science and Medicine* 167, 43 and Komlos J & Brabec M, 2011. The trend of BMI values of U.S. adults by deciles, birth cohorts 1882–1986 stratified by gender and ethnicity. *Economics & Human Biology* 9(3), 234

52 Mazzocchi M & Traill W B, 2011. Calories, obesity and health in OECD countries. *Applied Economics* 43(26), 3926

53 McKinsey Global Institute, 2014. Overcoming obesity: an initial economic analysis. *Discussion Paper*, 1

trying. For example, a recommended 'regulatory' menu (Text Box 2.1), represents a complete takeover of a child's life – from protecting breastfeeding to restricting unhealthy food in school tuckshops to forcing healthy food into low-income neighbourhoods. Such interference has other rationales. Some schools, for example, have initiated campaigns to remove red meat, poultry, pork, and seafood from the menu on one or more days of the week to (ostensibly) promote health and environmental stewardship. Unfortunately, while children are told red meat is unhealthy, they are not told that they are missing 'a protein- and micronutrient-dense whole food option.'[54] This is not smart. More broadly, the purview of health professionals is spreading to entire suburbs where people do not shop for fresh food. The lack of such produce, of course, is blamed on suppliers. Food deserts bring the classic bête noire, where commercial interests, geography and commerce are blamed.[55]

Text Box 2.1 'Smart' food policies for obesity prevention

Provide an enabling environment for healthy preference learning
- Protection and promotion of breastfeeding
- Reformulation to reduce the sugar content in foods targeted at children
- 'Zoning out' unhealthy food retail in places where children gather.

Overcome barriers to the expression of healthy preferences
- Initiatives to make specific healthy foods available in schools
- Community and homestead gardening projects
- Incentives to attract retailers of healthy foods into underserved low-income neighbourhoods.

Encourage people to reassess unhealthy preferences at point-of-purchase
- Health-related food taxes
- Targeted food subsidies implemented in the form of an incentive
- Standards that restrict foods from specific settings.

Source: Hawkes C et al, 2015. Smart food policies for obesity prevention. *The Lancet* 385(9985), 8

54 Kavanaugh M et al, 2025. Considering the nutritional benefits and health implications of red meat in the era of meatless initiatives. *Frontiers in Nutrition* 12(1525011)

55 Allcott H, Diamond R, & Dubé J-P, 2018. The geography of poverty and nutrition: food deserts and food choices across the United States. *Working Paper No. 3631*, Graduate School of Business, Stanford University

Healthy eating is increasingly becoming part of the workplace. The Victorian Department of Health has released a healthy eating guide for workplaces. Yet, it is more than just a gentle nudge. It is a rallying cry. The guide encourages workers to 'Seek management endorsement for implementing the Policy & Guide.' The Department urges workers to: 'Nominate a staff member, establish a new committee, or utilise an existing committee to assist in planning and managing the implementation of the Policy & Guide.'[56] A rallying cry, indeed, if the employer is willing to fund it. And since when has it been standard practice to instruct employers to dictate how employees should eat?

Would rationing be beneficial? A natural experiment stemming from the abrupt end of sugar rationing in the UK after World War II showed 'a protective effect of this rationing against the later development of type 2 diabetes and hypertension.'[57] Is rationing a viable option in reality? Would organised callisthenics help? Every morning, an alarm could ring to jolt citizens from their slumber and urge them into a rigorous round of exercise. Mass callisthenics were quite 'popular' in Hungary during Communist rule.[58] Governments could assign a nutritionist and a social worker to each citizen. Mind you, and wouldn't you know, some research hints that the intense activity to get you fit could make you unhappy. 'It is not clear that encouraging everyone to engage in higher intensity activity for longer will achieve the desired policy effect suggested by proponents of increasing the intensity of physical activity in the population.'[59] Having fun with friends in active leisure may be more effective. These various interventions aim to modify the environment in which people operate to enhance their health. The evidence is proving challenging.

---

56 Department of Health Victoria, 2016. *Healthy Choices: Healthy Eating Policy and Catering Guide for Workplaces*, 9

57 Gracner T, Boone C & Gertler P J, 2024. Exposure to sugar rationing in the first 1000 days of life protected against chronic disease. *Science* 386(6725),1043

58 https://muzeumkomunismu.cz/en/

59 Downward P & Dawson P, 2016. Is it pleasure or health from leisure that we benefit from most? An analysis of well-being alternatives and implications for policy. *Social Indicators Research* 126(1), 460

Is obesity a public health issue?

Obesity is not only poorly understood, but it may not be as harmful as many claim, certainly not enough to 'justify diverting scarce resources away from far more pressing public health issues.'[60] While the WHO is often keen to label something an epidemic—which, in this case, suggests exponential growth in obesity—it seems that, although there is significant weight gain among the heaviest individuals, the vast majority of people in the overweight and obese categories are only slightly above what they or their predecessors maintained a generation ago.[61] The WHO asserts that mortality rates increase with higher degrees of overweight, as measured by BMI. Still, most individuals classified as overweight and obese based on current definitions do not face any substantially increased risk of early death. Evidence showing that weight loss in obese individuals reduces mortality is lacking.[62] In other words, while maintaining a healthy body weight is a good thing, not having a healthy body weight is not necessarily the catastrophic public health crisis it is made out to be.

The thrifty gene hypothesis suggests that mutations favour fat storage and survival during famine but also increase the risk of diabetes. Consequently, obesity may be a symptom of diabetes rather than its primary cause. Health improvements are attributed to diet and exercise rather than any subsequent body fat loss as part of a program. Discussions surrounding obesity and being overweight as health risks often equate weight with health behaviour, paralleling smoking. Hence, overweight and obesity are frequently labelled as preventable causes of illness. However, the connection between behaviour and weight is closely linked to unchangeable factors such as genetics, body build, and shape. The average person's control over their weight is, at best, limited. As the authors conclude, 'it is a remarkable fact that the central premise of the

60 Campos P et al, 2006. The epidemiology of overweight and obesity: public health crisis or moral panic? *International Journal of Epidemiology* 35(1), 55

61 Campos P, 2006, 55

62 Campos P, 2006, 56

current war on fat — that turning obese and overweight individuals into so-called "normal weight" people will improve their health — remains an untested hypothesis.'[63]

An example of a modifiable risk factor is high body mass — fat. This can lead to heart disease, diabetes, and more. Many modifiable risks are linked to life history and behaviour; they are familiar and include alcohol, tobacco, drugs, unsafe sex, physical inactivity, childhood sexual abuse, domestic violence, and a diet low in vegetables. All these factors are heavily influenced by social class. However, the flaw in the association between health and class is that there may be other significant reasons why those who are poor tend to be unhealthy.

It will not come as any surprise, for example, that all these factors are intergenerational. Children whose parents exercise, do not smoke, or binge drink are more likely to consume more fruit and vegetables and fewer energy-dense (junk) foods. In contrast, children of mothers with poor habits tend to eat less fruit and vegetables. Unhealthy eating habits in children, often carried into adolescence and adulthood, are more prevalent among males, those from low-income families, single-parent households, rural areas, children of parents without a university degree, those who were not breastfed at six months old, and kids whose mothers have less healthy eating and lifestyle practices.[64] The same study found that children in single-parent households watched more television and consumed more high-fat and high-sugar foods while eating less fresh fruit and vegetables than children from dual-parent households. The findings suggest that an additive effect of dietary and activity variables may contribute to the higher rates of overweight and obesity in Australian children, with girls from single-parent households being particularly at risk.[65] A trial intervention to reduce

---

63 Campos P, 2006, 57

64 Daraganova G & Thornton L, 2013. Eating behaviour: socio-economic determinants and parental influence. *Longitudinal Study of Australian Children Annual Statistical Report 2013*, 91

65 Byrne L et al, 2011. Parental status and childhood obesity in Australia. *International Journal of Pediatric Obesity 6*, 415

sugar-sweetened drink consumption in disadvantaged schools showed no effect, suggesting that sustained change would require a massive intervention.

Obesity Australia observes, quite plausibly, that 'over the first two to three years after birth, a child's taste and food preferences are set, contributing to susceptibility in our current obesogenic environment.'[66] Obesity Australia argues that many individuals are prone to obesity in an era when food is plentiful and cheap. For Obesity Australia, as for nearly all advocates of preventive programs, the solution is to remake disadvantaged environments and teach children healthier habits than their parents. In some respects, this agenda is no different from that which established the public school system. That is, there are those who, if left to their own devices, would be unable to afford to learn or would lack sufficient insight or intelligence to acquire the skills and habits that would make them more capable of succeeding overall and less vulnerable to harm. The issue here concerns the allocation of resources to school curricula and related contexts. The various programs discussed would likely be ineffective or, at the very least, as ineffective as any school's programs have been in reducing differences in intelligence, personality, and income.

But to what extent can policies influence a person's chances of obesity? It appears not much. A heritability rate of 70 per cent for weight, for instance, suggests that, on average, the differences in weight among individuals are primarily due to inherited DNA variations, even when accounting for personal differences in diet, exercise, and lifestyle. For genetic reasons, some individuals find it far easier to gain weight than to lose it.[67] As Robert Plomin argues, 'although weight is a physical characteristic, ... weight is the result of behaviour – what we eat, how much we eat, and how much we exercise ... In many ways, the obesity epidemic is a psychological problem.'[68] The scope for changing

66 Obesity Australia, 2013. *Action Agenda*, 4

67 Plomin R, 2018, 10

68 Plomin R, 2018, 12

people's psychology is no simple matter and not be undertaken lightly. For example, public health wants people to lose weight, but it cannot engage in body shaming because public health campaigns insist that leads to stigma and mental ill health.

So what does all of this tell us about how public health sees genetics? Objectively, we can see that genetics are important – not just in terms of their role in people's body size and shape, or susceptibility to certain conditions, but because things like intelligence and personality affect a range of other behaviours and circumstances that in turn influence obesity. And genetics and their influence get passed on, creating an intergenerational cycle that is exceptionally resistant to change. Yet according to public health, banning school tuckshops from selling lollies will achieve something, because exposure to lollies is a social determinant that is just as, if not more, important than genetics and upbringing.

What is to be done?

Public health has latched onto social determinants and inequality not only to insert itself into an ever-widening range of issues, but to shift attention away from the reality of human existence – that being, we are not blank slates. In his study of family circumstances over generations, Gregory Clark concludes that individuals tend to return to the genetic norm. Nature persists across generations despite public investment in equality. 'Time and again, social mobility is inherited within families, and there is scant evidence that we can, through feasible social programs, significantly increase it.'[69] The tendency for genetics to assert itself across generations is not a condemning statement, but it does highlight the limits of interventions; only those that are direct, powerful, and affordable should be included in the policy toolkit. Rather than attempting to reinvent the world and using social determinants as a means of lamenting unfairness as if it were the root cause of disparities

69 Clark G, 2014. *The Son Also Rises: Surnames and the History of Social Mobility*. Princeton University Press

in health outcomes, we should focus on effective interventions. While Plomin has significantly highlighted the role of genes in health, he clearly states that 'heritability describes what is, not what could be.'[70] Genetic influences are powerful tendencies, not deterministic programming.

The scope for social intervention in health is very narrow. Three examples of interventions proposed in the differential epidemiology literature may be beneficial — emulating the lifestyles of those best positioned to manage their health, education, and the patient-doctor relationship.

It is not hard to notice how smart people take care of their bodies and health, and how they manage their illnesses. These strategies can be widely promoted and regarded as valid and helpful healthcare guidelines. The same applies to the behavioural choices of people with high conscientiousness.[71] Such modest interventions are a far cry from the change society, defeat inequality and defeat capitalist grocers typical of public health campaigns. Indeed, this idea harks back to an earlier era when it was expected to learn manners from those who, in turn, had been taught them. In socialising medicine and the school system, the idea of behaving well, perhaps in a middle-class manner, was eschewed.

There is the inevitable hope of better education. Efforts to enhance intelligence through education might be just as significant for public health.[72] The difficulty arises from the massive intervention required among some groups to get them to attend school, interventions that would offend the sensibilities of the public health mindset. Dragooning our Aboriginal children to school to overcome their poor parental examples to improve their health may be a good idea, but what public health official would have the heart for it?

The final string in this exceedingly thin bow of recommended interventions by the differential epidemiologists on how people interact with and communicate with health-care practitioners. Regarding

70 Plomin R, 2018, 154

71 Deary I J, 2010, 73

72 Anton C J, 2012, 398

cognitive abilities, one possibility is that more intelligent patients tend to have larger vocabularies and might have researched their condition before visiting a doctor. As a result, they may be better able to articulate their symptoms. Likewise, the broader vocabulary of more intelligent patients may enable them to understand better and apply advice for managing a health condition. Is it possible to prepare the less intelligent to ask better questions and to be more diligent in their health regimes?

Unfortunately, aspects of personality may influence how an individual interacts with others. Patients who display higher agreeableness may be more compliant, more inclined to trust their doctor, and more honest and open when discussing their condition. In contrast, individuals who are cynical and distrustful of medical practitioners might be more likely to resort to unorthodox and unproven treatments, which could be ineffective or even dangerous. Moreover, the effects of intelligence and personality on the relationship might be subtler, with intelligent and congenial patients possibly eliciting more empathy from their healthcare providers. [73]

Of the public health interventions in Figure 2.1, only one social determinant makes sense: health literacy. Individual health literacy involves personal skills such as the ability to find, understand, and use health information; for instance, completing healthcare forms or navigating the healthcare system. The health literacy environment is also considered, encompassing the policies, processes, and materials that influence how individuals interact with the healthcare system.[74] Here, and only here, the crucial attributes of individuals take centre stage, and interventions may be effective.

Individuals with low health literacy tend to experience poorer overall health outcomes and engage in adverse health behaviours,[75] such as higher

73 Deary I J, 2010, 67

74 Australian Commission on Safety and Quality in Health Care, 2014. *National Statement on Health Literacy*

75 Berkman N D et al, 2011. Low health literacy and health outcomes: an updated systematic review. *Annals of Internal Medicine* 155(2), 97

hospital readmission rates,[76] and challenges in self-managing illness.[77] For example, lower health literacy, diminished cognitive function, and a higher number of medications have each been independently linked to a reduced understanding of the preadmission medication regimen.[78] Clinicians should consider these factors when evaluating the accuracy of patients' reported medication regimens and advising patients on safe and effective medication use. Encouragingly, another study found that health literacy interventions significantly impacted adherence among lower-income groups and racial-ethnic minority patients compared to non-minority and higher-income samples.[79] Timing may also be influential. For example, in-hospital nutrition, following surgery, may be a time in which the limited intervention of the hospital can change a person's habits, and indeed, doctors are more entitled to influence their patients, as opposed to the public at large. Scale and timing are important in calculating interventions and payoffs.[80]

Conclusion

These few pointers to possibly effective interventions may seem inadequate compared to the extensive list of health determinants. However, it is better to possess a small list of interventions that genuinely understand humans than a lengthy list that treats them as mere pawns in vast sociological and ideological schemes. Yet this is what the social determinants model of public health does. The barriers to change are significant, the costs are high, and where is the payoff?

76 Mitchell S E et al, 2012. Health literacy and 30-day post discharge hospital utilization. *Journal of Health Communication* 17(3), 325

77 Geboers B et al, 2016. The association between health literacy and self-management abilities in adults aged 75 and older, and its moderators. *Quality of Life Research* 25(11), 2869

78 Marvanova M et al, 2011. Health literacy and medication understanding among hospitalized adults. *Journal of Hospital Medicine* 6(9), 488

79 Miller T A, 2016. Health literacy and adherence to medical treatment in chronic and acute illness: a meta-analysis. *Patient Education and Counseling* 99(7), 1079

80 Winter G, 2022. Nutrition and the surgical patient. *The Bulletin of the Royal College of Surgeons of England* 104(1)

The Tasmanian Government, for example, announced in 2015 that it aimed to make Tasmania the healthiest population in Australia by 2025. Tasmanians are among the least healthy Australians, and they are the oldest, second only to Northern Territorians, who, although the youngest, have high rates of chronic diseases and health risk factors such as smoking, obesity, poor nutrition, low levels of physical activity, and risky alcohol consumption. The Tasmanian strategy and push for this goal originated from the public health lobby, the Health and Wellbeing Advisory Council, and the Health Council of Tasmania.[81]

In 2016, the strategy was in development. Almost a decade later, there is an evaluation framework, but no evaluations have been conducted. They are planning various initiatives, showing enthusiasm for governance, and maintaining a grant fund for small community organisations, yet they lack evaluations and concrete data on health outcomes. Despite the absence of evidence, they are eager to promote the notion that there is a link between climate change and health. They have supported community food hubs, again without proof that anyone is healthier, engages in more bike riding, or develops stronger social connections, with no evidence of improved outcomes. The objective was merely to appear busy.[82] That, however, is how public health maintains its relevance. It has even turned the blatant shortcomings of the social determinants model into both an excuse for lack of outcomes and a rallying cry for its troops – change does not happen overnight, and just because something is hard to do does not mean it should not be done.

By emphasising the social determinants of health above all else, and — most importantly — by finding a constant supply of (increasingly distant and ephemeral) determinants, or new ways for old determinants

81 Will Hodgman Premier of Tasmania and Michael Ferguson, Minister for Health, A Healthy Tasmania. *Press release* 22 February 2015

82 Doherty T, Jose K & Cleland V, 2022. *Healthy Tasmania Research and Evaluation Framework*. Menzies Institute for Medical Research, University of Tasmania. Tasmanian Government Department of Health, 2023. *Healthy Tasmania Five-Year Strategic Plan 2022–2026 Report for Years 1 and 2*

to affect people, public health ensures that its work is never done. Had it not hitched itself to social determinants, public health may have withered decades ago.

3

Public Health Acts: instruments of oppression

Health regulation that... achieves a minimal health benefit with disproportionate human burdens is not tolerated in a society based on the rule of law.[1]

Lawrence Gostin, Professor of Public Health at Johns Hopkins University

Does Gostin's observation mean that Australia is no longer a society based on the rule of law? It was undoubtedly true in Victoria, where it is hard to forget the COVID-19-era footage of a distressed, pregnant woman in her pyjamas being arrested in her home in front of her partner and children, handcuffed by Victoria Police, for nothing more than making Facebook posts about lockdowns. The police charged Zoe Buhler with incitement to breach a public health order. She had created a 'freedom day' anti-lockdown protest event. During her arrest, she told police, 'I have no idea why you guys are doing this...My two kids are here. I have an ultrasound in an hour. I'm happy to delete the post.'[2] Police stated that 'any gathering of this nature is in blatant breach of the chief health officer's directions and puts Victorian lives at risk.' Two years later, Victoria Police withdrew the charge because it was 'not in

1 Gostin L O, 2000. *Public health law: power, duty, restraint.* University of California Press, 20

2 Michael McGowan, Pregnant woman arrested in Ballarat for creating anti-lockdown protest event on Facebook. *The Guardian* 2 September 2020

the public interest to continue with the prosecution.'[3] Why, then, was it in the public interest to arrest Ms Buhler in the first place?

This was just one prominent example of the massive infringements on civil liberties that Australia's public health laws encouraged, while human rights agencies stayed silent. Although it was easy at the time to blame the police for overreach and abuse of power — and that is undoubtedly true — the fact is that the police were applying the laws following the declaration of an emergency and the exercise of emergency powers under various Public Health Acts.[4]

During the COVID-19 era, emergency declarations, as well as State and Territory public health legislation and subsequent directions,[5] gave license to the many travesties.[6] Those powers were in place long before the pandemic declaration. Most importantly, they have not gone away. Public Health Acts continue to grant government officials astonishing powers. Lawmakers and large sections of society tolerated it, and some watchdogs were asleep. The Australian Human Rights Commission raised concerns about the increasing authoritarianism in response to COVID-19.[7] Unfortunately, the Victorian Equal Opportunity and Human Rights Commission seemed indifferent to Victorians confined for an unprecedented time under Victoria's *COVID-19 Omnibus (Emergency*

---

3 Lexie Jeuniewic, Police drop anti-lockdown incitement charge against Ballarat woman Zoe Buhler. *ABC News* 30 Aug 2022

4 Mclean H & Huf B, 2020. Emergency powers, public health and COVID-19. *Research Paper No. 2, August*. Research & Inquiries Unit Parliamentary Library & Information Service, Victorian Parliament

5 For example, the Chief Health Officer of Queensland gave 496 directions stemming from her powers under the Health Act. See, Revoked and superseded public health directions https://www.health.qld.gov.au/system-governance/legislation/cho-public-health-directions-under-expanded-public-health-act-powers/revoked

6 Although there is federal public health legislation, this concerns itself mainly with the Pharmaceutical Benefits Scheme and tobacco. While the latter is certainly relevant, this chapter focuses on state and territory legislation.

7 Croucher R, 2022. Executive discretion at a time of COVID-19: promoting, protecting and fulfilling human rights in the contemporary public health context. *11th Austin Asche Oration in Law and Governance*. Australian Human Rights Commission. And various statements by Commissioners as of April 2020.

Measures) Act of May 2020. The Commissioner prioritised workplace equality and addressed racism, but paid little attention to the widespread confinement of the population and the arrests of individuals for peaceful protests.[8]

Amnesty International displayed commendable courage in its submission to the Commonwealth Inquiry, saying that 'governments must not impose blanket vaccination mandates and should seek to ensure that vaccination is with full consent.'[9] Such human rights groups, however, are characterised by formulaic thinking, spouting such memes as 'the right to prior, free, and informed consent for any medical procedure', and that Aboriginal communities are affected disproportionately, as if individuals in any community do not count. They did not go so far as to point out the lack of consent inherent in a vaccine, or in vaccines developed in such a short time that long-term side effects could not be known. Putting aside the obsession with group sentiment, after all, the COVID-19 response adversely affected every person, there was some, but not much, resistance from human rights advocates to the powers governments wielded under the Public Health Acts in Australia. The Acts granted authorities the power to manage a pandemic. They were central to the oppressive treatment of those who questioned the COVID-19 responses, as well as specific measures such as employee vaccine mandates.

It is comforting to think that such powers could or would only ever exist in extraordinary times, and would be swiftly overturned at the earliest moment. In reality, the powers used during COVID-19 were in place long before the pandemic declaration. Most importantly, they have not gone away. This should not surprise us: the coercive powers of the state have long been a tool that public health relies on to advance its ideology.

---

8 Victorian Equal Opportunity and Human Rights Commission, 2020. Human rights and Victoria's *COVID-19 Omnibus (Emergency Measures) Act* May 2020 and Opening Statement for the Parliamentary Inquiry into the Victorian Government's Response to the COVID-19 Pandemic 26 August 2020

9 Amnesty International Australia, 2024. *Submission to the Commonwealth Government COVID-19 Response Inquiry*

Public health legislation covers just about anything

Public health gets its power from legislation, and using the law to advance its own ends is a favoured tool. Thanks to its social determinants focus, the legislative remit of public health is almost limitless, extending far beyond infectious diseases and physical conditions linked to pathogens. The Australian Capital Territory legislation, for example, defines public health as 'the health of individuals in the context of the wider health of the community; or the organised response by society to protect and promote health and prevent illness, injury and disability.'[10] In Western Australia, public health means 'the health of individuals in the context of the wider health and wellbeing of the community and the combination of safeguards, policies and programmes designed to protect, maintain, promote and improve the health of individuals and their communities and to prevent and reduce the incidence of illness and disability.'[11] In the Northern Territory and Tasmania, public health means 'the physical, mental and social wellbeing of the community.'[12] Wellbeing? Where, exactly, does that begin and end? And can there be any limit whatsoever on how far the nebulous idea of social wellbeing can reach?

An Act's objects provide a better understanding of how far public health can meddle in the life of citizens. In New South Wales, for instance, the objects of the Act are not solely about protecting the public from infectious diseases but to 'promote, protect and improve public health.'[13] From this broad base, the health Minister has considerable power. If the Minister considers, 'on reasonable grounds', a 'likely risk' to public health, the Minister may deal with the risk and its consequences.[14]

The objects of the South Australian and Western Australian Acts are significant for social engineering and reducing inequality. For example, in South Australia, 'to prevent disease, medical conditions, injury and

10 *Public Health Act 1997* (ACT) Part 3, 17

11 *Public Health Act 2016* (WA) Part 1, 10

12 *Public And Environmental Health Act 2011* (NT) Part 1, 4

13 *Public Health Act 2010* (NSW) Part 1, 2

14 *Public Health Act 2010* (NSW) Part 2, 7

disability through a public health approach; and to ensure … a healthy environment for all South Australians and particularly those who live within disadvantaged communities … and to encourage individuals and communities to plan for, create and maintain a healthy environment.'[15] In Western Australia, the objects are 'to encourage individuals and communities to plan for, create and maintain a healthy environment … and to facilitate the *provision of information to decision-making authorities* (emphasis added) about public health risks and benefits to public health that may result from certain proposals.'[16] Providing information to authorities is important, but providing the public with information about the advice to authorities is undoubtedly the most essential aspect of public health. No Public Health Act does so.

The Victorian Act explicitly embeds government in people's lives and has almost unlimited scope to do so. For example, The Parliament recognises that 'public health and wellbeing includes the absence of disease, illness, injury, disability or *premature death* and the collective state of public health and wellbeing' and that 'interventions should *reduce inequalities* in health'[17] (emphasis added). The addition of premature death is significant because although death does, of course, relate to health, premature death can be linked to almost anything. There is, after all, no shortage of public health academic papers claiming that X will take Y years off our lives, or public health lobbyists seeking funding in the name of (in their opinion) 'preventable' mortality. Victoria, unsurprisingly, also gives itself one of the broadest mandates 'to achieve the highest attainable standard of public health and wellbeing.'[18] Concepts, such as premature death, can extend to almost any lifestyle choice people may make. Promoting conditions that support people's health is very broad. Does that include, for example, silencing debate denounced as a risk of triggering distress, potentially leading to mental ill health? As for reducing inequality, the Act knows no bounds, because, courtesy of genetics, inequalities are

15 *South Australian Public Health Act 2011*(SA) Part 2, 8

16 *Public Health Act 2016* (WA) Part 1, 3

17 *Public Health and Wellbeing Act 2008* (Vic) Part 2, 36

18 *Public Health and Wellbeing Act 2008* (Vic) Part 2, 36

inherent to individual health.

When courts interpret laws, they examine these objects to determine what the laws are intended to achieve. This is not in itself unusual. Officials are, of course, meant to act in line with the law and advance its objectives. However, in the context of public health, advancing the broad and nebulous objects of the Acts gives Ministers and health officials license to take equally broad and nebulous actions. What these Acts say is that anything whatsoever that people do that might have some bearing on their (or someone else's) physical, mental, or social wellbeing, is an opening for government intrusion. If terms such as reasonably necessary or reasonably believes are scrutinised by the courts, it is difficult to argue that something was not reasonably necessary, or that an official did not believe that something was reasonable, given the sheer breadth of what public health acts are supposed to achieve.

Chief Public Health Officers have extraordinary powers under these Acts to undertake measures they consider effective in reducing or eliminating health risks. The Chief Public Health Officer may request the participation of any public authority whose intervention may help identify or respond to the circumstances.[19] Is it any wonder that we saw our army deployed against Australian citizens during COVID-19? During a public health state of emergency, the Chief Health Officer coordinates the activities of any public authority needed to respond to the emergency. The Chief Health Officer may direct any public authority to perform any function and appoint an officer of a public authority to have overall control of activities carried out by public authorities in response to the emergency.[20] Most disconcertingly, public health powers can encompass anything remotely related to people's health. The Minister may, by notice in the Gazette, declare a disease or medical condition to be a non-communicable condition if the Minister considers that the disease or medical condition is of significance to public health.[21]

19 *South Australian Public Health Act 2011* (SA) Part 3, 15

20 *Public Health Act 2016* (WA) Part 12, 157

21 *South Australian Public Health Act 2011* (SA) Part 7, 36

Given that medical conditions now include psychological conditions, and that reducing or preventing a condition can involve all manner of environmental and social interventions, this raises fundamental questions about precisely what public health is.

Risk and harm – magic words

The concepts of risk and harm provide the astonishing powers in each Act. Some jurisdictions primarily focus on the concept of risk as an activity that may involve the transmission of disease, as is the case with the Tasmanian Act.[22] However, this is the exception; most acts go further. In the ACT, for example, the Minister may declare an activity that may 'adversely affect the health of individuals in the context of the wider health of the community, to be a public health risk activity.'[23] Some jurisdictions leave the notion of risk so broadly defined that it could include almost anything. The Northern Territory and Western Australia, for instance, use the delightfully circular definition that 'public health risk means a risk of harm to public health.'[24] Given that a risk factor can now be anything that is even remotely statistically connected with some type of health outcome – up to and including premature death – it is hard to see where risk begins or ends.

To understand the legislative meaning of risk, then, we must also understand harm. Again, there is little clear definition of harm or what might give rise to harm. In most Acts, the meaning must be inferred from the context. In Queensland, for instance, harm appears in the context of police or ambulance officers attending a callout. The section applies if an ambulance officer or police officer believes 'a person is threatening to commit suicide.'[25] Indeed, suicide is an obvious harm. However, harm becomes far broader in the context of searching a person detained in a

22 *Public Health Act 1997* (Tas) Part 1, 31

23 *Public Health Act 1997* (ACT) Part 3, 17

24 *Public And Environmental Health Act 2011* (NT) Part 1, 4 and *Public Health Act 2016* (WA) Part 1, 11

25 *Public Health Act 2005 (Qld)* Section 157B, 139

public health facility. Here, harm means anything that may be used to 'threaten the security or good order of a public sector health service facility.'[26] Examples of harmful things are common enough, such as a dangerous drug, but 'provocative or offensive documents' seems far-fetched.[27] In the Western Australian Act, harm encompasses both physical and psychological harm to individuals, regardless of whether it has an immediate or long-term impact.[28] What this means is that being anxious about something, such as words someone has said or ideas put into the public domain, can be harmful. Nor is the definition of harm exhaustive. This does not rule out other things. Even the potential for something to be harmful is sufficient, for example, in South Australia, 'potential harm includes risk of harm and future harm.'[29]

Harm is not necessarily connected to any measures of risk seriousness, which is only sometimes defined, for example, high impact or on a wide scale or irreversible, but neither trivial nor negligible.[30] Serious risk to public health means a 'material risk' considering the number of persons likely to be affected, as well as the 'availability and effectiveness of any precaution, safeguard, treatment to reduce the risk to the health of human beings.'[31] Any harm can give rise to some form of risk, and if that risk is widespread or affects a few persons, it can easily become serious.

Many, but certainly not all, of the powers of Public Health Acts in Australia are framed around entirely sensible things like ensuring that the supply of drinking water is not contaminated, making sure food venues and health care facilities (and places like tattoo parlours) operate hygienically, and, above all else, controlling infectious diseases. Nobody wants to drink water that will make them sick, eat at a restaurant where rat droppings line the benches, or contract a serious illness from a minor medical or cosmetic procedure. It is the infectious diseases part that

26 *Public Health Act 2005 (Qld)* Section 157X, 152

27 *Public Health Act 2005 (Qld)* Section 157X, 152

28 *Public Health Act 2016* (WA) Part 1, 7

29 *South Australian Public Health Act 2011* (SA) Part 1, 8

30 *Public Health Act 2016* (WA) Part 1, 12

31 *Public Health and Wellbeing Act 2008* (Vic) Part 1, 27

gives the real bite to public health's coercive powers.

Infectious diseases are, by their very nature, frightening, and we tend to equate them with serious illness and death automatically. Those over the age of forty-five cannot help but recall the utterly terrifying Grim Reaper bowling alley commercials about AIDS, for instance. In the face of such fear, things that may otherwise seem intrusive can often be justified, even though in the AIDS cases, the infection was almost entirely confined to gay men and intravenous drug users. Given an outbreak of Ebola or bubonic plague, for instance, it could seem perfectly reasonable that a Minister should have the power to declare that disease to be a pandemic and, because of making such a declaration, may 'at any time on or after the making of a pandemic declaration, make any order (a pandemic order) that the Minister believes is reasonably necessary to protect public health.'[32]

It may even seem justifiable that the laws might not apply equally to everybody, or may create certain classes of people based on, say, a person's likelihood of being exposed to or spreading a disease. For example, a pandemic order may differentiate between people based on their vaccination status for 'a disease of pandemic potential',[33] by restricting the unvaccinated from 'engaging in specified activities unless they are exempt from vaccination.'[34] A Minister may only make a pandemic order that they believe is reasonably necessary to protect public health. Having done so, the Minister may delegate significant powers to the Chief Health Officer who may authorise the exercise of certain powers, who may extend the authorisation for the period of the pandemic declaration[35] and who has extensive public health risk powers to,[36] for example, take any action, or give any direction, the chief health officer considers to be necessary or desirable to alleviate the emergency

32 Pandemic Orders during COVID-19 were made under section 165AI of the *Public Health and Wellbeing Act 2008* (Vic)

33 *Public Health and Wellbeing Act 2008* (Vic) Part 8A, 181

34 *Public Health and Wellbeing Act 2008* (Vic) Part 8A, 191

35 *Public Health and Wellbeing Act 2008* (Vic) Part 8A, 207

36 *Public Health and Wellbeing Act 2008* (Vic) Part 10, 275

specified in the declaration, the reduction, removal or destruction of any threat to public health, the segregation or isolation of any person in an area; the evacuation of any person from an area; the prevention or permission of access to an area; place the property under the control, or at the disposal, of the chief health officer.[37]

Declaring something to be a public health emergency or pandemic triggers remarkable powers, including the power for officials to close premises to 'investigate, eliminate or reduce the risk to public health', direct people to leave premises and seize anything necessary for investigating, eliminating or reducing the risk to public health without a warrant.[38] Expectations of privacy rights fly out the window, too. The Information Commissioner may make a pandemic information determination if satisfied that the public interest in the organisation doing the act substantially outweighs the public interest in complying with the specified Information Privacy Principle.[39] This means that any data a government might want can be accessed with no obligation to comply with the types of laws that are usually applied stringently to protect personal information.

Given the astonishing powers triggered by a declaration, it should be difficult to declare a public health emergency or pandemic circumstances. Unfortunately, it is not. The Minister may declare a public health emergency if satisfied that it is justified in the circumstances,[40] even when there have been no cases of the disease,[41] or where the infectious disease has the potential to give rise to a pandemic.[42] The bar to declare something a pandemic and activate warrantless search powers, powers of detention, powers to restrict movement, powers to access highly sensitive personal information is not a difficult one to reach. If an official wished

37 For example, but these are generic to each Act in Australia, *Public Health Act 1997* (ACT) Part 7, 127

38 *Public Health and Wellbeing Act 2008* (Vic) Part 10, 275

39 *Public Health and Wellbeing Act 2008* (Vic) Part 8A, 222

40 *Public Health Act 1997* (ACT) Part 7, 126

41 *Public Health and Wellbeing Act 2008* (Vic) Part 1, 30

42 *Public Health and Wellbeing Act 2008* (Vic) Part 1, 31

to do so, they could reactivate all the powers used under COVID-19, based on a handful of cases or historical circumstances. Regardless of how politically likely or unlikely such an occurrence may be, the law allows it to happen with relative ease.

When police arrested Ms Buhler, she said that she did not know what she had done wrong. Unsurprisingly, people can fall foul of public health without realising it. It remains easy to sin without knowledge. For example, a person must take all reasonable and practicable steps to prevent or minimise any harm to public health. What is reasonable and practicable covers environmental, social, and economic implications. A person will not be in breach if they are acting within 'community expectations.'[43] Who, exactly, gets to decide what community expectations are, and whether an action falls within or outside those? The Acts lack clarity on the relevant environmental, social, and economic practices and standards.

It is not uncommon for people to find themselves before the courts due to public health laws, regulations, and orders. However, courts have little ability to intervene when public health orders affect entire groups rather than specific individuals. An order that somebody must, for example, undertake counselling regarding their infectious disease status can be challenged under standard administrative law provisions. An order that an entire population must do something, however, cannot be given the same legal oversight. Something a health official declares or an action they take remains outside any standard system of checks, balances, and independent oversight that would ordinarily apply to government decision-making. In any legal proceedings, a court or tribunal is not authorised to stay the operation of an emergency declaration or an action taken by the Chief Health Officer under some provisions.[44]

Disclosure – who knows why?

Legislation provides a framework for officials and politicians to act.

43 *Public Health Act 2016* (WA) Part 3, 30

44 *Public And Environmental Health Act 2011* (NT) Part 5, 31

Power is also exercised by the mere fact of assumed expertise: medical opinion, or the guise of medical opinion, no matter how ill-suited to society-wide harm, is hard to resist. One of the more fascinating aspects of the COVID-19 era was watching how submissive elected officials were to health officials who had no direct stake in how their decisions would affect the public's lives and activities. It is only years later that the educational, economic, and psychosocial impacts became known, which have implications that politicians were warned about at the time (by people other than health officials). The law upholds the unhealthy influence of health officials over Ministerial decision-making because, by statute, the Minister must request the advice of the Chief Health Officer about the serious risk to public health posed by the disease specified in the pandemic declaration and the public health measures that the Chief Health Officer considers are necessary or appropriate to address this risk.[45] A benign interpretation of this requirement is that expert, level-headed, apolitical public servants will give calm, measured advice to flighty, ill-informed, partisan politicians to head off any ignorant excesses and deliver balanced, moderate actions.

Sometimes that might be true, but it is as much the case that the allegation by former Deputy Chief Commonwealth Medical Officer Nick Coatsworth is generally closer to the truth —that groupthink took over and advice became path-dependent: that is, neither politicians nor officials wanted to contradict earlier advice in the face of new circumstances and evidence. For example, amendments to the *Public Health and Wellbeing Act 2008* (Vic)[46] provided for the management of pandemic emergencies. Although the Act, before its amendment, imposed obligations to disclose information to the public and Parliament on decisions, for example, in the Government Gazette, they were not obliged to produce evidence justifying the need or rationale for these decisions. Additionally, the Act does not require the publication of directions issued under emergency

45 An example is, Acting Chief Health Officer Advice to Minister for Health Advice relating to the making of Pandemic Orders as required by section 165AL of the *Public Health and Wellbeing Act 2008* 07 April 2022 at which the rationale for extensive further measures were made on masks, testing, quarantine and many more.

46 *Public Health and Wellbeing Amendment (Pandemic Management) Act* 2021 (Vic)

powers, nor does it require the publication of advice or analysis that has influenced this decision-making process.[47] There is a requirement that decisions be transparent[48] and provide access to reliable information, but this is often uncontested evidence that the Chief Health Officer or Minister determines. The Act does not impose a duty to disclose the sources of advice beyond the Officer, or to disclose health advice that informs decisions.[49] Decisions under uncertainty are complicated, and leaders do not want to share advice that may undermine their authority, but it is not a good approach to make the proof appear more certain than it is.

The Victorian Government spent many years attempting to block the release of documents revealing that politicians were willing to make sweeping decisions about lockdowns and curfews without seeking advice from their health department. An excellent example is the work of a Member of the Legislative Assembly in Victoria, David Davis's freedom of information win against the Victorian Department of Health in the Victorian Civil and Administrative Tribunal in April 2024,[50] which the Department unsuccessfully appealed.[51] It became clear from emails released under the Freedom of Information Act that the government had no medical advice to justify the curfew imposed on Victorian citizens during the COVID-19 pandemic. The now-infamous 'Document 34' was an email between the then-Chief Health Officer, Professor Brett Sutton, and the health department's public health commander, Dr Finn Romanes. Romanes wrote, 'the action of issuing a curfew is a mirror to the State of Disaster and is not occurring on public health advice but is a decision taken by Cabinet.'[52] Dr Romanes then asked his superior, Professor Sutton, for approval to issue curfew orders, which he granted.

47 Wolf G, 2023. How to manage a pandemic?: decision-making under the *Public Health and Wellbeing Amendment (Pandemic Management) Act 2021* (Vic). *Journal of Law and Medicine* May, 38

48 *Public Health and Wellbeing Act 2008* (Vic) Part 2, 37

49 Wolf G, 2023, 40

50 *Davis v Department of Health (Review and Regulation)* [2024] VCAT 490

51 *Secretary To the Department of Health V The Hon David Davis MLC* [2025] VSCA 40

52 ABC News, Emails show Melbourne COVID -19 curfew was not based on health advice, opposition says. 20 April 2025

Incidentally, the Supreme Court of Victoria ruled that the curfew did not contravene the Human Rights Charter.[53]

Mandatory vaccination

No decision was more savage, ill-founded, and wrong than that which made vaccination compulsory for employees. This is an example of legislative power and the hubris of public health officials, thinking they know best for everybody. Writing in October 2022, well into the COVID-19 response, the American Academy of Emergency Medicine Ethics Committee wrote that 'vaccine mandates for healthcare workers are ethically just and appropriate, and the benefit to society far outweighs the minor inconvenience to an individual's personal liberties.'[54] They knew at the time that the vaccines did not stop the spread of infection. The only benefit, if any, was to minimise the effects of a health worker falling ill and being unavailable for work. This is vastly different from arguing that an unvaccinated worker is a risk to other workers and patients. This is possibly the best illustration of abuse of power for power's sake. There was no medical reason to do this.

Three hundred police and paramedics who were unlawfully directed to get COVID-19 vaccines lodged class actions on 25 October 2024 in the Supreme Court of Queensland seeking compensation.[55] An earlier challenge in the Queensland Supreme Court before Justice Martin on 27 February 2024 was successful on a procedural point on the Queensland Government's vaccine mandates.[56] The police and paramedics are seeking compensation from the State of Queensland due to many losing their jobs, being injured by the COVID-19 vaccines and being unlawfully disciplined for not following the vaccine directions set by the

53 *Loielo v Giles* [2020] VSC 722

54 Myers M et al, 2023. An ethical analysis of the arguments both for and against covid-19 vaccine mandates for healthcare workers. *Journal of Emergency Medicine* 64(2), 246

55 United Australia Party, press release 25 October 2024

56 *Johnston & Ors v Carroll (Commissioner of the Queensland Police Service) & Anor; Witthahn & Ors v Wakefield (Chief Executive of Hospital and Health Services and Director General of Queensland Health); Sutton & Ors v Carroll (Commissioner of the Queensland Police Service)* [2024] QSC 2

Queensland police and ambulance services.

The February matter concerned directions issued by the Commissioner of Police requiring each police officer or staff member to receive a COVID-19 vaccine (the Sutton and Johnston matters). The third case concerns a similar direction given to employees of the Queensland Ambulance Service (the Witthahn matter) by the Director-General of Queensland Health. The court found that the Directions were not invalid but unlawful.[57] The Supreme Court found that the Directions limited the applicants' rights not to be subjected to medical treatment without their full, free and informed consent under section 17(c) of the *Human Rights Act 2019* (HR Act). This limitation was held to be demonstrably justified and compatible with human rights. While the decisions were compatible with human rights, the processes were unlawful.[58]

The *Mandatory Vaccination for Health Workers Act 2020* (Vic) enabled employers of high-risk workers (such as health care workers) to mandate COVID-19 vaccination.[59] In evidence to a parliamentary committee on the oversight of pandemic orders, Professor Sutton, as Victorian Chief Health Officer, said that his advice 'appropriately cites all literature, or most literature, that informs the advice.'[60] What advice was Professor Sutton relying on in January 2022 when discussing mandatory vaccination, including among children aged five to eleven? For example, he said that he had 'to consider what the immune evasion potential of any new variant may be and what that means in terms of what vaccines can provide as direct protection for the individual who is vaccinated, but also that [of] indirect protection or herd immunity protection.'[61] Was Sutton

57 *Johnston & Ors v Carroll* [2024] QSC 2, par 461

58 Crown Law, Supreme Court judgment on vaccination directions issued to Qld Police and Qld Ambulance officers https://www.crownlaw.qld.gov.au/about/news/supreme-court-judgment-on-vaccination-directions-issued-to-qld-police-and-qld-ambulance-officers

59 Kevat D, 2021. Medico-legal considerations of mandatory COVID-19 vaccination for high risk workers. *Medical Journal of Australia* 215(1), 22

60 Parliament of Victoria, 2022. Transcript. *Pandemic Declaration Accountability and Oversight Committee Review of Pandemic Orders*. Melbourne, 31 January, 4

61 Parliament of Victoria, 2022, 15

not aware of evidence of the absence of illness among the young as a lack of a medical reason to mandate vaccines?[62] Was Sutton unaware of evidence challenging the scientific rationale for vaccination mandates, including the inability of COVID-19 vaccines to prevent transmission or infection, similar viral loads among vaccinated and unvaccinated individuals, and significant evidence of serious adverse effects?[63] Was he not aware that booster doses temporarily restored effectiveness but that this effect declined over time, and that reinfection rates during the Omicron wave were unexpectedly high, particularly among younger adults, with those who received two or more vaccine doses having a higher risk of reinfection?[64]

A study on compulsory vaccine boosters for U.S. university students found that to prevent one Omicron-related COVID-19 hospitalisation over six months, between 30,000 and 40,000 students needed to be vaccinated with an mRNA vaccine.[65] The implementation of such policies, despite expert controversy, the lack of an updated publicly available risk-benefit analysis specific to Omicron, and the absence of methods subjected to public scrutiny, suggests a significant lack of transparency in scientific and regulatory policymaking. The researchers concluded, 'policymakers should immediately repeal COVID-19 vaccine mandates for young adults and ensure pathways to compensation for those who have suffered

62 Feldstein L R et al, 2025. Protection from COVID-19 vaccination and prior SARS-CoV-2 infection among children aged 6 Months-4 Years, United States, September 2022-April 2023. *Journal of Pediatric Infectious Diseases Society* 14, 121

63 Faksova K et al, 2024. COVID-19 vaccines and adverse events of special interest: a multinational Global Vaccine Data Network (GVDN) cohort study of 99 million vaccinated individuals. *Vaccine* 42(2200). Fraiman J et al, 2022. Serious adverse events of special interest following mRNA COVID-19 vaccination in randomized trials in adults. *Vaccine* 40, 5798-5805

64 Eythorsson E et al, 2022. Rate of SARS-CoV-2 reinfection during an Omicron wave in Iceland. *JAMA Network Open* 2022(5), e2225320

65 Bardosh K et al, 2024. COVID-19 vaccine boosters for young adults: a risk-benefit assessment and ethical analysis of mandate policies at universities. *Journal of Medical Ethics* 50, 135

negative consequences from these policies.'[66]

Should leeway have been granted to workers who had been infected?[67] Sutton must have been aware that 'patients could not give their informed consent…because the long-term side effects were (unknown).'[68] After all, it usually takes at least eight years for a vaccine to go from development to market.[69] The Australian Health Practitioner Regulation Agency (AHPRA) and National Boards released a statement on 21 March 2021, when the vaccine roll-out was getting underway, that 'There is no place for anti-vaccination messages in professional health practice, and any promotion of anti-vaccination claims, including on social media, and advertising, may be subject to regulatory action.'[70] This threatening release was part of the regimen at the time, but agencies and chief medical officers such as Sutton must have observed the dehumanisation and othering of the unvaccinated, and the social atmosphere of hatred and agitation against people who decided against COVID-19 vaccination.[71] A reasonable message would have been "vaccines are advisable for the vulnerable, that is, aged people or those with comorbidities, but any new vaccine may have long-term adverse side effects not known at this time."

A clear example of an oppressive action against an employee was Scott Morrison (Text Box 3.1). Sutton's lack of introspection, or lack of

66 Bardosh K et al, 2024, 136

67 McGonagle D G, 2022. Health-care workers recovered from natural SARS-CoV-2 infection should be exempt from mandatory vaccination edicts. *Lancet Rheumatol* (4), e170

68 Chaufan C et al, 2025. 'It isn't about health, and it sure doesn't care': a qualitative exploration of healthcare workers' lived experience of the policy of vaccination mandates in Ontario, Canada. *Journal of Public Health and Emergency* (9)16, 5

69 Zhang S et al, 2022. Why does COVID-19 continue to spread despite mass vaccination? *Frontiers in Public Health* Jul 25(10), 938108

70 Australian Health Practitioner Regulation Agency and National Boards. 2021. *Registered Health Practitioners and Students: What you need to know about the COVID-19 Vaccine Rollout.* 21 March. AHPRA's failure to warn vaccinators not to collaborate with COVID-19 vaccination mandates is subject of complaint to the National Health Practitioner Ombudsman.

71 Junger N & Hirsch O, 2024. Ethics of nudging in the COVID-19 crisis and the necessary return to the principles of shared decision making: a critical review. *Cureus* 2024(16), e57960

scholarship, was not alone. Various agencies, which should have known better, oppressed multiple people and were found to be wrong in doing so.

Text Box 3.1 Commonwealth – oppressive action against a vaccine mandate opponent

Scott Morrison

Commonwealth public servant

The federal government strongly encouraged though never mandated vaccinations. However, it allowed federal government agencies, such as the Australian Electoral Commission, to implement mandatory vaccination policies under the guise of work, health and safety.

Morrison participated in the 'consultation' process for vaccination and applied for an exemption under the interim policy. Exemption was denied and he was ordered to take leave. When he was allowed to return to work, he was subject to stringent additional hygiene measures. After the pandemic was declared over, he was subjected to a code of conduct investigation. It was determined he had breached the Australian Public Service Code of Conduct and sanctioned by fine (two per cent of his annual salary).

On appeal to the Merit Protection Commissioner, the sanction was reduced to one per cent of his annual salary. However, due to significant delays with the AEC decision, the MPC refused to review the initial breach determination. When he questioned an MPC delegate as to why any sanction remained in place, it was reminded that many others had lost their jobs.

Fortunately, Morrison has been able to secure an opportunity with an agency that did not introduce a mandatory vaccination policy.

He questions how it is reasonable for an employer to direct an employee, under an interim WH&S policy, to take a vaccine that the TGA acknowledges has killed Australians and caused significant adverse reactions in many others.

Source: Morrison S, 2024. *Submission to the Commonwealth Government COVID-19 Response Inquiry*

The Medical Board of Australia acted against a general practitioner whose evaluation of COVID-19 vaccines contradicted the official stance. He faced severe penalties, later receiving relief from the courts after being suspended for over two years (see Text Box 3.2).

Text Box 3.2 Medical Board - oppressive action against a medical practitioner[72]

Dr William Bay

General practitioner, Brisbane

On 17 August 2022, the Medical Board of Australia and the Australian Health Practitioner Regulation Agency suspended Dr Bray under Queensland's *Health Practitioner Regulation National Law.*

The Health Ombudsman for Queensland accused Bay of 'departing from acceptable professional standards' because on the Facebook page for the Queensland Peoples' Protest (a political organisation) Bay made claims that COVID-19 vaccination has caused harm. By the time the matter came to court Bay's registration had been suspended for more than two years.

The Supreme Court of Queensland set aside the decisions to suspend Bay's registration. The decision of the Medical Board of Australia to refer matters to the Queensland Civil and Administrative Tribunal was also set aside.

None of the allegations concerned his clinical practice. None could be characterised as a 'mandatory notification' under the National Law (Qld). The investigation decision was set aside on the grounds of having taken into account an irrelevant consideration (a contravention of legislation and a breach of a Code of Conduct that had not occurred) and of apprehended bias.

The Board's show cause letter identified as concerns that Bay had 'espoused and encouraged' views, including 'mistrust of vaccinations (in relation to COVID-19), of public health measures, of the health system generally, and of the regulation of the health care system.' and being 'in contrast with … public health directives.' No public health directive was found in the show cause letter.

The Board's 'combative approach' towards Dr Bay continued long after the epidemic had passed. The judge remarked, 'It must have been apparent from the outset that all the notifications concerned political conduct by Dr Bay.'

Source: Bay W, 2024. *Submission to the Commonwealth Government Covid-19 Response Inquiry* and *Bay v Australian Health Practitioner Regulation Agency* [2024] QSC 315

72 See also, Dr My Le Trinh, Dr Luke McLindon, Dr Mark Hobart.

The Australian Medical Professional Society's Human Cost of AHPRA survey of health practitioners conducted in 2024 indicated that more than half of medical practitioners have engaged with the Australian Health Practitioner Regulation Agency.[73] Of the 1,500 practitioners surveyed, 21.5 per cent reported experiencing unfair treatment by the regulator. In contrast, 83 per cent asserted that AHPRA is neither 'fair nor transparent' in its handling of complaints against practitioners. Among the 980 comments collected in the survey, the prevailing theme highlighted a perception of guilt rather than innocence regarding the claims made against practitioners. Although these results do not relate specifically to the COVID-19 response, it does suggest a breakdown between the regulator and the profession, some of which was attributable to the overbearing stance of AHPRA and chief health officials during COVID-19.

As if the unfair and intimidatory punishment of medically or scientifically trained individuals were not enough, workers who chose not to be vaccinated faced repercussions at work or worse, exclusion. Mandatory vaccination policies also undermined the doctor-patient relationship. Millions of doses of COVID-19 vaccines were distributed under a regime that did not guarantee informed consent. Governments intervened in a decision that should have been made between each patient and their doctor. Public health officials exaggerated the effectiveness of vaccines and sought to demonise those who refused vaccination by labelling them as part of the pandemic of the unvaccinated.

As the Australian toxicologist Phil Burcham stated concerning mRNA vaccines, 'someone with my scientific training ought not accept ex cathedra pronouncements from chief medical officers or local doctors concerning the safety of ambitious pharmaceuticals, especially those with problematic histories ... The ... primary purpose of a pharmacology department was to protect Australians against bastards in drug companies.' Someone had to evaluate the scientific claims of foreign

73 Australian Medical Professional Society, Survey of members supplied by the Association 31 December 2024.

pharmaceutical companies critically.[74] Burcham's suspicions were well-founded, considering Dr Fauci's inflammatory remarks about the unvaccinated, dismissing concerns about refusing vaccination as mere 'ideological bullshit' and suggesting that institutions should complicate life for the unvaccinated through vaccine mandates.

> *Once people feel empowered and protected legally, you were going to have schools, universities, and colleges are going to say, you want to come to this college, buddy? You're going to get vaccinated. ... Amazon and Facebook ... are going to say, you want to work for us, you get vaccinated.*[75]

Vaccine mandates were found to inflict considerable collateral damage.

> *We question the effectiveness and consequences of coercive vaccination policy in pandemic response and urge the public health community and policymakers to return to non-discriminatory, trust-based public health approached.*[76]

The leading case on vaccine mandates, *Kassam v. Hazzard*, did not overturn the NSW government's authority to legitimately restrict individuals from continuing to work at their places of employment unless they sought to receive the COVID-19 vaccine.[77] Employees should understand they cannot refuse to work if a colleague is unvaccinated against the coronavirus. This is because the employer may not have the authority to mandate vaccination, and the colleague may have a valid reason or exemption for not being vaccinated.[78] Nevertheless, in four cases, the Fair Work Commission upheld the right of employers to mandate COVID-19 vaccination and terminate the employment of employees who either fail to get vaccinated or do not have an applicable

---

74 Burcham P, 2025. An injured toxicologist on Covid vaccines, parts I, II and III. *Quadrant* April-June

75 U.S. House of Representatives, 2024, 343

76 Bardosh K et al, 2022. The unintended consequences of COVID-19 vaccine policy: why mandates, passports and restrictions may cause more harm than good. *BMJ Global Health* May 7(5), 1

77 *Kassam v Hazzard*; *Henry v Hazzard* [2021] NSWSC 1320, 15 October 2021

78 PH Solicitor, Can the COVID vaccine be made compulsory for employees? Unpublished advice.

medical exemption (supported by evidence).[79] Where a government health order is in place, making it an offence for employers to allow an unvaccinated employee (without an applicable medical contraindication supported by evidence) to enter the workplace to perform work, the Commission will accept that employers have no effective choice but to comply with the government order. The solution rests with the oppressive public health orders. Whether future legal challenges to the government's power to enforce vaccine mandates are successful is less significant than the political pressure to change laws that prohibit such regimes. There have been successful claims against employers for injuries resulting from refusal to be vaccinated and subsequent loss of employment.[80] Hopefully, this should serve as a warning about any legislation enacted in the name of public health.

The Nurses Professional Association of Victoria and the Australian Medical Professional Society submitted a plea to the Victorian Government to immediately revoke the Vaccination of Health Care & Ambulance Workers (COVID-19) Secretary Directions, arguing that there was no rationale for the mandates.[81] They contended that the Department's persistence in maintaining the Directions represented 'a fundamental misunderstanding or recklessness regarding the reality of COVID-19 vaccinations' and that the 'government must revert back to an advisory role, avoiding gate-keeping to employment and workers' medical decision-making.'[82] The Department contended that vaccine mandates were reasonable and lawful measures to minimise the transmission of SARS-CoV-2, protect the public, and ensure workers' health and safety. However, there was no evidence that the available therapeutics would significantly influence transmission. Victoria was the last jurisdiction to uphold the mandates, yet the question remains:

79 Byrnes M, 2024. Mandatory workplace vaccination: some recent COVID-19 vaccination cases. *Governance Institute of Australia Journal*

80 *Dawking v Secretary (Department of Education)* [2022] NSWPIC 611

81 Nurses Professional Association of Victoria, letter to the Minister for Health 27 August 2024

82 Nurses Professional Association of Victoria, letter to the Minister for Health 27 August 2024

why were these mandates allowed in any jurisdiction, given their lack of scientific basis? The obvious answer is: because the public health establishment wanted them, and because governments were too scared to say no.

WHO – pandemic prevention, preparedness and response agreement

The WHO — the international home of public health meddling, and the body whose policies and beliefs are invoked to justify all manner of domestic public health legislation — did not perform well during the COVID-19 pandemic. It was overwhelmed by panic and abandoned its trusted pandemic responses, which was to avoid lockdowns and masks. It was pressured into not thoroughly investigating the source of the pandemic. Accepting the Chinese government's suppression of information and delayed disclosure of critical data, not to mention silencing Chinese medical staff, damaged its credibility. Lack of transparency hindered the investigation into the origin of the virus and fueled the spread of the lab-leak or intentional manipulation hypotheses.[83] Why the WHO changed its mind on aspects of the response, and indeed, many governments followed a Chinese-style suppression, is a mystery born of conspiracy and panic. The most significant argument against the lab theory is that China and other nations suffered significant losses. If they were developing a virus as a weapon, they would conceivably develop a vaccine to protect themselves.

Controversy has not deterred the UN's intentions to be better prepared for the next pandemic. In December 2021, the World Health Assembly established an intergovernmental negotiating body (INB) to draft and negotiate a convention, agreement or other international instrument under the Constitution of the WHO 'to strengthen pandemic prevention, preparedness and response.' WHO Member States have adopted two other global, legally binding agreements to protect and promote

83 Yoo J H, 2025. On the controversies surrounding the *Lab-Leak* theory of COVID-19. *Journal of Korean Medical Science* 40(16), e153

people's health: the WHO Framework Convention on Tobacco Control and the International Health Regulations, which provide a public health response to the international spread of disease. Of course, how this new agreement fits with the myriad other priorities is anyone's guess. Bjorn Lomborg has pointed out that the long list of UN priorities amounts to no priorities. He offered a short list, some of which were health-related, including tuberculosis, malaria, and chronic diseases; others were education, trade, electronic government procurement (to slow corruption), and land tenure.[84]

Undeterred, the agreement was obsessed with 'inequities at national and international levels that hindered timely and equitable access to health products to address coronavirus disease (COVID-19).' Worryingly, the agreement states that an adequate pandemic response is part of a 'continuum to combat other health emergencies and achieve greater health equity through resolute action on the social, environmental, cultural, political and economic determinants of health', and 'the importance and public health impact of growing threats such as climate change.'[85] Other worrying elements are the One Health approach for pandemic prevention, which recognises 'that the health of humans is closely linked and interdependent with the health of domestic and wild animals, as well as plants and the wider environment (including ecosystems), aiming for a sustainable balance ... which contributes to sustainable development in an equitable manner.'[86] Whatever this means is almost certainly expensive and bound to slow progress and wealth creation. Indeed, it looks suspiciously like the spectre of another pandemic is just convenient – and emotionally powerful — window dressing for more of public health's usual cant.

The bottom line is, as always, the bottom line. The Agreement demands

---

84 Lomborg B, 2023. *Best Things First.* Copenhagen Consensus Center

85 World Health Organization, 2025. Intergovernmental Negotiating Body to draft and negotiate a WHO convention, agreement or other international instrument on pandemic prevention, preparedness and response *Report by the Director-General 14 May*, 5

86 World Health Organization, 2025. *14 May*, 7

additional monies to support 'developing country Parties implement the Agreement.'[87] The Agreement wants nations to 'take measures to enhance the availability of licences for pandemic-related health technologies to which it owns the rights, on a non-exclusive, transparent and broad geographic basis and for the benefit of developing countries, including contracting a proportion of vaccine and other therapeutics manufacture.[88] A Global Supply Chain and Logistics Network has been established to enhance access to pandemic-related health products, facilitate their distribution, and remove barriers to their use.

While the agreement does not derogate Australia's sovereignty, given the Albanese government's propensity to do whatever is fashionable at the UN, it is likely to be an enthusiastic adopter.[89] The Agreement provides one more pillar in the edifice of top-down decision-making, enhancing the appearance of unity in medical responses. One false move at the UN and the world panics. Conferences of the parties will be scheduled to maintain the conversation, similar to the panic and poor policy on climate change, with a rolling message of crisis and the need for regulation and funding. As for funding, the U.S. has withdrawn funds, and much of the remaining support comes from highly conflicted private sources. For example, most of the top 100 donors to the WHO's specified donations program were pharmaceutical companies or those aligned with pharmaceutical interests.[90] Public health disdain for commercial interests, seems to not extend to their supporters.

---

87 World Health Organization, 2025. *14 May*, 25

88 World Health Organization, 2025. *14 May*, 17 and 20

89 Department of Foreign Affairs and Trade, *Global Health Reform* https://web.archive.org/web/20250514201534/https://www.dfat.gov.au/international-relations/themes/global-themes/global-health-reform

90 Australian Medical Professionals' Society, 2025. *Follow the Money: WHO's Directing Global Health Policy?*, 4

Conclusion

Public health has long harnessed the coercive powers of the state and depends on them for its very existence. Emergency declarations, generally under Public Health Acts, took many by surprise during COVID-19. The scope of those powers came to light during COVID-19, but they existed long before then and still exist today. Indeed, legislation has obediently followed the social determinants model of public health, with increasingly nebulous concepts such as wellbeing finding their way into law. The expanding scope of public health powers, used in conjunction with the social determinants model of public health, gives public health almost unlimited power to intervene in people's lives – and to punish people who do not make the 'right' choices, or who raise their voices against the public health lobby.

That legislators have enabled this to happen – and even encouraged it – shows how truly unfettered the public health lobby's political ambitions have become. The application of those powers nevertheless could come at any time, especially given the desire of public health officials to operate on a very wide remit and campaign for a more equitable society: that is, a remit that knows no bounds and brooks little dissent. In recent times, mandatory vaccination was perhaps the greatest infringement on civil liberties without justification, although closely followed by lockdowns. It is time to review the powers of these Acts and assess the level of information shared with the public when these powers are invoked.

The history of these powers is opaque. They have rarely been discussed publicly. Instead, discussions have been held among officials as if in a hospital setting – again, using the appearance of medical credibility to push things that are decidedly unscientific. Society is not a hospital ward, nor should public health tsars have unlimited powers to meddle, and public health Acts must be reframed with that in mind.

4

Taxation: no cure-all

We will implement a further four annual 12.5 per cent increases in tobacco excise, with the first increase to take effect on 1 September 2017. The net impact of the tobacco measures will raise $4.7 billion over the next four years.[1]

- Hon. Scott Morrison, Treasurer of Australia, 2016

We will not be allowing organised crime to determine our health policy.[2]

- Hon. Tony Burke, Home Affairs Minister, Australia, 2025

Taxation is an instrument that the public health lobby especially likes to use to manipulate individual behaviour, and it is central to the public health approach to re-engineering society. The idea runs that if you make something too expensive for people to afford, they will stop doing it. Again, like most things in public health, much of today's approach replicates merely what has been done with tobacco over decades – so we use that example below. Of course, now that public health has introduced the concept of commercial determinants of health into its lexicon, this paves the way not just for punishing individuals for making choices the public health lobby disapproves of, but also for punishing

1 Delivered on 3 May 2016 on the second reading of the *Appropriation Bill (No. 1) 2016-17* by the Honourable Scott Morrison MP, Treasurer of the Commonwealth of Australia

2 Sarah Ison, Criminal gangs turn to extortion as blackmarket tobacco war intensifies. *The Weekend Australian* 4-5 October 2025

legal businesses for providing products that enable people to make those choices.

Politicians have come to rely on virtuous taxation as a source of revenue. When the Treasurer announced further swingeing, indeed gouging, taxes on tobacco in 2016, smoking rates had dropped from 25 per cent of the population in 1990 to 12 per cent (Figure 4.1). They had fallen further to eight per cent, and tobacco duty paid reached $16 billion in 2019-20, before dropping to $7 billion in 2024-25.[3] Most of the work had been done before the announcement. Presumably, a generational effect would have led to more enlightened individuals entering adulthood who did not wish to smoke because they were aware of its harm. As members of the government backbench cheered their Treasurer in 2016 at the news of more revenue, the Treasurer did not bother to tout any 'health' benefit from further taxing tobacco. Few will cease smoking because of the new taxes, because these come on top of many others and follow decades of programs to help change the culture of acceptability of tobacco. The Home Affairs Minister was disingenuous when, in 2025, he blamed organised crime for 'determining health policy'. His colleagues had done that.

And there are advocates whose ignorance of public policy and command of double-think is astounding. Dr Margaret Chan, then Director-General of the WHO, addressing a worldwide meeting of parliamentarians, berated them to 'Get your governments to raise taxes on tobacco products ... Above all, fight against tax policies ... that punish the poor.'[4] It is impossible to use tax policy to cut the demand for tobacco products and not punish the poor, who are its greatest consumers.[5] Even a surefire sin, such as tobacco consumption, has activists and regulators making errors and governments gouging. In Australia, despite the Minister's denial, the

3 Australian Taxation Office, 2024. *Tobacco Tax Gap: Compare the 2022 Previous Years* and Fei Gao and Andrew Terry, Tobacco excise revenue has tanked amid a booming black market. *The Conversation* 28 March 2025

4 Address at the 133rd Inter-Parliamentary Union Assembly Geneva, Switzerland, 19 October 2015

5 Hirono K T & Smith K E, 2018. Australia's $40 per pack cigarette tax plans: the need to consider equity. *Tobacco Control* 27(2), 229

taxation regime led directly to a massive problem with organised crime controlling an illegal tobacco trade because the price difference between legal (taxed) products and illegal ones was immense.

Figure 4.1 Daily smokers and key tobacco control measures in Australia, 1990 to 2023, per cent

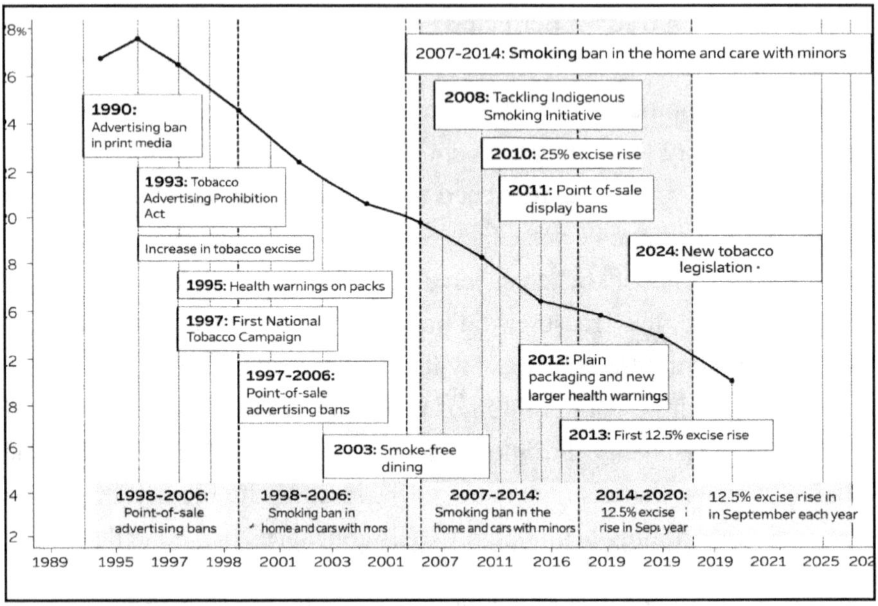

Source: Australian Institute of Health and Welfare, 2024. *Health promotion and health protection*

Figure 4.1 tracks the decline in smoking prevalence rates (for individuals aged 14 years and over) in Australia from 1990 to 2023, highlighting the critical policy initiatives implemented during this period. Smoking prevalence rates in the last two decades have declined substantially. Tobacco control measures implemented in Australia suggest the measures have had a substantial impact on the decline. They also indicate that a cultural revolution based on better information, advertising bans (combating presence of mind temptations) and inconvenience (banning indoor smoking) have been key measures.[6] Tax increases have come at the end of the culture change. And yet, in 2016, legislation was passed for

6 Greenhalgh E M et al, 2024. *Tobacco in Australia: Facts and Issues*. Cancer Council Victoria

four further increases in tobacco taxation, with smaller rises scheduled to take effect from 2023. And still, they want greater restrictions, with licence fees[7] and a tobacco endgame — its abolition.[8] Having a low smoking rate will never be enough for public health. In its pursuit of so-called optimal wellbeing for all, public health aims to abolish what it deems contrary to well-being. However, as we saw in the previous two chapters, its list of risks, harms, and determinants has no bounds and is growing, becoming increasingly broad and ill-defined. Coupled with politicians' penchant for revenue, public health's enthusiasm for taxation is ripe for abuse.

Taxation is not a cure-all; it incurs costs, and while it can be used to recover spillover expenses, it often overreaches, either gouging consumers or making only a minimal difference to their health, thereby creating a black market. It proves ineffective when the source of harm is widespread and can worsen inequality, the very issue that public health officials lament.

Tax is not cost-free

Most taxes result in some loss of economic efficiency as they distort usual economic behaviour. The deadweight loss from taxation arises from reduced incentive effects associated with additional taxation. This is because it drives a wedge between the prices paid and received for goods and services. This has been estimated to be, on average, 27.5 cents in the dollar. The Australia's Future Tax System Review (Henry review)[9] reported that the marginal welfare losses from major Commonwealth taxes included 24 cents in the dollar for personal tax and 40 cents for company tax. This means that for every $1 of personal income tax

7 Ziesing S et al, 2023. Is it time to increase the cost of tobacco licences after 10 years of stagnation? *Australian and New Zealand Journal of Public Health* 47(5)

8 Gartner C et al, 2023. International progress toward a commercial tobacco endgame is an opportunity for advancing tobacco control. *Australia Australian and New Zealand Journal of Public Health* 47(2)

9 Australia's Future Tax System, 2009. *Final Report*

raised, community welfare is reduced overall by 24 cents. Likewise, for every $1 of company tax raised, community welfare is reduced overall by 40 cents.[10]

Using the same logic and similar figures, Henry Ergas queried an estimate by the Grattan Institute of the costs of obesity shifted onto others. Over half of the estimated $5.3 billion a year arose from the loss of tax revenue owing to the lower earnings of people who are obese. That is the price they pay, a cost to them, not to anyone else. As Ergas pointed out, the cost to the community of reducing tax revenues by a dollar is not one dollar: it is, at most, that dollar's opportunity cost, which can be estimated as the economic damage caused by raising another dollar to replace it, with the rest of the fiscal loss being a transfer from one part of the community to another. 'On the report's assumptions, that net cost amounts to 25 cents. However, the report not only counts the 25 cents but also adds to it the original dollar, so that 25 cents in community costs becomes $1.25. The estimates of third-party costs are egregiously overestimated.'[11]

Further to Ergas' critique of the overestimation of community benefit, obesity is a public health problem in one respect only: if its harms affect others. Finding ways to claim that individual behaviours affect others and, therefore, should be subject to intervention is a common strategy in public health. In the case of obesity, the only way it affects others is because of pooled insurance, which is why public health advocates want obesity categorised as a disease.[12] For example, to be a Health Promotion Charity in Australia, it is not sufficient for a charity 'to promote appropriate weight reduction or increased physical activity, without identifying the disease(s) that are being prevented or controlled

10 ACIL Allen, 2014. *Counting the Costs of Alcohol Policy-relevant Costs to Australia*, 30

11 Ergas in a letter to the editor (*The Weekend Australian* 24-25 December 2016), the author of the Grattan report denies the Ergas critique of 'double counting'.

12 The NGO Obesity Australia's 2016 summit was titled, Is Obesity a Disease? Obesity Australia is a health promotion charity.

through this promotion activity.'[13] Awarding obesity disease status would allow obesity advocates to get on with their remedies without proving links to disease. Obesity would become everyone's problem, allowing such charities and other interested parties free rein to expand their remit. Such a stance would also be in the interests of commercial organisations interested in anti-obesity measures (and who also stand to benefit under the commercial determinants of health banner).

It also follows that Medicare would cover the condition (conditions caused by obesity would, of course, be covered in any event), and taxpayers would pay for it (which largely negates any of the claims to economic costs to society, used to justify classification/intervention in the first place). All semblance of personal responsibility would disappear. Guidelines for reporting obesity suggest that writers use the term "people with obesity" rather than "obese people" to guard against prejudicial statements such as 'the people who are overweight or obese have no self-control.'[14] Spot the difference: It is not my fault; my 'obesogenic environment' made me do it! It is not beyond possibility that, whether for good or bad, mandatory reporting of severe childhood obesity will lead to children being taken from their parents.[15] But that bespeaks parenting skills and genetics, not a universal call to arms to stop an obesity epidemic.

Smokers sometimes impose costs on others. The costs of passive smoking, for example, include the costs of disease and premature death caused by passive smoking, as well as the discomfort of those exposed to the smoke of others. It is possible to assess the cost of second-hand smoke, for example, which may have caused the deaths

---

13 Australian Charities and Not-for-profits Commission, 2015. Commissioner's interpretation statement: health promotion charities. *CIS 2015/01*, 4

14 Obesity Australia, 2015. *Rethink Obesity: A Media Guide on How to Report on Obesity*. Sydney, 13

15 Magnusson R, 2016. Is obesity a disease?: legal implications. *Obesity Australia Summit Papers*

of 149 Australians in 2004-05,[16] but this has to be considered among the total number of deaths, which was 132,500 in that year.[17] Babies of Australian women who smoke during pregnancy are twice as likely as other babies to have low birth weight and are more likely to require special care.[18] The Henry review, however, indicated that the social costs of tobacco consumption were low compared to the private costs: 'Spillover costs need to be taken into account but are small compared with the costs borne by smokers themselves.'[19] Taxation to recover the costs of smoking imposed directly on others should, therefore, be small.

The Henry review also considered that in any given year, a smoker's healthcare is likely to cost more on average than that of a non-smoker of the same age and sex. It is also thought that because smokers tend to die earlier than non-smokers, the lifetime healthcare costs of smokers and non-smokers in high-income countries might be similar.[20] Unfortunately, the review did not calculate the actual lifetime health costs or the pension costs for long-lived non-smokers, so a crucial part of the public health debate was not considered. This seems an odd omission.

In his submission to a 2016 parliamentary inquiry, Sinclair Davidson questioned the Henry review's acknowledgment of low spillover costs and support for higher taxation.[21] Davidson distinguished two forms of taxation. Because tobacco demand is relatively unaffected by taxation, simple revenue-raising could be a straightforward exercise, that is, seeking no change in behaviour. Alternatively, taxation could be used to discourage tobacco consumption. In the latter, the government wishes to impose a different set of preferences on those freely chosen by smokers.

---

16 Collins D & Lapsley H, 2008. The costs of tobacco, alcohol and illicit drug abuse to Australian society in 2004-05. Department of Health and Ageing. *Monograph Series no. 64*, 53

17 Australian Bureau of Statistics, 2007. *Deaths, Australia, 2004*

18 Laws P et al, 2006. Smoking and pregnancy. *Australian Institute of Health and Welfare, National Perinatal Statistics Unit* No. 33, x

19 Australia's Future Tax System, 2009. *Final Report*. Part 2, chapter, e6-3

20 Australia's Future Tax System, 2009, e6-1

21 Davidson S, 2016. *Submission to Parliamentary Joint Committee on Law Enforcement Inquiry into Illicit Tobacco*. Australian Parliament, 11

Davidson points out that this strategy risks destroying 'consumer utility' and can lead to adverse behaviour and costs, such as a black market in illicit cigarettes. Davidson was spot on. In 2024, approximately 18 per cent of all tobacco for sale was illicit. The duty value would have been $2.7 billion. This result was a net tax gap of 14.3 per cent.[22]

The Henry review concluded that Australia's tobacco taxes were modest compared to those of OECD countries. Davidson, however, demonstrated that excise in Australia was well above the world average on a measure of excise as a percentage of cigarette prices, and that Australian excise, at the time of his submission, comprised 60 per cent of the price.[23]

A second element of the critique consisted of assumptions about the inferred behaviour of smokers. This is an argument for government intervention in markets where consumers lack the knowledge to understand their preferences, due to factors such as limited product knowledge and health effects. The review examined the extent to which smokers value the present over the future, and the extent to which smokers can be described as 'sophisticated' or 'naive'. Sophisticated smokers understand that their future selves might wish to quit smoking and act consistently with that objective, while naïve smokers underestimate the preferences of their future selves. To justify its recommendation for a substantial increase in tobacco excise, the Henry review would have had to demonstrate that Australian smokers are both naïve and value the present substantially over the future.

Using the Henry review estimates, Davidson found that excise rates were (then) high enough to force even naive smokers to value the future over the present (they were not being irrational by consuming tobacco in the present). Davidson concluded that there was no market failure to justify government intervention, and no 'basis to argue that tobacco excise should be substantially increased – merely the anti-tobacco

22 Australian Taxation Office, 2024. *Latest Estimates and Findings: How we Combat Illicit Tobacco Behaviours with Help from other Government Agencies*

23 Davidson S, 2016, 6

prejudice of the Review itself.'[24] Davidson's critique was that the basis for government intervention was not revenue maximisation or social cost minimisation but, rather, paternalistic.

Or, makes little difference

Taxes are also unlikely to be an effective way of reducing the costs of other sin products, such as problem gambling – another thing public health now concerns itself with. The Henry review had the following observations on taxation and problem gambling. To the extent that existing gambling taxes recoup costs imposed on others, they do not affect the odds that gamblers face. But even when taxes do more than recoup 'economic rent', they can only mitigate the effects of problem gambling if they increase the average amount lost by a player per dollar bet, and if problem gamblers respond by reducing their losses.

The price of gambling for some games, such as many casino table games, is fixed by the game's rules and is not affected by gambling taxes (although businesses may be able to adjust the price by offering discounts or modifying the rules). In other games, such as TAB wagering, the price of gambling (the average player's loss) may be affected by gambling taxes, but this is not immediately apparent to the gambler. In such cases, increasing the price of gambling is not likely to affect the behaviour of problem gamblers.

Even where the price of gambling is affected by gambling taxes and is apparent to the gambler, problem gamblers may not markedly reduce their losses. If their gambling is constrained only by the amount of money available to them, their losses will not fall. If they face other constraints on their gambling, like the amount of time they can devote to gambling, higher prices may lead to higher losses and more severe problems.[25]

Approximately one per cent of the adult population are problem

24 Davidson S, 2016, 8

25 Australia's Future Tax System, 2009, E7–2

gamblers,[26] so using taxes to help counteract problem gambling imposes high costs on non-problem gamblers. Other policy interventions may help to address spillover costs and the costs borne by gamblers themselves. These interventions, some of which have been implemented in Australia, include limiting or prohibiting the advertising of gambling services.[27] None of the above has stopped the government from taxing gamblers. The most recent imposition in South Australia is an attempt to retain some taxation from the state.

The 2016-17 State Budget introduced a place of consumption tax of 15 per cent on the net wagering revenue of betting companies offering services to South Australia, effective from 1 July 2017. All bets placed in South Australia with Australian-based betting companies are subject to tax. South Australia is the first Australian jurisdiction to introduce a wagering tax based on the place of consumption. The place of consumption tax applies to bets on horse, harness, and greyhound racing, as well as bets on sports such as AFL, cricket, and soccer. It will also apply to other bets, such as those on the winner of the federal election or the Academy Awards.[28] Presumably, these taxes have the potential to drive gambling to offshore sites.

There is an expectation among anti-gambling public health campaigners that a significant portion of the revenue raised should be devoted to prevention. The logic is somewhat twisted, as the tax is often touted as reducing the risk of harm; in other words, the tax is the program, and sufficient to recoup spillover costs, including the sinner's costs shared by others. Whether taxes are the solution, a means of recouping spillover costs, or simply a means of raising funds is, in practice, difficult to determine. These funds should be returned to the general revenue. Nevertheless, governments often respond to lobbies, so it is common for some funds to be diverted to specific prevention and rehabilitation programs run by

26 It is 0.7 per cent in South Australia. South Australia Report of the Auditor General, 2023. *Gambling Harm Minimisation*, 17

27 Banks G, 2011. Evidence and social policy: the case of gambling. *Presentation to South Australian Centre for Economic Studies, Corporate Seminar*, Adelaide

28 Revenue South Australia, *Wagering Tax Announcement*. 7 July 2016

public health-aligned organisations. A cynic might even suggest that this is part of the reason why the public health lobby is so fond of sin taxes.

Gambling taxes accounted for approximately seven per cent of all state revenue in 2022-23, amounting to $9 billion.[29] State governments allocate part of gambling revenue to social programs such as problem gambling services and research into the impact of gambling on the community. In some states, substantial revenue is allocated to health services. In Victoria, for example, in 2022-23, taxes and levies paid to the state of Victoria totalled over $2.3 billion[30] and more than $1 billion per year from gambling revenue is allocated to various social programs: the Community Support Fund, the Hospitals and Charities Fund and the Mental Health Fund.[31] Gambling generated taxation revenue of $531 million for the South Australian government in 2021-22, representing 10 per cent of total State taxation revenue.[32] The Gamblers Rehabilitation Fund holds $9 million, most of which comes from gambling taxes and industry contributions.[33]

The U.S. Master Settlement Agreement, under which tobacco companies agreed to pay annual sums to the states to compensate them for healthcare costs related to smoking (a minimum of US$206 billion over the first twenty-five years), created and funded the National Public Education Foundation. The Foundation is dedicated to reducing youth smoking and preventing diseases associated with smoking.[34] There is, however, considerable complaint that those monies have not been sufficiently targeted toward prevention. From 2000 to 2009, the states received US$79 billion from the tobacco settlement (and US$124 billion from

29 Australian Bureau of Statistics, 2025. *Taxation Revenue, Australia 2023-23 Financial Year*

30 Victorian Gambling and Casino Control Commission, *Gambling Data*

31 Victorian State Government Department of Treasury and Finance, 2024. *Community Support Fund financial overview 2023-24*

32 South Australia Report of the Auditor General, 2023,17

33 South Australia Report of the Auditor General, 2023, 22

34 Michon K, 2015. Tobacco litigation: history and recent developments. *NOLO* 30 December

tobacco taxes). During this time, the states have allocated US$6.5 billion to tobacco prevention and cessation programs.[35]

Taxation can be costly, punitive, and ineffective in solving public health problems. It is also well to check which taxes are beneficial and which are exercises in gouging (i.e. taxation without benefit). Public health advocates do not help the cause by proclaiming the effectiveness of taxation and seeking to divert its income stream to their cause, for which taxation was meant to be a solution.

Or, creates a black market

In April 2025, the Commonwealth government advertised for the position of Illicit Tobacco and e-cigarette Commissioner. The role was established to counter the threat of illicit tobacco and e-cigarettes. These are two different 'threats'. One is taxation. Indeed, illicit tobacco is an indirect consequence of tobacco taxation. The second, e-cigarettes, are an indirect consequence of tobacco smoking regulation. Some advocates hope that smoking tobacco (and vaping) can be eliminated, despite years of swingeing taxation and bans on advertising. The price of a packet of cigarettes in Australia has risen considerably over the last forty years, primarily driven by increases in tobacco excise. For example, a packet of 25 Winfield Blue cigarettes cost $1.07 in 1980, but in 2023, it cost $46.95, with $31.00 of the total price comprised of excise and duty.[36] Smokers can avoid those taxes by buying under-the-counter products.

The illicit tobacco market has grown as higher tax excises have made legal tobacco prohibitively expensive for some sections of the community, especially when coupled with inflation and the resulting

35 Campaign for Tobacco-Free Kids, 2008. A decade of broken promises: the 1998 state tobacco settlement ten years later. *Robert Wood Johnson Foundation*. Litigation has not been a feature of the Australian debate, that which has been litigated can be found at Liberman, J. 2024. Litigation brought by Australian consumer and regulatory groups against the tobacco industry. In E M Greenhalgh et al (Eds) 2024, 16.2

36 Australian Taxation Office, 2024. *Excise Duty Rates for Tobacco*

cost-of-living pressures.[37] Smokers are disproportionately concentrated among lower socio-economic groups.[38] Many are unable or unwilling to pay the ever-increasing prices for cigarettes. KPMG estimates a packet of illicit cigarettes costs 47 per cent of the price of a legitimate major brand.[39] As a result, almost one-quarter of all people who smoke have smoked unbranded tobacco in their lifetime.[40]

The unintended consequence of taxation has been the rise of a lucrative and expanding black market for these products. Emerging black markets tend to attract established organised crime groups, which can use violence to enforce contracts, collect debts, and threaten competitors. Recently, for instance, there have been more than 40 fire bombings of stores selling illicit tobacco and vapes across Victoria. According to police, this serious criminal activity is being perpetrated at the behest of rival criminal networks engaged in a 'turf war' for control of the lucrative trade. From October 2024, police had searched nearly 70 stores believed to be involved in the illegal tobacco trade, seizing more than 100,000 vapes with an estimated street value of $3.2 million, along with 3.2 million cigarettes. While most of the violence associated with the black market seems to be occurring in Victoria, this is a national issue. In Sydney, in February 2024, health authorities seized 30,000 vapes and 118,000 cigarettes with an estimated street value of $1.1 million[41] and $8 million worth of illicit vapes located through collaboration between the Therapeutic Goods Authority and Victoria Police.[42]

The growth in illicit trade directly affects the collection of excises owed

37 Parliament of Victoria Public Accounts and Estimates Committee, 2024. *Vaping and Tobacco Controls*, xii

38 Australian Institute of Health and Welfare, 2024. *National Drug Strategy Household Survey 2022–2023: Alcohol, Tobacco, ecigarette and Illicit Drug use by Population Groups: Interactive data*

39 Parliament of Victoria Public Accounts and Estimates Committee, 2024, 22

40 Australian Institute for Health and Welfare, 2024. *Alcohol, Tobacco & other Drugs in Australia*

41 NSW Minister for Health, Sixty retailers targeted in major vaping blitz across Sydney. *Press Release* 6 February 2024

42 Therapeutic Goods Administration, *$8 million of illicit vapes located in collaboration between TGA and Victoria Police*. 30 October 2024

on tobacco and e-cigarettes, leading to lost revenue for the Australian Tax Office (ATO).[43] While the total value of the tobacco market in Victoria in 2023 was estimated at $6 billion, the proportion of illicit tobacco ranged from six per cent to 40 per cent.[44] The Commonwealth Government's estimates for tobacco excise revenue have recently been revised downwards. In the 2023–24 Budget, it was projected to increase to $14.7 billion by 2026–27, but in the latest 2024–25 Budget, the forward estimates indicate a decline in tobacco excise revenue to $10.7 billion by 2027–28.[45] The ATO estimates that $2.7 billion in duties were evaded from illicit tobacco entering the market.[46]

It is unlikely law enforcement agencies will be able to tackle the black market when the trade is so lucrative, and the penalties are so much less than those for illegal trade in hard drugs. The Australian Border Force is already stretched beyond capacity, tackling the booming illicit drug market.[47] While law enforcement agencies have made inroads with arrests of black marketeers and seizures of their products, these are often quickly replaced so that trafficking operations continue unabated.[48] Prohibition on alcohol and other substances, for example, has proven that the dangers associated with black markets extend beyond systemic violence. Additional harms are inferior and adulterated products, which can present even greater health risks than legal tobacco products.

Not satisfied with creating a black market in illegal tobacco and substitutes and treating the few remaining smokers as pariahs and taxing them massively, the National Health and Medical Research Council (NHMRC) has a Centre of Research Excellence on Achieving the Tobacco Endgame. The Centre boasts 30 professors spread over numerous

43 Parliament of Victoria Public Accounts and Estimates Committee, 2024, xiii

44 Parliament of Victoria Public Accounts and Estimates Committee, 2024, 21

45 Parliament of Victoria Public Accounts and Estimates Committee, 2024, 21

46 Australian Taxation Office, 2024. *Tobacco Tax Gap*

47 Australian Criminal Intelligence Commission, 2022. *Illicit Drug Data Report 2020–21*

48 Bouchard M, 2007. On the resilience of illegal drug markets. *Global Crime* 8(4), 325

universities.[49] The endgame is to achieve a smoke-free Australia. For example, the centre is developing new methods of estimating the size of the illicit tobacco market, such as wastewater analysis. But their advice caused it! The obsession with elimination is way out of line. Surely, after the black market fiasco and the COVID-19 response, the idea of elimination should be eliminated. As two criminologists have commented, 'Australia's tobacco and vaping policies have transformed two largely legal and peaceful markets into increasingly dangerous and uncontrolled ones.'[50] There exists a sweet spot in regulating the sale of harmful products – one that limits access and lessens harm without being so burdensome as to foster a significant black market or so ideologically puritanical as to pursue prohibition. The sweet spot has passed in Australia. Excessive regulation will mean that an irreducible proportion of the population will rely on nicotine or similar stimulants to get through their day, but an illegal market and the costs and consequences of it will have replaced the legal market. The call by some state ministers, including the NSW health minister, for the Commonwealth to lower its tobacco excise has fallen on deaf ears.[51]

Taxation is ineffective where the source of harm is diffuse

Many advocates argue that Australia should follow the lead of at least 54 countries that have taxes on sugar-sweetened beverages.[52] While there is evidence of reduced sugar consumption from that source, there is little to suggest reductions in obesity.[53] One of the leading papers cited by the

49 https://tobacco-endgame.centre.uq.edu.au

50 Martin J & Bright D, 2024. Australia's restrictive vaping and tobacco policies are fuelling a lucrative and dangerous black market. *The Conversation* 12 March

51 Mohammad Alfares and Lachlan Leeming, States attack federal Labor's tobacco policy. 12 November 2025 *The Australian*

52 Cobiac L et al, 2017. Taxes and subsidies for improving diet and population health in Australia: a cost-effectiveness modelling study. *PLoS ONE* 14(2), 1. Duckett S & Swerissen H, 2016. *A Sugary Drinks Tax: Recovering the Community Costs of Obesity*. Grattan Institute

53 Obesity Evidence Hub

Global Obesity Observatory (GOO)[54] was hardly a ringing endorsement of sugar taxes as a solution to obesity, concluding that taxing sugar-sweetened beverages would raise prices in markets with limited producers, thereby halting further increases in obesity prevalence. However, it would not result in permanent weight reduction for the population.[55] As for other ways of intervening, such as community-based, another of GOO's reviews concluded that 'the strength of evidence is moderate that a combined diet and physical activity intervention conducted in the community with a school component is more effective at preventing obesity or overweight.'[56] Sugary drink taxes are regressive, hitting hardest those for whom the tax is meant, the poor.[57] Public health taxes on less healthy food and beverage products may be effective; however, it is not clear whether reductions in the quantity of taxed products result from price increases due to the tax or from accompanying messaging.[58] A Saudi study of a sweetened drinks tax, introduced without adequate public information, noted a decline in volumes, but this does not necessarily translate into a long-term decline in obesity-related disease.[59]

Why does the WHO recommend an excise tax on sugar-sweetened beverages, knowing that sugar is a single nutrient and obesity is caused by excess calories from any nutrient?[60] Sugar can weaken appetite control and lead to increases in weight gain and a greater risk of obesity. Sugar is added to an enormous array of processed foods, but taxing a single source

---

54 Global Obesity Observatory

55 Nakhimovsky S et al, 2016. Taxes on sugar-sweetened beverages to reduce overweight and obesity in middle-income countries: a systematic review. *PLoS ONE* 11(9), 1

56 Bleich S N et al, 2013. Systematic review of community-based childhood obesity prevention studies. *Pediatrics* 132 (1), 201

57 Kao K et al, 2020. The health and financial impacts of a sugary drink tax across different income groups in Canada. *Economics and Human Biology* 38,100869

58 Doble B et al, 2020. The effect of implicit and explicit taxes on the purchasing of 'high-in-calorie' products: a randomized controlled trial. *Economics and Human Biology* 37, 100860

59 Alsukaita R et al, 2020. Evaluating Saudi Arabia's 50% carbonated drink excise tax: changes in prices and volume sales. *Economics and Human Biology* 38, 100868

60 World Health Organization, 2022. *WHO Calls on Countries to Tax Sugar-sweetened Beverages to Save Lives*

of a single ingredient in obesity-causing foods might not yield significant results. Taxing junk food, or a component of it, to reduce consumption is more complex than taxing tobacco or alcohol. Unlike those products, there is no universally agreed-upon definition of what constitutes healthy or harmful food. As a result, public health advocates criticise opponents of taxation for arguing against differential tax rates for different food types, because the implementation of food taxes in real-life settings is limited, and the analysis of their effectiveness is even more restricted.[61] However, the advocates are mistaken; there is sufficient evidence from real-life settings to suggest that a sugar tax, or indeed other food taxes, is not a valuable tool for combating obesity.

The worldwide increase in obesity and related chronic diseases has primarily been driven by 'nutritional transitions in low-income and middle-income countries [that] are typically characterized by increases in the consumption of animal fat and protein, refined grains, and added sugar.'[62] Obesity is multi-faceted. Sugar is but one source of energy, and sugary drinks are one source of sugar. Most free sugars consumed in Australia, for example, are from the energy-dense, nutrient-poor discretionary foods and beverages. Just over half (52 per cent) of free sugars in the diet are consumed from beverages, with the leading beverages being soft drinks, sports and energy drinks (19 per cent), fruit and vegetable juices and drinks (13 per cent) and cordial (4.9 per cent). The leading food categories are confectionery and cakes/muffins (each contributing 8.7 per cent).[63]

Meanwhile, there is evidence in Australia that while obesity's incidence has increased, and diabetes prevalence has increased from three per cent in 2001 to five per cent in 2022,[64] the proportion of people aged two years and over who consumed sweetened beverages decreased from 49 per cent

61 Comans T et al, 2013. The cost-effectiveness and consumer acceptability of taxation strategies to reduce rates of overweight and obesity among children in Australia: study protocol. *BMC Public Health* 13(1182), 4

62 Malik V S et al, 2013. Global obesity: trends, risk factors and policy implications. *National Review of Endocrinology* 9(1), 13

63 Australian Bureau of Statistics, 2016. *Australian Health Survey: Consumption of Added Sugars 2011-12*, 6

64 Australian Bureau of Statistics, 2023. *National Health Survey 2022*

in 1995 to 42 per cent in 2011-12. This was primarily driven by a decrease in cordial consumption, with a corresponding decline in consumption among children from 35 per cent in 1995 to 11 per cent in 2011-12. The most significant decrease in consumption of sweetened beverages was observed among children, with the proportion of children aged 2-3 years who consumed sweetened beverages decreasing by more than half (from 67 per cent to 31 per cent).[65] While there has been no inoculation for tobacco (although nicotine substitutes help), nor for alcohol, there may be some relief for food. Big Pharma may be able to come to the rescue. Ozempic became available in Australia in 2020 and was initially used for diabetes sufferers, but has since been found to have a much broader applicability. Whether its use at scale can make an appreciable difference to global obesity,[66] and overcome warnings of side effects, is debatable.[67] But this also raises an interesting question: if a drug turns out to have greater impacts on obesity than all the years of public health campaigns, then what is public health really achieving?

Does taxation save lives?

A recent study estimated the consequences of an additional 20 per cent tax on sugar-sweetened beverages on health and healthcare expenditure in Australia. The researchers were eager to demonstrate that the tax would generate an estimated $400 million in annual revenue. The primary health consequence, however, was that an estimated 1606 additional

65 Australian Bureau of Statistics, 2014. *Australian Health Survey: Nutrition First Results: Foods and Nutrients, 2011-12*

66 Stein M, 2025. The Ozempic effect: how one drug reshaped health, hype and regulation in Australia. *Hall & Wilcox* lawyer's website 29 August

67 Therapeutic Goods Administration, 2025. Product warnings updated for GLP-1 RA class. Safety alert. Includes high-profile medicines used to treat diabetes and obesity. 1 December. See also weight gains on cessation of treatment, West S et al, 2026. Weight regain after cessation of medication for weight management: systematic review and meta-analysis. *BMJ* 392:e085304

people would live as a result of the tax.[68] Given that at least 190,000 Australians died in 2022, 1606 across the lifetime of the scheme seems aminimal return on a considerable taxation measure.[69] Indeed, Australia has had a de facto sugar tax since 2000, with the introduction of the Goods and Services Tax, which taxes processed foods while leaving fresh foods untaxed. Meanwhile, obesity rates have continued to rise.

A U.S. case study on a sugar tax offers little comfort to its proponents. Nearly two-thirds of all states currently tax soft drinks using excise taxes or sales taxes. An analysis of the impact of changes in states' soft drink tax rates from 1990 to 2006 on body mass index (BMI) and obesity suggested that weight responds to changes in soft drink tax rates, though the response is not significant. A one percentage point increase in the state soft drink tax rate was associated with a 0.003-point decrease in BMI. Extrapolating, the results suggested that increasing the soft drink tax to 58 per cent would decrease the mean BMI in the United States by 0.16 points – a meaningless change. In comparison, the average gain in BMI between 1990 and 2006 was more than 2.3 points. Increasing the tax rate comparable to that of cigarettes yielded a decrease in the proportion of the population who are obese or overweight by nearly 0.7 percentage points. The conclusion: 'Although increasing the tax rate on soft drinks to be comparable with cigarettes will not halt the obesity epidemic, the impact on population weight would likely be non-negligible.'[70] This is not a lot to look forward to.

In addition to the lack of impact on health, several further problems are associated with a food tax. Several problems were experienced with the recent brief experiment with a fat tax in Denmark. In October 2011,

68 Veerman L et al, 2016. The impact of a tax on sugar-sweetened beverages on health and health care costs: a modelling study. *PLoS ONE* 11(4), 1. Two of the authors are employed by the Obesity Policy Coalition, which the Victorian Department of Health funded.

69 In 2022, 190,939 deaths were registered in Australia, so a crude measure of 25 multiplied by that number could underestimate the rate. Australian Institute of Health and Welfare, 2024. *Deaths in Australia*

70 Fletcher J et al, 2010. Can soft drink taxes reduce population weight? *Contemporary Economic Policy* 28(1), 24

Denmark introduced the world's first tax on fat. The tax included meat, dairy, animal fat, oils, margarine and butter blends as well as composed foods containing these products. The taxation rate was DKK 16 per kilogram of saturated fat, excluding a 25 per cent value-added tax. A threshold limit of 2.3 per cent saturated fat exempted all types of regular drinking milk and milk-based yoghurts. The tax was imposed on anyone producing or importing foodstuffs for commercial purposes and was expected to be passed on to consumers at retail outlets, restaurants, and fast-food outlets.

Research on the tax concluded that Denmark's fat tax proved economically damaging and did not change the habits of 80 per cent of Danes. The tax led to a tiny 0.4 per cent reduction in fat consumption in seven months, while food prices increased by 14 per cent. The tax led to some strange behaviour on purchases. The sale of butter blends and margarine decreased, while the sale of butter, oils, cream, chips and snacks increased. The decrease in sales of cookies and biscuits, combined with an increase in sales of chips and snacks, indicates a shift among consumers from sweet to salty between-meal foods during the fat tax.

In addition, a tax that targets explicitly saturated fat can lead to a simultaneous reduction in the intake of unsaturated fat, since some of those foods high in saturated fat are also high in unsaturated fat, e.g. butter blends and margarine, which can potentially outweigh the positive health benefits of a tax on saturated fat. The changes in consumption patterns caused by the fat tax, therefore, had only a marginal effect on the population's risk of ischaemic heart disease.

The avowedly pro-fat-tax researchers pressed on, concluding that governments should raise tax rates. This, they conceded, 'involves a risk of increasing economic inequalities, as food taxes are regressive, i.e. burden low-income households proportionately more than high-income households.'[71] To compensate, researchers suggest a tax subsidy and hope

71 Bødker M et al, 2015. The Danish fat tax: effects on consumption patterns and risk of ischaemic heart disease. *Preventive Medicine* 77, 203

that politicians do not use food taxes to generate revenue.[72] But would the poor spend the subsidy on junk food? The problems associated with the Danish fat tax —economic damage, lack of effect on people's health, increased economic inequality, and government overreach —may not deter public health advocates, but they certainly turned off everyone else. It was repealed in January 2013 after only 15 months.[73]

Inequality exacerbated

A small-sample study of 160 French women simulated the effect of a five per cent value-added tax on 22 food items. The study concluded that a fat tax policy is unsuitable for substantially affecting the nutrients purchased by French households and yields ambiguous effects. Although it would generate significant tax revenue, the fat tax is highly regressive. Somewhat bizarrely, the researchers were more interested in health inequality than in any health benefit, providing further insight into the perspectives of certain advocates. For instance, attempts to improve the health of the overall population may 'increase health disparities between social groups because those who were formerly at a lower risk of exposure derive more benefits than those who were formerly at a greater exposure to risk.'[74] The researchers viewed this as a significant issue, not because some were harmed, but because not everyone benefited. This differs notably from, for instance, a tax that penalises the poor and has little effect on health.

Another study suggested that food price policies, such as subsidies for fruits and vegetables combined with appropriate taxes, could improve certain aspects of diet quality, but only with a 30 per cent price increase. As the researchers acknowledged, 'it is unlikely that actual policies would

72 Bødker M et al, 2015. The rise and fall of the world's first fat tax. *Health Policy* 119, 737

73 Bødker 2015, The rise and fall, 737

74 Darmon N et al, 2014. Food price policies improve diet quality while increasing socioeconomic inequalities in nutrition. *The International Journal of Behavioral Nutrition and Physical Activity* 11(1), 66

use such high rates, which could be judged politically unacceptable.'[75] To achieve modest health gains among the poor, not only would there likely be riots in the streets over a 30 per cent price rise and subsidies on foods they do not favour, but there might also be a reaction from the food industry to maintain their market share. The food industry may respond to tax changes by altering the nutritional quality of taxed products —for example, by substituting more expensive ingredients and/or introducing new processes —which could make the modified products less affordable. This could lead to shifts in demand from high-end supermarkets to low-end discount stores, a shift that seems to have been exploited by discount chains to raise butter and margarine prices by more than the pure tax increase.[76] Taxation would be succeeded by regulation in a cycle of heightened imposition and surveillance. These strategies may worsen class disparities in the nutritional quality of food selections. Heaven forbid, a fat tax might have unintended consequences as it could 'exacerbate nutritional disparities among consumers.'[77]

Substitution

While the public health lobby strives to alter the consumption habits of the recalcitrant consumer, the consumer continually undermines their efforts. A U.S. study combined soft drink tax data from 1989 to 2006 with the National Health Examination and Nutrition Survey to explore the effects of soft drink taxes on child and adolescent soft drink consumption, substitution patterns, and weight outcomes. The study overall found evidence of moderate reductions in soft drink consumption resulting from current soda tax rates. Still, it also revealed that reductions in calories from soda were entirely offset by increases in calories from other beverages. Hence, 'soda taxes do not reduce weight in children and

75 Jensen J D & Smed S, 2013. The Danish tax on saturated fat: short run effects on consumption, substitution patterns and consumer prices of fats. *Food Policy* 42, 26

76 Allais O et al, 2010. The effects of a fat tax on French households' purchases: a nutritional approach. *American Journal of Agricultural Economics* 92(1), 243

77 Fletcher J et al, 2010. The effects of soft drink taxes on child and adolescent consumption and weight outcomes. *Journal of Public Economics* 94, 968

adolescents and are, therefore, likely an ineffective obesity tax.'[78]

In seemingly more controlled environments, such as schools, substitution emerges as a barrier to behavioural change. During the 2011-12 school year, a district in Oregon, U.S., removed chocolate milk from the menu for students in kindergarten to grade five, offering skim milk instead. The rationale was that chocolate milk could contain up to twice as much sugar as white milk. Thus, removing chocolate milk from school cafeterias may help lessen childhood obesity. However, milk is a source of nutrients crucial for bone growth and development; in that context, any milk is better than none. A study analysing the impacts of eliminating chocolate milk yielded striking results: among participating schools, its removal correlated with a 10 per cent decline in average daily milk sales, a 10 per cent rise in the cost of milk consumption, and a 30 per cent increase in milk waste.[79]

Alongside these potentially harmful changes to the selection, the researchers inquired whether altering the availability of chocolate milk affected other behaviours, such as within-meal compensation, after-school snacking, or reduced lunch sales. The research did not examine whether students compensated for their lunch or after-school snacks by consuming higher-calorie beverages. Still, they were quite suspicious that this might be the case. They concluded, 'drinking chocolate milk is better than drinking an alternative caloric drink, such as a sports drink, or even skipping a school lunch.'[80] Consumers change their habits when goods are taxed. Taxes on sugary drinks can slow their purchase, but not slow growth in waistlines.

Some studies suggest that substitutions and compensations may occur, moderating any effect on consumption; however, there is considerable variation in these findings.[81] The following study (Text Box 4.1) tried to

---

78 Hanks A et al, 2014. Chocolate milk consequences: a pilot study evaluating the consequences of banning chocolate milk in school cafeterias. *PLoS ONE* 9(4), 1

79 Hanks A et al, 2014, 1

80 There is some propensity for like with like substitution, bad or good substitution. See Miao Z et al, 2013. Accounting for product substitution in the analysis of food taxes targeting obesity. *Health Economics* 22, 1318

81 Edwards R, 2011. Commentary: soda taxes, obesity, and the shifty behavior of consumers. *Preventive Medicine* 52(6), 417

unravel the extent to which consumers switch under a new tax, in this case, from soft drinks to beer.[82]

Text Box 4.1 From Coke to Coors

> Could taxing calorie-dense foods like soft drinks help reduce obesity?
>
> A six-month field experiment was conducted in a 62,000-person city in America. Half of the 113 households recruited for the study were subjected to a 10 per cent tax on calorie-dense foods and beverages, while the other half were not.
>
> The tax caused a short-term decline in soft drink purchases for one month; however, there was no reduction over the three- or six-month periods. Moreover, in households that buy beer, this tax resulted in an increase in beer purchases.
>
> In line with the existing literature, the evidence indicated that consumers substituted products due to specific food taxes. Households that regularly purchased beer bought even more, while those that frequently bought soft drinks did likewise. The tax prompted an increase in water sales, but any potential health benefits were completely offset by the extra calories gained from soft drinks.
>
> Taxes on less healthy foods may not effectively lower soft drink consumption or overall calorie intake. More worrying is the potential that such a tax could result in increased alcohol consumption in some households.

Source: Hanks A et al, 2013. From Coke to Coors: a field study of a fat tax and its unintended consequences. *Journal of Nutrition Education and Behaviour* 45(4), S40, 26

A more horrifying substitution has emerged in remote Australia, where Aboriginal drinkers have started consuming kava,[83] and worse, hand sanitiser, which became common during COVID-19, mixing it with low-alcohol beer and soft drinks.[84] We know that consumers will shift their demand towards cheaper foods in response to fat taxes. Taxing sugary drinks will likely decrease their consumption. Still, it is also likely to

82 Hanks A et al, 2013, S40

83 National Drug and Alcohol Research Centre UNSW, 2025. Kava. *NDARC Fact Sheet*

84 Liam Mendes, Alice mother killed after hand sanitiser drinking session. *The Australian* 15 January 2025

increase consumption of closely related substitutes, such as diet soft drinks, fruit and vegetable juices, milk, water, and possibly alcoholic beverages. Such a tax might also increase demand for complementary goods, such as salty snacks. The overall impact of a sugary drink tax on obesity thus depends not only on how responsive demand for these drinks is to price changes, but also on how responsive demand for a wide range of substitutes and complements is. The net effect on calorie intake from this shift is not guaranteed to be negative, as consumers choose foods for various reasons beyond caloric content alone. Some taxes on certain types of food might even increase obesity if close substitutes have higher caloric content. As for alcohol, some substitutes can be deadly.

Much of the taxation argument rests on the assumption that the target individual will change behaviour sufficiently to avoid the harm associated with smoking, alcohol, food, or gambling. In addition to the arguments canvassed, the salutary observation is that some people will not change. The most striking aspect of the AIDS pandemic's history, for example, is that behaviour changed only partially after the recognition of a new and deadly disease transmitted through sex and needle sharing. A U.S. report noted 'rapid, profound, but … incomplete alterations in the behaviour of both homosexual/bisexual men and intravenous drug users [as well as] considerable instability or recidivism.'[85] By 1998, 19 per cent of all U.S. adults reported some change in their sexual conduct in response to the threat of AIDS.[86] The introduction of combination antiretroviral therapy in 1996 somewhat lessened the fear factor. However, a 2017 paper revealed that fewer than half of at-risk men had used a condom during their last time they had sex.[87]

85 Becker M H & Joseph J G, 1988. AIDS and behavioral change to reduce risk: a review. *American Journal of Public Health* 78(4), 394

86 Feinleib J A & Michael R T, 1998. Reported changes in sexual behavior in response to AIDS in the United States. *Preventive Medicine* 27(3), 400

87 Nasrullah M et al, 2017. Factors associated with condom use among sexually active U.S. adults, national survey of family growth, 2006–2010 and 2011–2013. *Journal of Sexual Medicine* 14(4), 541 See also Zhu W, Bazzi S A & Bazzi A R, 2019. Behavioral changes following HIV seroconversion during the historical expansion of HIV treatment in the United States. *AIDS* 33(1), 113

Conclusion

Public health does not like people making choices it disapproves of, and taxation is its go-to strategy to modify behaviours. People make bad choices, and some interventions, such as banning tobacco advertising and sponsorship and taxation to discourage a habit that can kill, seem reasonable. Maybe new measures to stem drunkenness in nightspots to prevent violence, or removing ATMs from poker machine outlets to curb problem gamblers, also seem sensible, but controlling the eating habits of adults and children? There is a challenge. Banning, taxing, forbidding, and many other tools from the government's regulatory arsenal are potent interventions. However, applying these to food, despite recent breakthroughs in medication, is bound to provoke a reaction and have unintended consequences. Worse still, the evidence on how much of the wrong food causes harm is unclear.

Observing the poor state of those who purchase their tobacco at the shop counter reinforces the harsh measure that tobacco taxation is. The criminal gangs setting fire to tobacco outlets indicate that a black market has led to serious criminal activity. Tobacco consumption does kill, but beyond that product, alcohol, gambling, sweet drinks, and junk food are simply not amenable to taxation fixes and their downsides. Taxation is no cure. But it is certainly necessary to advance public health's ideology of prohibiting sinful behaviour.

Case studies

The previous chapters looked at some of the key strategies public health uses to get what it wants, and how its efforts are all too frequently focused on ideology rather than genuine, long-term health outcomes.

In the following sections, we provide case studies to show how these strategies – and many other elements of public health, such as overblown fear campaigns, othering, and the self-interested pursuit of power by a few – look in practice. The examples are just a handful of instances that have gained considerable public attention in recent times. COVID-19, of course, features large.

Sadly, to compile a case study for every piece of public health over-reach would require thousands and thousands of pages. Such is the state of Australia under the public health thumb. However, selective though these case studies are, they show the true face of public health in Australia today, and further demonstrate just how little public health is concerned with people's lives.

All public policy is a display of power, and public health is no different. In the pursuit of the best health outcomes, those who recommend a course of action can be wildly off course.

It was true for the COVID-19 response; it is true of the dominant response to gender dysphoria and Aboriginal health. The response to those who suffer from mental ill-health risk over-promoting their cause, as is now abundantly clear with the NDIS.

5

COVID-19: society is not a hospital ward

By focusing on population health, public health officials and scholars value health over other values, such as happiness, fun, religious compliance, cultural traditions, or freedom.[1]

Professor Jessica Flanigan

You have to have the courage when you're a public health official to say, 'I don't know when you don't know' rather than 'I didn't think the public was ready to hear that'.[2]

Dr Robert Redfield, Director of the U.S. Centers for Disease Control and Prevention

Panic-demic: the politics of fear remain alive and well

Despite Dr Redfield's rare insight into the astoundingly conceited mindset of some public health officials, the script for the next pandemic response has already been written: 'Lock 'em up and wait for a vaccine.' This strategy has been devised by politicians who, on the back of intense fear campaigns, took on a 'wartime mentality'[3] and harvested votes in Queensland, Western Australia, and Victoria, and were advised by Chief Medical Officers who enjoyed the limelight, as well as media owners

1 Flanigan J, 2024, 509

2 U.S. House of Representatives, 2024. *Final Report of the Select Subcommittee on the Coronavirus Pandemic Committee on Oversight and Accountability*, 335

3 Macedo S & Lee F, 2025. *In Covid's Wake: How Our Politics Failed Us*. Kindle Edition, 7

and journalists who thrived on a fearful and locked-down audience during the COVID-19 pandemic.[4]

There is little reason to believe the response to the next pandemic will differ unless the influence of such individuals changes, creating space for alternative views. The COVID-19 response is a case study in the abuse of power by health officials who read their political leaders' fear of the unknown and innate desire for control. Politicians were afraid to be seen to contravene public health advice, but also sensed an opportunity in gathering votes in the fear of the moment. The wider medical profession, which should have been a countervailing voice of caution, was either reluctant to speak up or cowed. Far from a fulsome analysis of the use of power, the Australian Commonwealth's Inquiry into the COVID-19 response was an exultation in the abuse of power. The Inquiry asserted, for example, that interventions from the Commonwealth, such as JobKeeper, and from the states and territories, like rent relief and eviction moratoriums, mitigated the pandemic's impact; for instance, the Inquiry accepted as truth that the number of households facing housing affordability stress would have surged by 74 per cent without these interventions.[5] But had the lockdowns, school closures, and mandated vaccinations not closed businesses and caused job losses (accounting for any net increase in illness without these measures), would affordability stress have been as severe? Is the 74 per cent a sign of success or failure?

As noted elsewhere, vaccines have saved countless lives, and promoting people's understanding of their role is a success for which science in the service of public health deserves credit. However, this does not mean that all claims about vaccines are accurate. What the pandemic response showed was that public health ideology now prioritises the concept of vaccination over evidence about specific vaccines' impacts (or, indeed, their necessity for those unlikely to become seriously ill). The claim that COVID vaccines save lives has come under intense,

4 One television outlet ran a continuous COVID-19 program, knowing the audience was in lockdown or working from home.

5 Commonwealth Government, 2024. *COVID-19 Response Inquiry*, 450

devastating scrutiny. Public health authorities were aware that they were withholding evidence of vaccine efficacy when they recommended mass vaccinations. The early narrative was that vaccines were effective against infection and transmission. It was the basis for a national rollout of vaccinations across Australia. That assertion collapsed in August 2021, and a new justification emerged. The vaccines could not prevent infection but offered 'robust and sustained protection against severe illness and death' – thus placing them firmly within the public health framework. That claim was being undermined as early as October 2020. The coup de grâce was the finding in 2021 that vaccines did not prevent death. The emergence of these false narratives of vaccine salvation rested on flawed research methodologies, the misrepresentation of results in scientific communication, the misinterpretation of findings by public health authorities, and the systematic suppression of dissenting voices.[6] The one fleeting, semi-credible observation that the vaccines were effective against severe illness overrode a host of problems,[7] revealing just how closely intertwined public health and politics are. Public health authorities were aware that they were withholding evidence of vaccine efficacy when they recommended mass vaccinations.

Oblivious of those scientific discussions and evidence, or not, three state premiers were rewarded for locking down or locking in their voters with lockdowns that may 'go down as one of the greatest peacetime policy failures in modern history.'[8] Western Australia Premier Mark McGowan delighted in his state's isolation while resisting the Commonwealth's call to open up.[9] Queensland Premier Annastacia Palaszczuk denied entry to NSW residents living near the border who were in dire need of emergency services.[10] Victorian Premier Daniel

6 Ophir Y et al, 2025. A step-by-step evaluation of the claim that COVID-19 vaccines saved millions of lives. *ResearchGate preprint*, 20

7 Ophir Y et al, 2025, 29

8 Allen D W, 2021. Covid-19 Lockdown cost/benefits: a critical assessment of the literature. *International Journal of the Economics of Business* 29(1), 21

9 Natalie Oliveri, "An odd thing to say": WA Premier hits back at PM's Croods comparison. *Nine News* 25 August 2021

10 Kelsie Wilkie & Tita Smith, Only for our people. *Daily Mail* 28 August 2020

Andrews oversaw the world's longest lockdowns.[11] Lockdowns have been hailed as lifesavers, with the UK Inquiry claiming 23,000 deaths could have been averted had the lockdowns in the UK occurred one week earlier.[12] In Australia, some claimed that 18,000 deaths were avoided because of border controls instituted by the Australian state and federal governments.[13] These were projected saved lives, not *confirmed* saved lives, and many deaths may have occurred later, regardless. Another study concluded that 'the short-term trends in the number of COVID-19 cases, hospitalisations, and ICU patients in Australia, Canada, and the United Kingdom showed that closures resulted in reduced trend growth and openings resulted in increased trend growth.'[14] This conclusion is significant because it pertains to short-term and trend growth, without suggesting that COVID-19 was eradicated or that lives were saved that would not have been lost later. Additionally, neither study considered the age of those affected or the medical and other costs incurred by everyone else. International border closures from China effectively delayed the widespread transmission of COVID-19, but there was no evidence that they reduced long-term mortality rates.[15]

A meta-analysis of 24 studies on the effects of lockdowns on COVID-19 mortality found that lockdowns had little to no impact on mortality while imposing significant economic and social costs. The authors concluded, 'lockdown policies are ill-founded and should be dismissed

11 Judd Boaz, Melbourne passes Buenos Aires' world record for time spent in COVID-19 lockdown. *ABC News* 3 October 2021

12 UK COVID Inquiry, 2025. *A Report by The Rt Hon The Baroness Hallett DBE, Chair of the UK Covid-19 Inquiry on the Core Decision-Making and Political Governance*

13 Duckett S, 2022. Public health management of the COVID-19 pandemic in Australia: the role of the Morrison government. *International Journal of Environmental Research and Public Health* 19, 2

14 Chu L et al, 2024. Submission to *Response to Commonwealth Government COVID-19 Response Inquiry*

15 Constantino V, Heslop D J & MacIntyre C R, 2020. The effectiveness of full and partial travel bans against COVID-19 spread in Australia for travellers from China during and after the epidemic peak in China. *Journal of Travel Medicine* 27(5). Adekunle A et al, 2020. Delaying the COVID-19 epidemic in Australia: evaluating the effectiveness of international travel bans. *Australian and New Zealand Journal of Public Health* 2020, 44(4)

as a pandemic policy instrument.'[16] Professor Sunetra Gupta, a signatory of the Great Barrington Declaration and an eminent Oxford epidemiologist, was politely scathing of the UK Inquiry's claim that deaths were caused by delays in lockdown, or indeed that lives were saved because of lockdown.[17] Sabhlok argues that short-term excess deaths are an incomplete measure of human welfare losses. During 2020-2021, lockdowns likely reduced some deaths that might have occurred for other reasons, such as car accidents, other accidental deaths, and medical mishaps. In his reflection on the Victorian response, Dr Brett Sutton, the adviser to the government that imposed the world's longest lockdown, described lockdowns as part of an 'elimination strategy'.[18] It is more likely that, 'At best, [lockdowns] provided a small number of mostly elderly and sick individuals a few more years of life on average, at a tremendous cost borne by both the surviving elderly and the rest of society – a cost equivalent to many times the number of life-years 'saved' by lockdowns.'[19] The extent of the impact is only now becoming clear.[20]

Premiers knew—or their pollsters told them—that those voters preferred the promise of safety over freedom. Given the concerted politico-public health effort to terrify people into compliance, is it any wonder? In contrast, a longitudinal study of 1,211 non-voting students in years 11 and 12 during 2020 and 2021 found that, among those who had experienced extended lockdowns in Melbourne, 20 per cent experienced mental

16 Herby J, Jonung L & Hanke S H, 2022. A literature review and meta-analysis of the effects of lockdowns on COVID-19 mortality. *Studies in Applied Economics* 200(January), 2. Early lockdown can 'decelerate' contagion. Amuedo-Dorantesa C et al, 2021. Early adoption of non-pharmaceutical interventions and COVID-19 Mortality. *Economics and Human Biology* 42 (101003)

17 Professor Sunetra Gupta, The lost lessons of lockdown. *UnHerd* 22 November 2025

18 Sutton B, 2024. Pandemic lessons learned and future public health strategies. *Microbiology Australia* 45(1), 39

19 Foster G & Sabhlok S, 2023. Response to understanding the impact of lockdowns on short-term excess mortality in Australia by Philip Clarke and Andrew Leigh. *BMJ Global Health* 29 August, 9

20 Australian Human Rights Commission, 2025. *Collateral Damage: What the Untold Stories from the COVID-19 Pandemic Expose about Human Rights in Australia*

health issues for the first time, compared with pre-pandemic years.[21] The long tail effect of lockdowns is apparent in student attendance in Australian schools, which fell 20 per cent points after restrictions ceased and has recovered by only 10 percentage points.[22] The societal cost was enormous, estimated at 68 times the benefit in Australia,[23] and 141 times in Canada.[24]

It could have been different. What was primarily a pandemic affecting the elderly (see Figure 5.1), indeed, those in aged care facilities,[25] morphed into a panic-demic for everyone. It might have played out differently had the public health advice been more temperate, and if political leaders had, using this more measured guidance, brought media editors into their confidence in a way that highlighted the damage done by treating society like a hospital ward. However, adopting a more prudent mindset is not easy and comes with costs[26] – or, perhaps more accurately, *risks*, the acceptance of which public health's enthusiastic adoption of the precautionary principle forbids. Indeed, its concepts of prudence and caution are precisely what brought about the catastrophic policy failures that we are still struggling to deal with. Gupta makes the points that the most certain outcome of lockdowns was societal harm. That should have been the precautionary part. Instead, the precaution related to spread, and there was no certainty that there were benefits to the lockdowns where some had to move around the keep the economy running and others were barred from doing so. There had to be a release of all at some stage, a

21 Mundy L K et al, 2023. Adolescents at risk of mental health problems in the COVID-19 pandemic: a prospective population-based study of the effects of government mandates and school closures. *Australian Journal of Social Issues* 58(1), 85

22 Australian Curriculum, Assessment and Reporting Authority, 2025. *Student Attendance: Key Facts*

23 Foster G with Sabhlok S, 2022. *Do Lockdowns and Border Closures Serve the Greater Good?* Connor Court, 222

24 Allen D W, 2021, 21

25 Inacio M C et al, 2024. Excess mortality in residents of aged care facilities during COVID-19 in Australia, 2019–2022. *International Journal of Epidemiology* 53(1), 168

26 Ludvigsson J F, 2023. How Sweden approached the COVID-19 pandemic: summary and commentary on the National Commission Inquiry. *Acta Paediatrica* 112(1),19

spread of the virus at some stage, and herd immunity at some stage.[27]

The Swedish exceptional response to the pandemic may have stemmed more from epidemiologists' overreaction to the swine flu in 2009-10 than from their foresight during the COVID-19 pandemic. The Swedish population was vaccinated in 2009-10. The flu was mild, but hundreds of children and young people developed narcolepsy, allegedly because of the vaccine.[28] A similar occurrence was the single death from Swine Flu in the U.S. and a panic response from the Centres for Disease Control (CDC), estimating 80 per cent of the population would need to be vaccinated to avoid an epidemic. The flu strain was less virulent than thought, and an epidemic did not eventuate. Of those vaccinated, however, there were 450 cases of Guillain-Barré Syndrome (GBS). The vaccinated group were found to have a significant, but small, increased risk of developing GBS.[29] The CDC's memory did not seem to affect its behaviour in 2020 amid the COVID-19 pandemic. This does not mean that vaccines do not save lives, but that in the rush to provide certainty, vaccines may be brought on too quickly, and false hope of a total solution is used to justify horrendously invasive non-pharmaceutical measures in society.

The national plans and WHO advice, which at that time were reasonable, were disregarded during the pandemic.[30] Government leaders chose not to downplay fear; some were encouraged to instil it. The then Chief Medical Health Officer of Queensland, now Governor, Dr Jeanette

27 Gupta, S, The lost lessons of lockdown. *UnHerd* 22 November 2025

28 Anderberg J, 2022. *The Herd: How Sweden Chose its Own Path Through the Worst Pandemic in 100 Years.* Scribe Publications

29 Liester M et al, 2025. A narrative review of the COVID-19 infodemic and censorship in healthcare. *Secrecy and Society* 3(2), 4 and Schonberger L B et al, 1979. Guillain-Barre syndrome following vaccination in the national influenza immunization program, United States, 1976–1977. *American Journal of Epidemiology* 110(2), 105

30 Australian Government Department of Health, 2019. *Australian Health Management Plan for Pandemic Influenza* and 2020 *Australian Health Sector Emergency Response for Novel Coronavirus (COVID-19).* World Health Organization, 2019. *Global Influenza Program Non-Pharmaceutical Public Health Measures for Mitigating the Risk and Impact of Epidemic and Pandemic Influenza*

Young, recommended that the Premier shut down schools in March 2020, reasoning, 'If you go out to the community and say, this is so bad … all schools have got to be closed, you are really getting to people … So sometimes it's more than just the science and health; it's about the messaging.'[31] Messaging has consequences. For example, Victoria is experiencing the highest levels of youth crime in that state's history, following the world's most extended lockdown and school closures.[32] The alternative was obvious and already planned, not to lock down.

Greg Hunt worked diligently as Health Minister during the COVID-19 pandemic, consistently adhering to the guidance of Commonwealth medical officials.[33] The advice frequently changed, starting with the declaration of a pandemic. The WHO criteria for declaring a pandemic initially included a measure for severity but shifted to a standard where a virus emerges to which the population has little or no immunity,[34] representing a lower threshold. This debate over criteria has altered the proportionality of pandemic responses.[35] There is a risk in implementing a severe response to mild disease, as seen in Sweden during 2009-10. Of course, the opposite can happen, but opting for a severe response complicates efforts to scale back once a decision has been made and path dependency is established. The Queensland Chief Health Officer, Dr John Gerrard, appointed after COVID-19, has acknowledged that future strategies will shift from a 'mandate' approach to simply providing as much information as possible to the public regarding the issue, rather than penalising them for not following directions.[36] The Commonwealth Inquiry recognised the narrow focus of the response, noting that politicians received a constant stream of disease-control advice without accounting

---

31 Lydia Lynch, Jeannette Young: who is the woman leading Queensland's fight against COVID-19? *Brisbane Times* 30 April 2020

32 Crime Statistics Agency, Victoria, 2025. *Key Figures: Year Ending March 2025*

33 Hunt G, 2024. *Submission to Commonwealth Government Covid-19 Response Inquiry*, 1 and 12

34 World Health Organization, 2019, 3

35 Doshi P, 2008. The elusive definition of pandemic influenza. *Bulletin of the World Health Organization* 89(7), 532

36 The Editor, *The Courier-Mail* 16 August 2024

for all relevant costs. It recommended establishing mechanisms for the National Cabinet to obtain additional integrated expert advice for comprehensive societal emergencies, including insights on social issues, human rights, economic factors, and broader health impacts.

Figure 5.1 Australia, COVID-19 deaths by age, 2020 to 2023

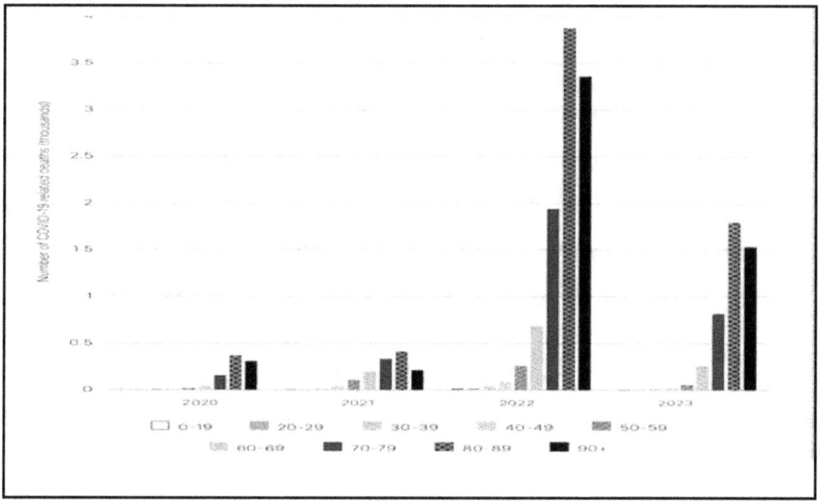

Source: Australian Government, 2024. *Covid-19 Response Inquiry Report,* 380

The WHO debate on immunity was crucial to the subsequent strategy of restricting societies in anticipation of vaccines. In June 2020, its advice stated, 'indirect protection from an infectious disease ... occurs when a population is immune through vaccination or immunity developed through previous infection. The threshold for establishing herd immunity for COVID-19 is not yet clear.'[37] In November 2020, the WHO revised its definition to exclude natural immunity and emphasised vaccination as the only method to achieve herd immunity and protect the vulnerable. 'Herd immunity exists when a significant percentage of the population is vaccinated, impeding the spread of infectious diseases due to fewer

37 World Health Organization, 2020, 9 June

people who can be infected.'[38] Following complaints from the scientific community, in December 2020, the WHO reinstated natural immunity as a contributing factor to herd immunity while strongly advocating vaccination.[39]

The WHO also made the unfounded statement, 'Vaccinated people are protected from getting the disease in question and passing on the pathogen, breaking any chains of transmission.'[40] COVID-19 vaccines do not prevent infection or stop its transmission.[41] As Angus Dalgleish remarked, 'U.K. Chief Medical Officer Chris Whitty provided the laughable rationale that children needed to be vaccinated to protect their parents and grandparents. With this one sentence, he demonstrated that he was not fit for purpose or his office, as you do not vaccinate people to protect others.'[42] As Former White House Coronavirus Response Coordinator Dr Deborah Birx admitted in July 2022, 'I knew these vaccines were not going to protect against infection.'[43] As Nyberg and others reported, 'previous SARS-CoV-2 infection offered some protection against hospitalisation and high protection against death in unvaccinated individuals.'[44] Natural immunity is a genuine phenomenon. Vaccines could offer immunity to more people, but if the spread was not contained and most were not falling ill, it was a futile exercise.

Although evidence suggests that COVID-19 vaccinations may have

38 World Health Organization, 2020, 13 November

39 World Health Organization, 2020, 31 December

40 World Health Organization, 2020, 31 December

41 Altman P M, 2024. COVID-19 vaccines: a failure of the drug regulatory system, in *COVID Revisited Lessons Learned, Challenges Faced, and the Road Ahead.* Australian Medical Professionals Society, 78

42 Dalgleish A, 2024. The cost of ignoring science. In C H Klotz & P McCullough (Eds) *Canary In a (Post) Covid World: Money, Fear and Power*. Canary House Publishing

43 *Fox News interview* 22 July 2022

44 Nyberg T et al, 2022. Comparative analysis of the risks of hospitalisation and death associated with Sars-Cov-2 Omicron and Delta variants in England: a cohort study. *The Lancet* 399(10332),1303

long-term adverse effects on the population,[45] the extent of these reactions remains contested. While readers can check the debate on adverse consequences,[46] these vaccinations were mandated, particularly in the early stages when knowledge about side effects was limited, and they were imposed on individuals who were at minimal risk of serious illness from infection, which is unconscionable. In Canada, mandates remained in effect until July 2024, a similar story occurred in Victoria, Australia, more than a year after the WHO had declared the end of its global health emergency.[47] Equally troubling was the neglect of medical opinions that diverged from those endorsed by government authorities, as well as the oppressive measures taken against dissenting voices. Stories of oppression are manifold, but a recent compendium suffices.[48]

Part of instilling fear involved recommending mask wearing. In June 2020, the WHO recommended that the public wear masks, even though it concluded that 'there is no direct evidence … on the effectiveness of universal masking of healthy people in the community to prevent infection with respiratory viruses, including COVID-19.'[49] It should have investigated the issue more thoroughly. Evidence published in 2020 indicated that trials did not show an apparent reduction in respiratory viral infection with the use of medical/surgical masks during seasonal influenza,[50] which aligned with other findings that did not observe associations between mask mandates or usage and reduced COVID-19

45 Sy W, 2023. Early indication of long-term impact of COVID injections. *Medical & Clinical Research* 8(10), 1

46 Australian Government Department of Health and Aged Care Therapeutic Goods Administration, 2023. *COVID-19 Vaccine Safety Report.* Also, *React19* is a not-for-profit organisation co-funded by two vaccine-injured persons. Available online: https://react19.org

47 Chaufan C, Hemsing N & Moncrieffe R, 2024. Covid-19 vaccination decisions and impacts of vaccine mandates: a cross-sectional survey of healthcare workers in British Columbia, Canada. *medRxiv* 10 December, 3

48 Clancy R & McCann M (Eds) 2025. *Covid Through Our Eyes: An Australian Story of Mistakes, Mistreatment and Misinformation.* Halstead Press

49 World Health Organization, 2020. Advice on the use of masks in the context of COVID-19. *Interim Guidance* 5 June

50 Jefferson T et al, 2020. Physical interventions to interrupt or reduce the spread of respiratory viruses. *Cochrane Database Systematic Reviews* 11, 3

spread in U.S. states.[51] Later studies found 'no apparent reduction in respiratory viral infections associated with using medical/surgical masks during seasonal influenza.'[52] As one Australian nurse and infection control consultant submitted to the Commonwealth Inquiry, 'Please do not make staff in hospitals and aged care wear masks. The masks are hell to wear while you work and will not prevent 'bugs' passing through them. Also, they need to be changed every 20 mins … Do not make children in school wear them! Read the microbiology reports of bacteria that grow inside masks, making children sick.'[53]

Once the notorious Imperial College London projection stating that 'the public health threat [COVID-19] represents is the most serious seen in a respiratory virus since the 1918 H1N1 influenza pandemic'[54] was published, the media fueled panic. Politicians were motivated to appear decisive, chief medical officers sought to present themselves as heroes, editors pursued sales, and vaccine companies targeted large markets with government backing. Fear, the pressure to conform, and deference to supposed expertise combined to suppress dissent and broader perspectives on the costs and benefits. Once committed to an elimination strategy, leaders had to recognise the mistakes made regarding masks, tracing, lockdowns, and everything else, or wait for a vaccine.

Path dependent

Nicholas Coatsworth, former Deputy Chief Medical Officer of the Department of Health and Aged Care, was insightful. Although his

---

51 Guerra D G & Guerra D J, 2021. Mask mandate and use efficacy for COVID-19 containment in U.S. states *medRxiv*, 11. Also, Alfano V, Cicatiello L & Ercolano S, 2023. Assessing the effectiveness of mandatory outdoor mask policy: the natural experiment of Campania. *Economics and Human Biology* 50(101265)

52 Jefferson T et al, 2023. Physical interventions to interrupt or reduce the spread of respiratory viruses. *Cochrane Database of Systematic Reviews* 1, 2

53 Sharp C A, 2023. *Submission to the Commonwealth Government COVID-19 Response Inquiry*

54 Ferguson F et al, 2020. Impact of non-pharmaceutical interventions to reduce COVID-19 mortality and healthcare demand. *Imperial College COVID-19 Response Team Report 9* 16 March

submission to the Commonwealth Inquiry on COVID-19 was not utilised in the report, he made two astute observations.

> *There was a notable absence of agreed ethical framework to discuss and evaluate decisions. This allowed the creation of a 'disease-control at all costs' policy path dependence, which, whilst suited to the first wave, was poorly suited to the vaccine-era.*[55]

An illustration of Coatsworth's first observation was that by Dr Francis Collins, the director of the National Institutes of Health, who highlighted this fact to the U.S. Congress Select Subcommittee on the Coronavirus Pandemic.

> *You attach infinite value to stopping the disease and saving a life. You attach a zero value to whether this ... disrupts people's lives, ruins the economy, and has many kids kept out of school in a way that they never quite recovered [: it] is a public health mindset.*[56]

Coatsworth criticised the Commonwealth Inquiry's recommendation to establish an Australian Centre for Disease Control, stating

> *The creation of a separate institution risks ... institutional group think and single-minded pursuit of disease-control over all other priorities ... There is no evidence at all to suggest that nations with CDC's performed any better during the pandemic.*[57]

The Centre for Disease Control will serve as a new label for existing institutions – the Doherty and Burnet Institutes and the University of Melbourne – foundational partners of the Australian Institute for Infectious Diseases.[58] Their recommendations for COVID-19 included lockdowns, border closures, masks, testing, tracing, isolation, quarantine, and vaccines. They also advocate ongoing vaccinations, testing, tracing,

---

55 Coatsworth N, 2023. *Submission to the Commonwealth Government COVID-19 Response Inquiry*, 2

56 U.S. House of Representatives, 2024. *Final Report of the Select Subcommittee on the Coronavirus Pandemic Committee on Oversight and Accountability*, 392

57 Coatsworth N, 2023. *Submission to the Commonwealth Government COVID-19 Response Inquiry*, 9

58 Burnet Institute, 2023. *The Burnet Institute's Response to the Commonwealth Government COVID-19 Response Inquiry*

and isolation efforts. An Australian CDC will embed exactly the kind of thinking that drove panic-fuelled responses and ensure a comparable response in future pandemics unless alternative sources of advice emerge. An institution will equally likely serve to lock in bad advice as good, and will build new ways to intervene and interfere with society with the same narrow focus that caused such damage during COVID-19.

The Commonwealth Inquiry divided the pandemic response into four phases: alert, suppression, vaccine rollout, and transition/recovery.[59] From January to April 2020, the Alert stage saw governments introduce comprehensive public health orders, including the declaration of an emergency on 18 March to ensure Australia's health system could treat those who would become seriously ill. State governments declared emergencies at a similar time, except NSW, which did not, as under its existing *Health Act 2010* (NSW), the minister could impose extensive health restrictions without a state of emergency declaration. These various declarations lasted from between 754 days (Commonwealth) and 1006 days (Queensland).[60]

From May 2020 to January 2021, the suppression stage involved an extended effort to keep the virus out and maintain low case numbers, ensuring care and access to intensive care units, and maintaining ventilator availability. The Great Barrington Declaration, issued on 5 October 2020, went unheeded. The vaccine rollout stage commenced on 22 February 2021, and path dependency became apparent when it was recognised that vaccines had become less effective in preventing infection or transmission with the Delta variant, yet the vaccination of most Australians continued. The transition/recovery stage, from November 2021 to the present, witnessed many more deaths due to the first community-wide exposure and infection, despite a lower case fatality rate with Omicron infections, particularly in a highly vaccinated population. This occurred despite the measures, vaccinations, and natural immunity already in place for those who were infected.

---

59 Australian Government, 2024. *COVID-19 Response Inquiry Report*, 74

60 Australian Human Rights Commission, 2025, 109

Preeminent researchers John Ioannidis, Jay Bhattacharya, and others concluded in April 2020, during Australia's alert phase, that most infectious respiratory viruses often go undetected. They stated, 'Contact tracing a small portion of the population is a waste of resources. … it was clear that SARS-CoV-2 was widespread around the globe, and reported cases did not reflect the magnitude of the spread.'[61] Many individuals who contracted the virus were not ill but immune. Yet in June 2020, the WHO asserted that it was rare for an asymptomatic person to transmit the virus to others.[62] Consequently, they recommended a policy of containment.

> *We don't even talk about containment for seasonal flu — it's just not possible. But it is possible for Covid-19. We don't do contact tracing for seasonal flu — but countries should do it for Covid-19 because it will prevent infections and save lives. Containment is possible.*[63]

Contact tracing is very effective for highly infectious diseases that spread through physical contact, such as Ebola. An asymptomatic case can be isolated to prevent further transmission to others and halt the spread. This was not the situation for COVID-19. The Commonwealth Report acknowledged that, with a partially vaccinated population, changes in the virus and increased case numbers meant that previously successful 'test, trace, and isolate' measures began to falter. But was it effective at all? The large-scale testing and contact tracing attempted early in Australia's COVID-19 response were significantly disruptive and costly. Yet, they were not subject to specific analysis regarding their effectiveness,

61 Ioannidis J P A, Bhattacharya J et al, 2020. COVID-19 antibody seroprevalence in Santa Clara County, California. *medRxiv* April

62 WHO, Asymptomatic spread of coronavirus is 'very rare'. 8 June 2020 *CNBC*

63 WHO, Director-General's opening remarks at the media briefing on COVID-19 3 March 2020

despite clear evidence of their inaccuracy.[64] It likely accomplished its purpose: to instil fear in those who need not be afraid. Australia's reopening coincided with the emergence of the more transmissible Omicron variant in December 2021. In New South Wales and Victoria, test, trace, and isolate measures were scaled back because they could not adequately control the spread of this new variant.[65] Should they have been abandoned earlier?

Medical advice did not change when the world's most eminent scientists published the Great Barrington Declaration.

> *As infectious disease epidemiologists and public health scientists we have grave concerns about the damaging physical and mental health impacts of the prevailing COVID-19 policies, and recommend an approach we call Focused Protection.*[66]

The authors expressed their concerns in the Declaration about the COVID-19 strategies that disproportionately affected children, the working class, and the poor. The lockdowns, contact tracing, and isolation led to significant and preventable health costs for individuals. They argued that, in the long term, this approach would result in higher mortality rates from both COVID-19 and non-COVID-19 causes compared to the focused protection plan. A study comparing early response strategies, including lockdowns in various countries from March 2020, indicated that mitigation strategies such as case isolation, quarantining household members, limiting large gatherings, social distancing in public spaces, border controls, and restrictions specifically targeting high-risk groups were far more beneficial than lockdowns in terms of quality-adjusted

---

64 Mouliou D S & Gourgoulianis K I, 2021. False-positive and false-negative COVID-19 cases: respiratory prevention and management strategies, vaccination, and further perspectives. *Expert Review of Respiratory Medicine* 15(8), 993. Borger P et al, 2020, External peer review of the RTPCR test to detect SARS-CoV-2 reveals 10 major scientific flaws at the molecular and methodological level: consequences for false positive results (Review Report - Corman-Drosten). *Eurosurveillance*. Günther M, Rockenfeller R and Walach H, 2025. A calibration of nucleic acid (PCR) by antibody (IgG) tests in Germany: the course of SARS-CoV-2 infections estimated. *Frontiers in Epidemiology* 5(1592629)

65 Australian Government, 2024. *Covid 19 Response Inquiry Report*, 63

66 *Great Barrington Declaration*, 2020. https://gbdeclaration.org

life years.[67]

Why was the advice in the Declaration ignored? One reason is the influence of U.S. regulators on their Australian counterparts. Dr Francis Collins wrote to Dr Anthony Fauci, U.S. Director of the National Institute of Allergy and Infectious Diseases, stating that a policy other than national lockdowns would require a swift and devastating public takedown. Collins referred to The Great Barrington Declaration as 'a fringe component of epidemiology… not mainstream science' and 'outright dangerous'.[68] International media outlets, including *Wired*, *The Wall Street Journal*, *The Guardian*, The *Independent*, and *The Telegraph,* as well as leftist groups such as the *Union of Concerned Scientists* and *The Conversation,* dismissed the Declaration. The Commonwealth Inquiry report did not mention the Declaration. This was an egregious and probably deliberate exclusion of 'expert' advice, that would disturb the path of earlier decisions made with less reliable information. Another factor was the stance of the WHO, which advocated lockdowns contrary to previous advice, seemingly influenced by China's approach. 'In the face of a previously unknown virus, China has rolled out perhaps the most ambitious, agile, and aggressive disease containment effort in history,' and 'Achieving China's exceptional coverage and adherence to these containment measures has only been possible due to the deep commitment of the Chinese people to collective action in confronting this common threat.'[69] Surely, Australian CMOs were not swayed by the authoritarian tactics of Collins and Fauci or the harsh regime's treatment of citizens in China, or perhaps their decisions were 'driven by mimicry of neighbouring countries'?[70] It is as if public health bureaucrats treated policymaking as a contest, to see who could be the toughest.

From early on, possibly at the suppression stage, keen observers knew

67 Lally M, 2022. A cost-benefit analysis of COVID-19 lockdowns in Australia. *Monash Bioethics Review* 40, 62

68 U.S. House of Representatives, 2024, 334

69 World Health Organization, 2020. *Report of the WHO-China Joint Mission on Coronavirus Disease 2019 (COVID-19)* 16-24 February

70 Lally M, 2022, 90

that the infection was potentially deadly for the very elderly and those with co-morbidities. The survival rate for the infection among individuals over 70 was 96 per cent, while for everyone else, it was greater than 99 per cent.[71] The WHO noted that most people would experience mild to moderate illness in the early stages.[72] Initially, the WHO overstated numbers by confusing the case survival rate with the infection survival rate.[73] A case is defined as a person with a positive test result who exhibits clinical symptoms of illness. The Commonwealth Inquiry appeared to make the same mistake by referencing infection rates based on positive tests without necessarily accounting for the number of people who were ill.[74] Instead, individuals without symptoms were counted as cases. This confusion not only made the pandemic seem more dangerous but also fueled the obsession with testing asymptomatic individuals and, subsequently, contact tracing. The inflation of case numbers continued because those who died *with* COVID-19 were counted alongside those who died *from it*. For example, data on deaths in aged care facilities in 2022 included both deaths with and from COVID-19, even when COVID-19 may not have been the cause of death.[75]

The seemingly straightforward issue of understanding excess deaths and attributing them to probable causes remains a contentious topic. Two aspects warrant consideration: whether a pandemic indeed occurred, as the scale of fatalities was hardly discernible in the excess deaths data, and whether any deaths can be attributed to vaccines. The implications of the death toll have been explored elsewhere – in the nothing-to-see-

---

71 Axfors C & Ioannidis J P A, 2022. Infection fatality rate of COVID-19 in community-dwelling elderly populations. *European Journal of Epidemiol*ogy 37, 235. Pezzullo A M, 2023. Age-stratified infection fatality rate of COVID-19 in the non-elderly population. *Environmental Research* 216(114655)

72 WHO, *Coronavirus Disease (COVID-19)* (undated), https://www.who.int/health-topics/coronavirus#tab=tab_1

73 Tedros Adhanom Ghebreyesus, WHO Director-General's opening remarks at the media briefing on COVID-19. 3 March 2020

74 Australian Government, 2024. *Covid 19 Response Inquiry Report*, 216

75 Australian Government, 2024. *Covid 19 Response Inquiry Report*, 475

here camp[76] and the highly suspicious camp.[77] The Commonwealth Inquiry views serious adverse events from vaccines as rare;[78] however, there is increasing evidence of significant concern.[79] The second phase of the New Zealand Royal Commission, for example, will delve into vaccine safety and harm, which were excluded from the scope of Phase One. Phase Two will report in early 2026.[80]

Contrasting inquiries

The Canadian province of Alberta's inquiry into the Alberta COVID-19 response was true to its motto: strong and free.[81] In contrast, the Commonwealth of Australia's inquiry was weak and captured by public health single-mindedness. Masks, lockdowns, infection-acquired immunity, rapid testing, and the shaming of medical professionals who questioned the orthodoxy were challenged in Alberta; yet, these issues

---

76 Australian Bureau of Statistics, 2024. Measuring Australia's excess deaths during the COVID-19 pandemic until December 2023. Actuaries Australia and Australian Institute of Health and Welfare submissions to the *Senate Inquiry into Excess Mortality 2024*

77 Corfield C, 2024. *Submission to the COVID-19 Response Inquiry*. O'Connor M, Adair T, Australian Medical Professionals Association, and Australians for Science and Freedom, 2024. Submissions to *Senate Standing Committees on Community Affairs Inquiry into Excess Mortality 2024*. Strecker J, 2023. Pandemic survivors and the silent victims of excess mortality. *The Spectator* 6 January. Sorli A S, 2025. The discrepancy between the number of saved lives with COVID-19 vaccination and statistics of our world data. *Journal of Clinical Trials* S32(001)

78 Australian Government, 2024. *Covid 19 Response Inquiry Report*, 257

79 Wucher M et al, 2024. *COVID-19 Spike Protein Pathogenicity Research Library*. Kim, H J et al, 2025. Broad-spectrum adverse events of special interests based on immune response following COVID-19 vaccination: a large-scale population-based cohort study. *Journal of Clinical Medicine* 14, 1767. Malhotra A, 2022. Curing the pandemic of misinformation on COVID-19 mRNA vaccines through real evidence-based medicine - Part 1. *Journal of Insulin Resistance* 5(1), a71. Malhotra A, 2022. Curing the pandemic of misinformation on COVID-19 mRNA vaccines through real evidence-based medicine - Part 2. *Journal of Insulin Resistance* 5(1), a72. Kelly T, 2024. Beyond blame: dissecting the systemic roots of societal disease exposed by the covid era. *The Hope Accord*. Craig C (Health Advisory and Recovery Team), 2023. Unsafe and Defective, 2024. *Submission to the People's Vaccine Inquiry UK*

80 Aotearoa New Zealand Royal Commission Covid-19, 2024. *Lessons Learned: Main Report*, 20

81 Alberta COVID-19 Pandemic Data Review Task Force, 2025. *Alberta's Covid-19 Pandemic Response Final Report*

were largely set aside in Australia. This lack of enquiry had nothing to do with the Commonwealth's terms of reference, which protected the states. It stemmed from an unquestioning public health mindset. Alberta scrutinised each contentious aspect of the COVID-19 response and challenged beliefs. Alberta embraced science. The Commonwealth consulted with stakeholders.

The Commonwealth began by 'acknowledging country' and 'recognising lived experience' (everyone has their truth). It included 'intersectional' warnings that addressed the layers of inequality and social disadvantage, language warnings for people with disabilities and those from culturally and linguistically diverse (CALD) backgrounds, and content warnings for anyone who might feel distressed by the material presented. Seven chapters focused on the standard checklist of allegedly vulnerable minorities – Aboriginal and Torres Strait Islanders, children and youth, CALD individuals, people with disabilities, the homeless, older Australians, and women. Who died from COVID-19? Very old people with comorbidities. Few others died.

The Commonwealth recommended support for children's mental health but did not criticise the lockdowns that caused it. They proposed new bureaucrats in the form of a Chief Paediatrician and a National Children's Commissioner to oversee the next pandemic, but did not mention closing schools, requiring children to wear masks, or mandating vaccinations.[82] What did the Alberta Inquiry do? It examined the evidence and asked questions, as inquiries are meant to. It scrutinised the modelling used to alarm the public, the necessity of lockdowns and closures, and the basis for their decisions. It questioned masking, testing, infection-acquired immunity, vaccines, and therapeutics. It asked why the existing pandemic response plan was abandoned and why decisions were made despite evidence suggesting they were unnecessary.

82 The effects may not have been severe or long-lasting, but the Commonwealth failed to engage in debate. Fayaz Farkhad B & Albarracín D, 2021. Insights on the implications of COVID-19 mitigation measures for mental health. *Economics and Human Biology* 40(100963)

During the COVID-19 pandemic, the Alberta government and its advisers employed the precautionary principle,[83] Under this principle, any potential environmental risk, known or unknown, leads to a lockdown. In the case of COVID-19, every measure was taken to combat the virus, while no precautions were taken against other risks. The precautionary principle failed to provide any guidance on the level of caution and the harm it caused. The Alberta Inquiry questioned why the government employed the precautionary principle, despite being aware of the potential harms associated with stringent measures. It also raised concerns about why most of the measures lacked scientific evidence for their efficacy.

The Alberta Inquiry questioned why public health officials in the province imposed their views on the medical profession and tolerated no dissent, why medical professional societies held the party line, and why doctors hesitated to voice their opinions. It also explored why the medical societies disregarded their independent duty to take measures against COVID-19 and complied submissively with directives. The Alberta Inquiry questioned why vaccinations were aggressively promoted to everyone, including infants and minors, despite their low risk of severe COVID-19 infection. The Alberta Inquiry understood comorbidities. The Commonwealth was mired in bureaucratic jargon. Clearly influenced by a public health mindset,[84] it obscenely referred to a One Health perspective—a need to 'optimise health for people, animals, and our environment and mitigate converging health threats relating to climate change, biodiversity collapse, stressed ecosystems, antimicrobial resistance, and ageing and increasingly comorbid population.'[85]

The Alberta Inquiry concluded that COVID-19 forecasts were ineffective. It recommended avoiding, at all costs, making the results of

83 Armstrong J S & Green K C, 2022. *The Scientific Method: A Guide to Finding Useful Knowledge.* Cambridge University Press, 4

84 Taylor J et al, 2023. Council of Academic Public Health Institutions Australasia, public health education for a sustainable future 'Call to Action', 2021. *Australian and New Zealand Journal of Public Health* 47(2)

85 Australian Government, 2024. *Covid 19 Response Inquiry Report*, 83

simulation models public. It argued that 'even meaningless mathematics can create the illusion of high-quality analyses' and 'generat[e] a false sense of control over complex, dynamic phenomena.'[86] The Australian Commonwealth must have been aware of the folly of modelling, but it remained silent.[87] The Alberta Inquiry questioned why public health officials enforced mask mandates without evaluating the harm, particularly in children who were at low risk from COVID-19. The Commonwealth faithfully followed the WHO, which later changed its stance to a pro-face-mask position without any scientific basis.

The Commonwealth paid little attention to herd immunity. The Alberta inquiry revealed that infection-acquired immunity, obtained through prior infection, can provide 'durable and protective immune responses.' More importantly, 'infection-acquired immunity should not be overlooked or downplayed in public health messaging and policies.' What was the Commonwealth's view? It was vaccines or nothing. As Alberta stated, 'recognising that infection-acquired immunity is superior to vaccine-acquired immunity does not equate to advocating infection over vaccination.'[88] Why were vaccines promoted as the solution to curtail the pandemic and restore normality? The Commonwealth was too fainthearted to enquire.

Alberta recommended an immediate halt to COVID-19 vaccinations and advised against vaccinating healthy children and teenagers. The Commonwealth did not raise relevant concerns regarding the vaccines. Indeed, the Commonwealth Department of Health now recommends that the COVID-19 vaccine not be administered to healthy infants, children, or adolescents without underlying medical conditions that increase their risk of severe illness.[89] Alberta presented scientific evidence on the effectiveness of hydroxychloroquine, ivermectin, and several other

---

86 Alberta COVID-19 Pandemic Data Review Task Force, 2025, ch 3

87 Winsberg E & Harvard S, 2024. *Scientific Models and Decision Making, Elements in the Philosophy of Science.* Cambridge University Press

88 Alberta COVID-19 Pandemic Data Review Task Force, 2025, ch 7

89 https://immunisationhandbook.health.gov.au/recommendations/healthy-infants-children-and-adolescents-aged

readily available medications. The Commonwealth stated that the prohibition of these medications only 'served to further fuel conspiracy theories.'[90] It adopted a tactical perspective on the matter, finding retrospective justification for bad public health decisions. The Alberta Inquiry employed a scientific approach and scrutinised the basis of each element of the response. The Commonwealth Inquiry focused on rollout processes without questioning efficacy. Why was the Commonwealth so afraid to question public health's influence?

Can government cope in a complex liberal society?

A keen observation of the COVID-19 response in the UK is that its complexity undermined it. While medically qualified officials may have guided Australian decision-makers, their early path became a template they chose not to depart from. Policy should have adapted as new information emerged. Instead, 'decision-makers and the … scientific elite shift[ed] subtly from caution to conviction.'[91] The combination of conviction and complexity resulted in many ineffective and harmful impositions.

The Commonwealth[92] and the states enacted thousands of new laws during the COVID-19 response.[93] Redfern Legal Aid estimated that in New South Wales, between 15 March 2020 and 31 January 2022, 266 principal and amending public health orders were issued, averaging a change in the law every 2.5 days. Each public health order included numerous directions, making it nearly impossible for the public and police to comprehend the laws, leading to many people being fined

90 Australian Government, 2024. *Covid 19 Response Inquiry Report*, 282

91 Pawson R, 2023. Do lockdowns work? Evidence from the UK. In P Eliadis, I Naidoo, & R Rist (Eds) *Policy Evaluation in the Era of COVID-19*. Taylor and Francis, 141

92 Australian Law Reform Commission, 2022. *Law Making During the COVID-19 Pandemic*

93 For example, Queensland Health, 2023. *Chief Health Officer Public Health Directions and Revoked Public Health Directions*

incorrectly.[94] For instance, movement and contact with others were permitted unless expressly prohibited by the orders' provisions. However, the Minister for Police and Police Commissioners asserted that individuals exploited loopholes in the public health orders while going about their daily activities. By late 2022, more than 33,000 fines — over half of those issued for alleged breaches of the public health orders — were cancelled by the government due to a lack of specificity under the *Fines Act 1996* (NSW).[95]

The Shopping Centre Council of Australia's submission to the Commonwealth Inquiry is another excellent illustration of complexity.[96] The National Code of Conduct for Commercial Tenancies — Leasing Principles was officially announced in April 2020 as a hibernation measure. While the Council developed the Code, the Commonwealth commandeered it, made several problematic changes, and transferred it to State and Territory Governments. The Code underwent national re-regulation 27 times, remaining effective for 2,472 days, while the lockdown lasted for just 555 days. A six-page, 11-provision document expanded to over 60 pages of regulations and complex provisions in the worst-case scenario, particularly in Victoria, which significantly exceeded its intended purpose as a hibernation policy. Furthermore, the rules governing shopping centres and their tenants, set out in Public Health Orders and other guidance materials, changed on average every few days.

In NSW, stay-at-home orders were issued in late June 2021, requiring residents of Greater Sydney to stay home unless they had a reasonable excuse to go out. In stay-at-home areas and areas of concern, most publicly accessible premises were closed, including swimming pools,

94 Redfern Legal Centre, 2024. *Submission to the Commonwealth Government Covid-19 Response Inquiry*

95 Sherry C, 2023. All about the land: the (mis)application of public health orders to strata schemes during the delta variant COVID-19 outbreak in Sydney, Australia. *Sydney Law Review* 45(2), 279

96 Shopping Centre Council of Australia, 2024. *Submission to the Commonwealth Government Covid-19 Response Inquiry*

gyms, shops, and hair salons. The public health rationale for shutting down these facilities was that they allowed multiple unrelated households from diverse geographic regions to interact, thereby heightening the risk of virus transmission. However, gyms and pools within strata and community schemes were exempt from these restrictions, as they were not considered open to the public. For instance, it was not illegal for a COVID-positive resident of a strata scheme to exit their apartment and mingle with unrelated households in communal areas.

Similar issues emerged with mask mandates, restrictions on close contact, and the authorisation of workers to enter residential premises.[97] Problems occurred in public housing, where extensive rules isolated residents from the community regardless of their COVID-19 status. This heightened the risk of the virus spreading within the building, as COVID-19 positive residents and their close contacts were not obligated to stay in their apartments.[98]

The Australian Catholic Bishops proposed a cautious approach to reopening churches as part of the Framework for National Reopening published by the Commonwealth government in November 2020 to safeguard the health and safety of parishioners and the broader community. In their submission to the Inquiry, they voiced concerns that several states and territories in Australia 'placed unreasonable restrictions on churches and places of worship compared to other public establishments such as pubs, restaurants, and hairdressing salons.' A notable example occurred in New South Wales in May 2020, where churches were restricted to 10 worshippers while the maximum permitted in clubs, restaurants, bars, and other venues was increased to 50. Additionally, there were confusing rules regarding whether patrons could be seated or standing. In Melbourne, Stage Two restrictions allowed for the reopening of pet groomers, cafés, restaurants, and

97 Sherry C, 2023, 279

98 Victorian Ombudsman, 2020. *Investigation into the Detention and Treatment of Public Housing Residents Arising from a COVID-19 'Hard Lockdown' in July 2020*

swimming pools, but did not permit places of worship.[99] Such is the convoluted, incoherent nature of public health.

Conclusion

Given the complexity of society, each pandemic intervention must be justified by its effectiveness and societal costs. The Commonwealth Inquiry's post-justification was a pathetic non-analysis, embarrassing in contrast to Alberta's. As Professor Coatsworth submitted to the Commonwealth Inquiry, the mindset among decision-makers was path-dependent and characterised by a herd instinct. Politicians were running scared of their advice, which was running scared with overwrought scenarios. The Commonwealth and the States were not thinking of disaggregated publics nor of an overall sense of harm. They got it wrong at both scales.

The voices that urged the panic response, both within and outside the public health cohort, were rewarded — and are likely to react similarly at the next opportunity unless significant barriers are put in place. The Australian response also leaves us with the question: why are our politicians so afraid to question public health?

99 Australian Catholic Bishops Conference, 2024. *Submission to the to the Commonwealth Government Covid-19 Response Inquiry*

6

Transgender Affirmation: a profession duped

No child is born in the wrong body ... it's their emotional life that needs attention and healing.[1]

Dr Miriam Grossman

Does it make sense to medically cement the child's pre-pubertal sense of self?[2]

Martha Wexler

Political activists have transformed the treatment of gender dysphoria into a public health issue by recruiting medical specialists to the cause and linking any dissent or debate with that greatest of all public health bogeymen – suicide risk. Gender dysphoria is not a disease, but it is contagious, stemming from a social contagion that has adversely affected many confused, unhappy, or mentally ill individuals. The political struggle over its existence and medical interventions illustrates that the principle of 'do no harm' in medical ethics has been disregarded in the pursuit of ideology.

The fatal technique employed in this particular public health intervention is the loss of rationality in the understanding of sex as a biological concept, in favour of the sociological phenomenon of gender. Medical

1 Grossman M, 2023. *Lost in Trans Nation: A Child Psychiatrist's Guide out of the Madness*. Skyhorse Publishing, 270

2 Wexler M, 2025. The shifting tide: part 1. *Democrats for an Informed Approach to Gender*. 11 August Substack

intervention based on sociology is hazardous. An explanation for the gender dysphoria loss of rationality may be attributed to a 'new pseudoscience … the sex spectrum.' The 'science' holds that sex exists on a continuum, that male and female are socially constructed, and the sense of self is the most accurate measure of sex. Proponents believe the two sexes are constructed categories, created by society, to oppress and control sexual minorities. As in so many other parts of culture wars, some agree out of compassion for those minorities, despite the lack of proof and the harm caused by such labelling. Proponents believe 'that male and female must be superseded by a subjective, feeling-based reality, where one's internal sense of self is prioritized over the truthful and important reality of our sexed bodies.'[3] The harm of the denial of biological sex and the elevation of feelings is that it 'erodes scientific progress' and opens the floodgates to 'alternative truths.'[4]

The extent of gender dysphoria — the distress felt by people whose sense of gender does not align with their natal sex — is a recent phenomenon. The causes are debatable, but it is almost certainly the case that social contagion is involved, judging from the rapid onset of symptoms in some cases among young people.[5] It reflects a belief, influenced by a peer group, that non-specific symptoms (such as a teenager being confused) are proof of dysphoria and that any who disagrees with this self-assessment is transphobic and should be cut off, i.e. parents. The epidemic is also fanned by social contagion in an era when gender is fluid, because it is made up, and social media makes its spread more virulent. Littman argues that rapid-onset dysphoria (which has become apparent in teenagers in recent years) has numerous possible causes, but is a social contagion event, especially among young females. Parents in online discussion groups such as *4thwavenow* in the U.S., who describe

---

3 Elliott Z, 2023. *Binary: Debunking the Sex Spectrum Myth*. Paradox Press, 3

4 Goymann W, Brumm H & Kappeler P, 2022. Biological sex is binary, even though there is a rainbow of sex roles. *BioEssays*, 45(2), 1

5 Littman L, 2019. Correction: parent reports of adolescents and young adults perceived to show signs of a rapid onset of gender dysphoria. *PLoS ONE* 14(3), e0214157. Also, Hakeem A, 2023. *Detrans: When Transition is Not the Solution*. Independent, 49

themselves as paediatric transition sceptics,[6] and *Transgender Trend* in the UK,[7] who call for evidence-based healthcare for children and young people suffering from gender dysphoria, discuss their children's perceived rapid onset of gender dysphoria. Parents describe a process of immersion in social media, such as 'binge-watching' YouTube transition videos and excessive use of Tumblr, immediately preceding their child becoming gender dysphoric, which raises the question of whether 'social influences may be contributing to or even driving these occurrences of gender dysphoria in some populations of adolescents and young adults.'[8] The gender ideology sweeping society also plays its part. Schools' obsession with safety from bullying and protection of LGBTQ students creates an 'enticing' climate for vulnerable students to experiment.[9] Like most revolutions, it eats its own, so the argument is that there is no such thing as a 'tomboy' anymore, 'lesbians do not exist; girls with more masculine presentations are "really" boys.'[10]

Adults can do as they wish with their bodies, but the now-prominent and controversial response to gender dysphoria, particularly in minors, the affirmation model, represents a very dark chapter of medical practice. Gender affirmation therapy begins with unquestioning social 'validation' towards the opposite sex, followed by gonadotropin-releasing hormone analogues in children to delay puberty and cross-sex hormone therapy to achieve the desired masculinisation or feminisation. Potential surgical procedures include breast reduction or augmentation, hysterectomy/orchiectomy, and vaginoplasty/phalloplasty. Other interventions that may be used to change secondary sex characteristics include liposuction/lipofilling, electrolysis, and voice surgery.[11] Professor John Whitehall

6 https://4thwavenow.com

7 https://www.transgendertrend.com

8 Littman L, 2018, e0202330

9 Shrier A, 2021. *Irreversible Damage: Teenage Girls and the Transgender Craze.* Swift Press, 61

10 Shrier A, 2021, 35

11 Goodman M & Nash R, 2019. Examining health outcomes for people who are transgender. *Patient-Centred Outcomes Research Institute*, 8

has described the result as an 'ersatz similarity with the opposite sex.'[12] The power of the 'therapeutic ritual' between patient and doctor — a force strong enough to create a placebo effect regardless of both diagnosis and cure — has been evident in the affirmation model popular in the treatment of gender dysphoria, especially among the young.[13] Science is the least important aspect. Accounts of the lives of those with gender dysphoria are often manipulated, rehearsed and recited and taken on face value. 'Individuals enter a retrospective examination of their lives to look for clues that might fit the transgender hypothesis: that they were born into the wrong body.'[14]

Dr Jillian Spencer, an experienced psychiatrist addressing gender dysphoria and other adolescent mental health issues, was suspended from her public health role at a Brisbane hospital for calling out the gender-affirming model of care. Importantly for our understanding of how public health is an unhealthy conceit, she observed that her colleagues felt more positive within the affirmation model, but it amounted to little more than narcissistic validation in an otherwise gloomy field of work.[15] The fightback against the affirmation model of 'care' is in its infancy, at least in Australia,[16] although in the U.S., 27 states have enacted laws restricting gender affirming paediatric care.[17] In the UK, a commission

12 Whitehall J, 2025. A review of the physiology and side effects of puberty blockers and cross sex hormones, *Proceedings: The Future of Youth Gender Medicine Seminar*. NSW Parliament House, 19

13 Clayton A, 2023. Genderaffirming treatment of gender dysphoria in youth: a perfect storm environment for the placebo effect: the implications for research and clinical practice. *Archives of Sexual Behavior* 52, 483

14 Hakeem A, 2023, 69

15 Dr Jillian Spencer, Lecture at *Moving Forward*, Sunshine Coast 23 March 2025, which Gary Johns attended.

16 A hopeful sign is the National Association of Practising Psychiatrists Guide. Managing Gender Dysphoria in Young People 8 June 2025 *Media Release* 'While respecting young people's views about their gender identity, it does so as part of the totality of their developmental and holistic clinical picture and incorporates these into the clinical formulation.'

17 Tennessee's ban on gender-affirming care for minors was affirmed by the U.S. Supreme Court *U.S. v. Skrmetti* 23-477 18 June 2025, which refused an argument that the law violated the Equal Protection Clause of the Fourteenth Amendment of the U.S. Constitution.

by NHS England, chaired by Dr Hilary Cass, reviewed gender-affirming clinics seeking to understand the reasons for the rising number of those presenting with gender identity problems, but also a change in the case-mix. Many more birth-registered females have been referred in adolescence, a shift from birth-registered males presenting in childhood, on whom the previous clinical approach to care was based. Clinicians also noted that these young people often had other issues that they were having to manage alongside their gender-related distress. Among the findings were that

> *Clinicians are unable to determine with any certainty which children and young people will go on to have an enduring trans identity.*
>
> *For the majority of young people, a medical pathway may not be the best way to manage their gender-related distress. For those young people for whom a medical pathway is clinically indicated, it is not enough to provide this without also addressing wider mental health and/or psychosocially challenging problems.*[18]

In April 2024, Professor Louis Appleby, University of Manchester Department of Health and Social Care examined claims by campaigners of a significant rise in suicides by young patients of the gender services at the Tavistock and Portman NHS Foundation Trust following the cessation of services. The claims were led by the Good Law Project, which challenged the decision by the Health Secretary to end the prescription of puberty-blocking drugs by private clinics to children and young people with gender dysphoria.[19] The data did not support the claim that there has been a significant rise in suicide in young gender dysphoria patients at the Tavistock.[20] This jettisons the entire public health premise on which the affirmation model relies.

---

18 Cass H, 2024. *Independent Review of Gender Identity Services for Children and Young People: Final Report*

19 *Bell and another v The Tavistock and Portman NHS Foundation Trust* [2021] EWCA Civ 1363 The minister ordered cessation of puberty blockers for those under 16. The decision was overturned on appeal on the basis that the courts should not interfere. The initial case was sufficient to have the clinic stop the practice.

20 https://www.gov.uk/government/publications/review-of-suicides-and-gender-dysphoria-at-the-tavistock-and-portman-nhs-foundation-trust

A more comprehensive and up-to-date review of pediatric treatment of gender dysphoria undertaken in the U.S. found that

> *The 'gender-affirming' model of care, as practiced in U.S. clinics, is characterized by a child-led process in which comprehensive mental health assessments are often minimized or omitted, and the patient's "embodiment goals" serve as the primary guide for treatment decisions. In some of the nation's 14 leading pediatric gender clinics, assessments are conducted in a single session lasting two hours.*

And scathingly of the trans affirmation mindset, the most egregious example of a public health approach:

> *The principle of autonomy in medicine establishes a moral and legal right of competent patients to refuse any medical intervention. However, there is no corollary right to receive interventions that are not beneficial. Respect for patient autonomy does not negate clinicians' professional and ethical obligation to protect and promote their patients' health.*[21]

Mental health matters, except when it's inconvenient

A study of 11,442 transgender people in the U.S. assessed their morbidity in general and after gender-affirming treatments. Disconcerting findings were notable associations in the transfeminine cohort of an elevated risk of venous thromboembolism and ischemic stroke. The increase in risk was particularly pronounced after six years of follow-up in the estrogen initiation sub-cohort. Another notable finding was the high prevalence of mental health conditions among transgender people, particularly children and adolescents. The prevalence of estimates for suicidal ideation and self-inflicted injuries was orders of magnitude higher in transgender children and adolescents than in the matched reference groups of the same age.[22] Of course, this suits the public health narrative well: claiming connections between 'something' and suicide is the

21 U.S. Department of Health and Human Services, 2025. *Treatment for Pediatric Gender Dysphoria: Review of Evidence and Best Practices*,14,15

22 Goodman M & Nash R, 2019, 6

trusted schtick that public health falls back on whenever it wants to push its latest ideological preoccupation. As soon as something is linked with suicide, it immediately goes beyond medical science and turns into a public health matter (even when it is medical doctors talking about it).

As always with suicide, it is never as simple as activists claim. A study of 641,860 individuals who completed information on gender, neurodevelopmental and psychiatric diagnoses, including autism, and measures of traits related to autism (self-report measures of autistic traits, empathy, systemising, and sensory sensitivity) found that transgender and gender-diverse individuals were three to six times as likely to be autistic as were cisgender individuals.[23] Transgender and gender-diverse individuals scored significantly higher on self-report measures of autistic traits, systemising and sensory sensitivity and scored substantially lower on empathy traits compared to cisgender individuals. Transgender and gender-diverse individuals had elevated rates of multiple other neurodevelopmental and psychiatric conditions. Transgender and gender-diverse individuals also had elevated rates of Attention Deficit Hyperactivity Disorder, bipolar disorder, depression, Obsessive Compulsive Disorder, learning disorders, and schizophrenia compared to cisgender individuals.[24] Causality is always a difficult thing to establish, and of course, conditions such as depression can certainly come *after* a person experiences gender dysphoria (as public health activists like to point out). However, claiming that a person's gender identity (or, how they are treated due to that identity) causes things like learning disorders, autism, and schizophrenia is a much harder sell. And – completely unsurprisingly – these are also things that tend to elevate a person's suicide risk.

Using legislation to implement medical affirmation for those suffering from gender dysphoria, among other ailments, may mark the first instance in history where doctors have lost control over a diagnosis, entrusting

23 Where gender corresponds with sex.

24 Warrier V et al, 2020. Elevated rates of autism, other neurodevelopmental and psychiatric diagnoses, and autistic traits in transgender and gender-diverse individuals. *Nature Communications* 11, 3959

it instead to a small, radical group of clinicians guided by those with lived experience — that is, transgender activists — who propose an alternative diagnosis and clinical response. Transgender affirmation is the only medical condition with laws compelling doctors to recommend a medical 'solution' desired by the patient. Sick kids demand trans conversion. At the same time, the government prevents doctors from exercising their professional judgment. This is wrong, it is an instance of conceit to have doctors subsume their obligation to the health of the patient in pursuit of a political goal that affirms a patient's misguided beliefs. As the psychiatrist Dr Andrew Amos observed, gender-affirming treatment might achieve some of the desired outcomes in appearance, but the claims in the affirmation model to improve mental health and quality of life are weak. Transgender affirmation represents an abuse of medical authority.[25] But it sure feels good to the public health types who vociferously endorse it.

Professor John Whitehall regards affirmation as an unregulated experiment with widespread evidence for maleficence. He points out the dangers when blockers obstruct the natural process of puberty.[26] Affirmers make claims that puberty blockers are reversible despite ample evidence to the contrary.[27] Affirmers claim to be saving distressed youths from suicide despite evidence that the link occurs after transition.[28] Affirmers are confident that disturbed youths can consent to affirming procedures despite Dr Eithan Haim's observation that you can't provide

---

25 Amos A, 2025. The landscape of gender affirming services in Australia. *Proceedings: The Future of Youth Gender Medicine Seminar*. NSW Parliament House, 37

26 Whitehall J, 2025, 31

27 Baxendale S, 2024. The impact of suppressing puberty on neuropsychological function: A review. *Acta Paediatrica* 113, 1156 and Koener B et al, 2025. Managing gender dysphoria in minors: what insights does evidence-based medicine offer in 2024? *Disease Biology, Genetics, and Socioecology* 1(1), 3

28 Kenny D, 2025. Psychotherapy for gender dysphoria in adolescents: a comprehensive and ethical approach. *Proceedings: The Future of Youth Gender Medicine Seminar*. NSW Parliament House, 68. Also, Kenny D, 2024. *Gender Ideology, Social Contagion, and the Making of a Transgender Generation*. Cambridge Scholars Press

consent by 'blackmailing them with the threat of their own suicide.'[29] As a patient of Dr Az Hakeem remarked, 'I was destined to kill myself if I was not affirmed, or so I was told.'[30] As others argue, while gender-affirming surgery may be beneficial in affirming identity, it increases the risk of harm to mental health.[31]

The gender dysphoria epidemic is also an overdiagnosis epidemic,[32] part of a broader critique of diagnostic overreach, explained by Allen Francis in his master work on the Diagnostic and Statistical Manual (DSM), *Saving Normal*.[33] Professor Philip Morris observed that DSM-5, in 2015, introduced the diagnosis of Gender Dysphoria. The WHO in 2019 removed gender incongruence from the mental disorders category in ICD-11, posing the question, if transgender identity is to be a 'normal variant' alongside, for example, homosexuality, 'does it necessitate medical intervention, particularly when such interventions carry significant risks?'[34] The two aspects, medicalisation and destigmatisation, worked to explode the prevalence of gender dysphoria/incongruence.

The magnitude of the problem

Trans is big business, and growing by the day. Accounts of the magnitude of gender dysphoria are now flowing thick and fast. Not only the number

29 A whistleblower & a former trans teen expose the medical establishment's radical gender ideology. https://www.youtube.com/watch?v=OYWBJFu3z3w

30 Hakeem A, 2023, 102

31 Lewis J E et al, 2025. Examining gender-specific mental health risks after gender-affirming surgery: a national database study. *The Journal of Sexual Medicine* 22(4), 1

32 Parry P, 2025. How did we get to where we are today? *Proceedings: The Future of Youth Gender Medicine Seminar*. NSW Parliament House, 5 and 8. Note, gender incongruence replaced gender dysphoria in International Classification of Diseases 11th revision (ICD-11).

33 Frances A, 2013. *Saving Normal: An Insider's Revolt Against Out-of-control Psychiatric Diagnosis, DSM-5, Big Pharma, and the Medicalization of Ordinary*. William Morrow

34 Morris P, 2025. Rebalancing diagnosis and clinical treatment: the contribution of NAPP to clinical discourse on youth gender medicine. *Proceedings: The Future of Youth Gender Medicine Seminar*. NSW Parliament House, 74

of those referred to affirming clinics, but also the number damaged by the experience, and the number of individuals who have de-transitioned. The harm to families who 'lose' their children to the affirmation process is additional. Kirralee Smith of Gender Awareness Australia has compiled case studies of the story of parents affected by their child's struggles with gender dysphoria and the affirmation pathway.[35] These harrowing stories, especially Tess's, are well worth reading. Her story, as told by her mother, is reminiscent of those being written throughout the Western world. The U.S. appears to be the epicentre of the epidemic. The group, *Do No Harm*, analysed insurance claims to assess which sex change procedures hospitals and healthcare facilities administered to minors. They found that between 2019 and 2023, 13,994 minors underwent sex change treatments, 5,747 minors had sex change surgeries, 8,579 minors received hormones and puberty blockers, and 62,682 sex change prescriptions were written for minors.[36]

The number of referrals to Spanish clinics increased 10-fold, from 18 in 2012 to 189 in 2021.[37] The number of referrals has increased throughout the 2010s in Finland, Norway, Sweden and the UK. Incidence rates rose from one per 100,000 to 17 per 100,000.[38] The number of referrals to the London Gender Identity Development Service increased from four in 1989 to 3,585 in 2021.[39] Referrals to the Royal Children's Hospital Gender Service in Melbourne increased from one in 2003 to 253 in 2017.[40] A further indication of scale was an Australia-wide self-identifying online

35 Smith K, 2024. *Devastated: How Gender Ideology is Tearing Australian Families Apart.* Gender Awareness Australia Limited

36 Stop the Harm Database. https://stoptheharmdatabase.com/about/

37 Expósito-Campos P et al, 2023. Evolution and trends in referrals to a specialist gender identity unit in Spain over 10 years (2012-2021). *The Journal of Sexual Medicine* 20(3), 377

38 Kaltiala R et al, 2020. Time trends in referrals to child and adolescent gender identity services: a study in four Nordic countries and in the UK. *Nordic Journal of Psychiatry* 74(1), 41

39 Grossman M, 2023, 1

40 Tollit M A et al, 2021. The clinical profile of patients attending a large Australian pediatric gender service: a 10-year review. *International Journal of Transgender Health* 24(1), 59

survey that collected data from 928 trans people.[41] The gender ratio is equally intriguing, with the number of girls seeking help far outweighing that of boys, as demonstrated in the Dutch example (Figure 6.1) and in other studies. An Australian clinician observed in his practice, 'in busy child & adolescent work, involving supervisory oversight of community teams, inpatient units and emergency departments since 1995, I don't recall ever seeing a single female-to-male gender dysphoric patient until the late 20teens.'[42]

Figure 6.1 Dutch transgender clinic-referred adolescents, 2000 to 2016

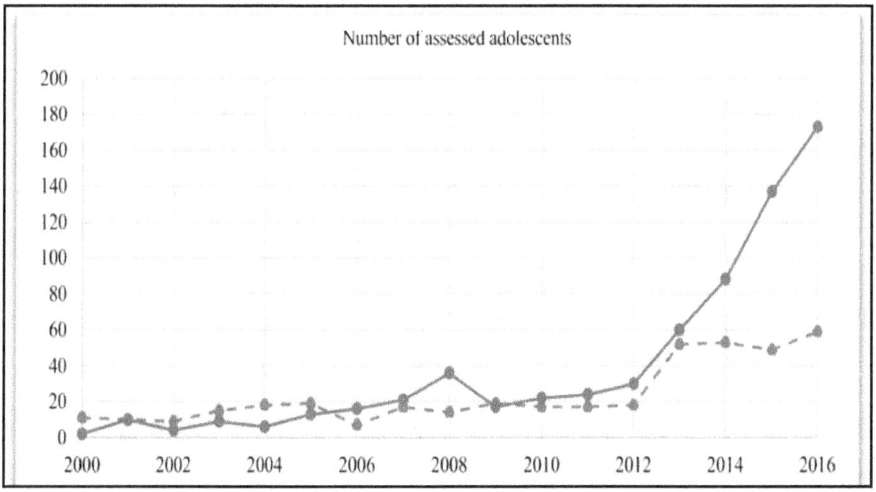

Source: Arnoldussen M et al, 2020. Re-evaluation of the Dutch approach: Are recently referred transgender youth different compared to earlier referrals? *European Child and Adolescent Psychiatry* 29, 803

The pro-transition group Transcend Australia and the Australian Professional Association for Trans Health (Auspath) worry that 're-identification' or de-transitioning is prone to misinformation and sensationalism. They reassure their people that 'Current high-quality research shows rates of re-identification remain low.'[43] Low is in the

41 Bretherton I et al, 2021. The health and well-being of transgender Australians: a national community survey. *LGBT Health* 8(1), 42

42 Parry P, 2025, 7

43 Transcend Australia and Auspath, 2024. Evidence brief: detransition. *Briefings on Trans Healthcare*

eye of the beholder. A U.S. five-year study of social transitioners among 300 children found that seven per cent had retransitioned.[44] If seven per cent of the relevant cohort did something that public health activists did not like (for example, smoking), they would be up in arms about that number, rather than pretending it was inconsequential. Clayton cites and discusses discontinuance rates in a U.S. cohort,[45] which reported for those who had started cross sex hormone treatment before age 18, a 4-year discontinuation rate of 25 per cent. For a Dutch cohort,[46] the treatment discontinuation rates in adolescents who had commenced puberty blockers before age 18 were one per cent at a median follow-up of 2.3 years, and those 'assigned male at birth' had a four per cent discontinuation rate at a median follow-up of 3.5 years. A weakness in the study was that the Dutch group reported an average time to detransition of more than 10 years. The Dutch study's short follow-up time and young follow-up age provide no insight into discontinuation rates over time. Clayton also observed that 75 per cent of the Dutch youth who discontinued hormone treatment had undergone gonadectomies. Still, at follow-up, they were receiving neither cross sex hormones nor sex hormones consistent with their birth sex.[47]

A recent study described treatment trajectories, detransition and mortality rate among children and adolescents referred to the Norwegian National Center for Gender Incongruence over twenty years. Almost 40 per cent of the female patients who were under age 18 when referred to Norway's national gender clinic from 2000 to 2020 went on to have mastectomies as adults. Of the 1,258 patients of both sexes referred over that period, one per cent were registered as dead by the end of 2023. While they

44 Olson K R et al, 2022. Gender identity 5 years after social transition. *Pediatrics* 150(2), 1

45 See Roberts C M et al, 2022. Continuation of gender-affirming hormones among transgender adolescents and adults. *The Journal of Clinical Endocrinology & Metabolism* 107(9), e3937

46 van der Loos M et al, 2022. Continuation of gender-affirming hormones in transgender people starting puberty suppression in adolescence: a cohort study in the Netherlands. *The Lancet Child & Adolescent Health* 6(12), 869

47 Clayton A, 2023, 486

did not report, this is probably higher than for the population, but not necessarily higher than for those with mental health conditions. Of 783 patients who began cross-sex hormones as minors, 18 females (2.3 per cent) detransitioned, stopping testosterone. The paper noted higher cessation rates of gender-affirming hormonal treatment in a Finnish study at eight per cent and acknowledges estimates of almost 30 per cent. It further remarked that the numbers at Norway's clinic 'could potentially be the beginning of an increase in persons transitioning back to their birth-assigned gender.'[48]

This raises the issue of the needs of those who detransition, which can involve medical changes such as stopping or changing hormone therapy and undergoing reversal surgeries and social changes such as presenting as one's birth sex again, changing one's post-transition name or going back to using the pronouns associated with one's birth sex.[49] An online international survey of 237 detransitioners conducted in 2021 found a high prevalence of comorbidities, with over half of participants reporting at least three diagnosed comorbid conditions. The most prevalent diagnosed comorbid conditions were depressive disorders and anxiety disorders, including PTSD. The most common reported reason for detransitioning was that they realised their gender dysphoria was related to other issues. The second one was health concerns, followed by different factors such as the fact that the transition did not help the dysphoria, they found alternatives to deal with dysphoria, were unhappy with the social changes, and 43 per cent who replied that they had 'a change in political views'.[50]

Symptomatic of the politics involved in this field are the comments among some detransitioners of the ilk, 'Only lesbians and feminists helped me. The trans and queer community demonized me and

48 Nyquist C B et al, 2025. Treatment trajectories among children and adolescents referred to the Norwegian National Center for Gender Incongruence. *Acta Paediatrica* 114, 1012

49 Vandenbussche E, 2022. Detransition-related needs and support: a cross-sectional online survey. *Journal of Homosexuality* 69(9), 1602

50 Vandenbussche E, 2022, 1606

ostracized me for my reidentification.' Politics, which in this account infuses the medical professionals involved is also a factor, 'When I first brought up wanting to stop T[estosterone] to my doctor, they were very dismissive and condescending about it.' Another detransitioner reported, 'I struggled to find a therapist who supported questioning my trans identity and considering alternatives to transitioning; most only knew how to encourage transitioning and reinforced the harmful ideas that led to my wrongly identifying as FtM in the first place.'[51]

The psychiatrist Dr Az Hakeem, who established a dedicated adult gender dysphoria specialist psychotherapy service within the UK National Health Service, has written a stunning account of the madness of transition from the eyes of detransitioners. As a result of his work, he became 'increasingly concerned that any psychosis ('madness') … around the trans phenomenon in our society, … has relinquished all … rationality in favour of the cult of Gender Ideology and erased the legitimacy of women's rights and the original concept of homosexuality,'[52] He describes the 'transing away the gay' phenomenon. Many gender dysphoric boys and girls who would otherwise have grown up to be homosexual or lesbian would become adults without gender dysphoria.[53]

> *What is presumed to be a progressive situation of acceptance of trans people has ... become a sanctioned resurgence of societal and organisational homophobia where any signs of gender non-conformity ... are subject to a 'transification' where future homosexuals are turned into 'heterosexual' trans adults.*[54]

Political actors

Arguably, the primary actor in the trans affirmation drama has been the Harry Benjamin International Gender Dysphoria Association. Formed in 1978, it later became the World Professional Association for Transgender Health (WPATH), which advises healthcare providers to use the WHO's

51 Vandenbussche E, 2022, 1611

52 Hakeem A, 2023, 18

53 Hakeem A, 2023, 45

54 Hakeem A, 2023, 45

International Classification of Diseases (ICD-11) classification of gender incongruence instead of the DSM-5's gender dysphoria. The reasoning is that the ICD-11 diagnosis is categorised as a 'condition related to sexual health' and not a mental disorder, which de-stigmatises transgender people. It also, entirely coincidentally, places transgender issues more in the realms of public health than a diagnosis of mental illness would necessarily achieve. A diagnosis of gender incongruence is arguably easier to obtain than one of gender dysphoria because there is no requirement for distress as a criterion, meaning a patient's embodiment goals can be deemed medically necessary care. All the patient needs to experience is a marked incongruence between their internal sense of self and their biological sex.

WPATH's Standards of Care 8 recommends that adolescents who have received a diagnosis of gender incongruence have access to puberty blockers, cross-sex hormones, and surgeries, so long as the young person demonstrates the emotional and cognitive maturity required to provide informed consent/assent for the treatment. However, members from a WPATH panel titled Identity Evolution Workshop, held on 6 May 2022, admit to the impossibility of obtaining proper informed consent for hormonal interventions from their young patients.[55] WPATH-affiliated healthcare professionals confess that their practices are based on improvisation, that children cannot comprehend them, and that the consent process is not ethical.[56]

This madness is a prominent part of a larger phenomenon in gender politics. In Australia, witness the question posed by Senator Antic at Senate Estimates on 7 April 2022 to Professor Murphy, former Commonwealth Chief Medical Officer and Secretary of the Department of Health: 'Can someone please provide me with a definition of what a woman is?' Murphy responded that there were 'a variety of definitions'. Antic asked Murphy to provide a simple one, and Murphy replied, 'I

55 Hughes M, 2024. The WPATH files pseudoscientific surgical and hormonal experiments on children, adolescents, and vulnerable adults. *Environmental Progress* 4 March, 10

56 Hughes M, 2024, 8

think perhaps to give a more fulsome answer, we should take that on notice.' Some 78 days later, the Department provided the following.

> *The frameworks adopted to define a person's gender include chromosomal makeup, the gender assigned at birth, and the gender with which a person identifies.*

Public health crusades have always thrived on legislative intervention. The reason the Department found the once straightforward answer difficult is due to an ideology of gender identification, written into law by the Commonwealth in 2013, which made gender a protected characteristic in the *Sex Discrimination Act 1984* (Cth) by removing the definition of biological sex.[57] As Justice Bromwich stated in *Tickle v Giggle*, 'amendments to the SDA all point forcefully to an understanding of sex, … that is changeable'.[58] Indeed, the states and Territories have headed down the same path, adding the ability to change sex on a birth certificate. For example, in Queensland, with varying provisos in any state or territory, a sixteen-year-old 'identifier', or a parent of a child under 16, can change the sex on the birth certificate.[59] In Victoria, a sex record can change no more often than every 12 months – changeable indeed. This insanity ran in the background while children were being 'treated' by clinicians determined to send them down a path of non-medically justified bodily mutilation on the non-evidence that they would commit suicide without the intervention. Remove public health claims about suicide, and would any of the arguments for embracing gender fluidity through changes in medical practice and the law be taken seriously?

There is some light in the issue of gender and sex, which appears to be driving some of the dysphoria, and the affirming response in a recent decision of the UK Supreme Court, which ruled that transgender women

57 https://www.ag.gov.au/rights-and-protections/human-rights-and-anti-discrimination/australian-government-guidelines-recognition-sex-and-gender

58 *Tickle v Giggle for Girls Pty Ltd (No 2)* [2024] FCA 960, 59

59 *Births, Deaths and Marriages Registration Act* 2023 (Qld), Part 5 Acknowledgement of Sex https://www.legislation.qld.gov.au/view/whole/html/current/act-2023-017

with gender-recognition certificates who assert that they are female do not share women's legal protections. The meaning of the terms sex, man and woman in the *Equality Act 2010* (UK) is biological and not certified sex. Gender reassignment and sex are separate bases for discrimination and inequality. This did not mean that trans people do not have protections under the Equality Act.[60] The Scottish government had created two sub-groups within those who share the protected characteristic of gender reassignment, giving trans persons who possess a certificate, greater rights than those who did not.[61] That interpretation would also seriously weaken the ability to have lesbian-only spaces and associations. Other provisions requiring a biological interpretation of sex include separate spaces and single-sex facilities (such as changing rooms, hostels, and medical services), as well as communal accommodation.[62] The scope of the UK decision, albeit limited, might at least give heart to those who wish to remove gender identity as a protected characteristic from the Sex Discrimination Act 1984 (Cth) in Australia.[63]

Returning to gender dysphoria, to add insult to injury, the prohibition of conversion practices legislation in Victoria, NSW and Queensland stands in the way of a rational approach to treating those suffering from confusing their sex and their gender. The legislation was heavily influenced by a Latrobe University paper written by activists on the 'religious LGBT conversion therapy movement'.[64] Gay and lesbian activists were concerned that conservative religious activists were trying to talk their flock out of being gay or lesbian. This putsch became warped as the trans issue emerged. Trans people, by and large, do not identify as gay or lesbian. Rather than come to terms with that, they

---

60 *For Women Scotland Ltd (Appellant) v The Scottish Ministers (Respondent) UKSC/2024/0042*, par 265 (xviii)

61 *For Women Scotland Ltd (Appellant)*, par 265 (xii)

62 *For Women Scotland Ltd (Appellant)*, par 265 (x)

63 *Sex Discrimination Act 1984* (Cth) - Sect 5b Discrimination on the Ground of Gender Identity

64 Jones T et al, 2018. *Preventing Harm, Promoting Justice: Responding to LGBT Conversion Therapy in Australia.* Melbourne: Gay and Lesbian Health Victoria, Australian Research Centre in Sex, Health and Society and the Human Rights Law Centre

want to convert to the opposite sex — how heteronormative is that? The legislation reeks of the battle against conservative religion, and indeed smacks of religious suppression,[65] but is a weapon against doctors who want to recommend a non-affirming path in their care of gender dysphoric patients. The prohibition on conversion became a compulsory conversion to affirmation.

Under Chapter 5B of the *Public Health Act 2005* (Qld), a health practitioner in Queensland is prohibited from performing conversion practices.[66] The Act defines conversion practices, which it refers to as 'conversion therapy', as any practice that attempts to change or suppress a person's sexual orientation or gender identity or expression.[67] For example:

> *techniques or interventions that are based in ideology that being LGBTQA+ is a defect or disorder that needs 'fixing'.*[68]

The difficulty is that while being same sex attracted is not a medical condition, gender dysphoria may well be (or, at least, a mental health condition). In any event, the affirmation fix is neither a fix nor risk-free. The definition does not include practices that provide support to persons dealing with sexual orientation or gender identity and expression, or reasonable clinical practices, even if these practices do not proactively affirm or support a person's sexual orientation or gender identity and expression. These exemptions are sensible, but the problem arises when some psychiatric professionals have opted to exclude practices that are not proactively affirming. The wording seems generous and careful, but

---

65 See Moens G, 2025. An abominable law. *Quadrant* April 26 https://quadrant.org.au/news-opinions/religion/an-abominable-law/

66 *Public Health Act 2005* (Qld)

67 Gender identity is the person's internal and individual experience of gender, whether it corresponds with the sex assigned to the person at birth. It includes the person's personal sense of the body; and if freely chosen modification of the person's bodily appearance or functions by medical, surgical or other means; and other expressions of the person's gender, including name, dress, speech and behaviour.

68 Conversion therapy is a practice that attempts to change or suppress a person's sexual orientation or gender identity, for example, by inducing nausea, vomiting or paralysis while showing the person same-sex images.

it is limiting and threatening in practice. Only affirmers need apply.

There are many good reasons why conversion therapy should not be practised, and most people would (hopefully) agree that a person should be able to live as they wish, without fear of discrimination because of their gender or sexuality, or coercion to behave as somebody they are not. But is 'shaming' somebody about gender identity really a matter for public health legislation? If you say that denying a person's gender identity, or disputing it in the 'wrong' way, can elevate the risk of suicide, then apparently so. Of course, this is precisely what activists say. The proof is Dr Jillian Spencer's trials and tribulations for suggesting caution in the approach to those suffering from gender dysphoria, for which she was summarily suspended from her Brisbane hospital.

The Australian Medical Association Queensland opposed amendments to the Act, fearing they could lead to the prosecution of health professionals providing evidence-based practices and limit therapeutic approaches supporting children and adolescents who present with gender dysphoria.

> *Gender Clinics who do comprehensive evaluations of family and dynamic drivers of the child's gender feelings could be vulnerable, especially if they identify powerful parental dynamics heavily influencing the child's expression.*
>
> *The bill as it currently is written, does not provide sufficient protection for therapists to assist young people ... to explore possible family, psychological or social dynamic causes of their gender dysphoria.*[69]

The fight within the profession is far from over. A letter dated 29 May 2024 to the President of the Royal Australian and New Zealand College of Psychiatry from members, regarding the College's response to the Cass Review, stated, 'We believe our serious professional concerns regarding the gender interventions being provided to Australian children and adolescents are not being adequately represented by the College.' They were right. The College president responded,

69 Dr Dilip Dhupelia, Australian Medical Association (Queensland). Letter to Mr Aaron Harper, Chair Health, Communities, Disability Services and Domestic and Family Protection, 31 January 2020

> *Being Trans or Gender Diverse is not a mental health condition.*
>
> *The College does not recommend that the Government commission an Inquiry following the release of the Cass Review.*
>
> *The College emphasises that assessment and treatment should be patient centred, ... and that psychiatrists have a responsibility to counter stigma and discrimination directed towards trans and gender diverse people.*[70]

The heart of the College position is that being trans or gender diverse does not represent a mental health condition, but 'stigma, discrimination, trauma, abuse, and assault contribute to this mental distress.' As such, 'psychiatrists have a responsibility to counter stigma, discrimination and violence directed towards TGD people.'[71] Few suggest that being trans or gender diverse is, of itself, a mental health condition. It may be that such people encounter stigma, but to assume mental ailments are external is an ideological statement. To argue that psychiatrists have a responsibility to counter stigma and discrimination is a political statement. One of the authors of the letter to the College, Andrew Amos, found a disturbing feature of gender affirming care was that his profession had 'completely failed to correct the lie that trans identity does not involve mental illness. Basic psychodynamics illustrate there is always a component of mental illness in any of the gender identities described by gender affirming care advocates.'[72]

Further evidence of the College's radical identity stance is their statement on the New Zealand parliament's rejection of New Zealand First Bill to amend Definitions of Woman and Man, which sought to define woman and man in law as 'adult human biological female' and 'adult human biological male' as an attack on the rights of trans people.

> *Intersex, trans and gender diverse people in Aotearoa [New Zealand]*

---

70 https://www.ranzcp.org/news-analysis/a-letter-from-members-regarding-the-cass-review-and-the-college-s-response

71 https://www.ranzcp.org/clinical-guidelines-publications/clinical-guidelines-publications-library/role-of-psychiatrists-working-with-trans-gender-diverse-people

72 Amos A, 2025, 40

> *already face significant mental health disparities due to stigma, discrimination, and lack of access to culturally safe and affirming healthcare. This bill, if progressed, will only deepen those harms and their impact.*[73]

The RANZCP maintains a radical stance despite evidence of harm in the affirmation model of care. Jillian Spencer ran as president in April 2025, and although she failed to win, she at least fired a shot across their bow.

Science fights back

The non-medical approach of the trans lobby, so illustrative of a public health approach, is under considerable attack from more traditional medical sources. Numerous changes have encouraged the hope that the College of Psychiatry and its associated entities, which currently support the affirmation model of care, will soon adopt a more considered approach. A tentative but positive move is the Queensland government's pause of puberty blockers and gender affirming hormones for young people at one clinic,[74] and the Commonwealth's very tentative and reluctant review by the NHMRC.[75]

In addition to the Cass Review, there has been considerable reconsideration within medical circles of the prevailing view of care, including in the literature.[76] There has been a dearth of research on psychotherapeutic approaches to managing gender dysphoria in children and adolescents. This is due in part to the mischaracterisation of such approaches as conversion therapy. Fortunately, Dianna Kenny has devoted a considerable part of her career to alternative models of

73 https://www.ranzcp.org/news-analysis/psychiatrists-reject-proposed-member-s-bill-targeting-trans-and-gender-diverse-new-zealanders

74 Hon Tim Nicholls, Independent Review into puberty blockers released. *Media Release* 19 December 2025

75 Assistant minister, Ged Kearney, sang the praises of the affirmation model at the time the minister (Mark Butler) announced the review. Hon Mark Butler. Healthcare for trans and gender diverse children and adolescents. Department of Health and Aged Care, *Minister Butler's Media.* 31 January 2025

76 Cohn, J. 2025. Censorship of essential debate in gender medicine research. *Journal of Controversial Ideas* 5(3)

care. While the gender-affirming model is advocated as best practice, two other models of care—gender reparative and gender explorative—are also available. The difficulty is that they have been 'deceptively conflated and subject to conversion therapy prohibition', which Kenny regards as 'an ideologically and politically driven state of affairs that is detrimental to the well-being of minors.'[77]

In 2023, the Norwegian Healthcare Investigation Board declared gender medicalisation of minors to be experimental. In a report, Patient Safety for Children and Young People with Gender Incongruence, the Norwegian Healthcare Investigation Board said, 'We know little about the long-term effects of puberty blockers and side effects of treatment with [opposite-sex] hormones.' On the question of informed choice, the report concluded that 'patients must be informed about this, and patients must be able to understand the consequences of the choices.' However, the board concluded that it was unclear what was required to determine that a young person is mature enough to consent to the sought interventions. 'There is no Norwegian comprehensive overview or systematic mapping of the patients' history, [of] how many are refused [treatment], who withdraws during treatment, [who] completes the treatment, or how patients with gender incongruence and gender dysphoria fare after treatment.'[78]

In 2024, a statement by the European Society of Child and Adolescent Psychiatry outlines the key principles that must be guaranteed in the work with minors with gender dysphoria.

- Non-maleficence: do not use interventions with unknown long-term consequences
- Beneficence: adopt medical interventions with a favourable benefits-to-harms ratio and consider the ratio of not providing medical interventions
- Autonomy: assess the capacity of minors to consent; consider the rights of parents and guardians to be fully informed; offer adequate support and resources to those who decide to de-transition to their assigned sex
- Justice: ensure access to reliable and up-to-date information for gender

77 Kenny D, 2025, 69

78 As reported in https://genspect.org/norway-takes-a-step-forward-in-ending-experiment-in-youth-gender-medicine/

dysphoria, and during transition or de-transition.[79]

In 2025, Justice Strum of the Federal Circuit and Family Court of Australia Division 1 in a parenting matter, excoriated the gender affirmation model of care, in particular two 'expert' witnesses for the mother who gave evidence where the father sought to restrain the mother from allowing their son to begin a course of puberty blockers, at age 12.[80] The judge found that the mother contended the child was gender dysphoric or incongruent and had pushed him along this path, attending the Royal Children's Hospital Gender Clinic in Melbourne, from the age of six. The mother's first expert, Associate Professor Michelle Telfer, described herself as an advocate for trans rights, to which the judge responded, 'Advocacy in a court is for lawyers, not witnesses, neither lay nor expert.'[81] The mother's other expert witness, Dr N, who found the father's case 'hard to … read', meaning upsetting, was reminded by the judge that the 'difficulty experienced by her is … hard to reconcile with her obligations, as an expert.'[82]

The judge also excoriated counsel for the mother for submitting 'for background context only' the *Change or Suppression (Conversion) Practices Prohibition Act 2021* (Vic) because 'it may explain some of the difficulties encountered by the father and the Independent Children's Lawyer who oppose the mother's case, … to obtaining both expert evidence for these proceedings and alternative treatment proposals for the child.'[83] Indeed, the father gave evidence that, 'to garner evidence in support of his case …, he had contacted very many (in fact, he said, because of the Change or Suppression (Conversion) Practices Prohibition Act and like pressure, "hundreds" of) therapists who were not interested

79 Radobuljac M D, 2024. ESCAP statement on the care for children and adolescents with gender dysphoria: an urgent need for safeguarding clinical, scientific, and ethical standards. *European Child & Adolescent Psychiatry* 33, 2012

80 Re: Devin [2025] FedCFamC1F 211

81 Re: Devin [2025], par 11

82 Re: Devin [2025], par 12

83 Re: Devin [2025], par 18

in treating children with gender issues.'[84]

The judge also noted that Telfer argued that the gender-affirming treatment standards of care guidelines issued by the hospital were 'best practice'. However, as she was the author, it was 'tantamount to her agreeing with herself'.[85] Dr Alison Clayton revealed the poor quality of the standards and guidelines at the Royal Children's Hospital, Melbourne, having obtained documents under the *Freedom of Information Act 1982* (Vic).[86] She questioned how the untrustworthy treatment guidelines of the hospital were approved by the hospital's governance processes, endorsed by health departments and medical bodies across the nation and are used to guide clinical practice at Australia's public youth gender clinics. The treatment protocol of the 2018 hospital guidelines is 'a series of poorly evidenced, novel interventions that pose numerous serious health risks to patients for a poorly understood condition.' Clayton argued that the protocol should have only been introduced as part of a hospital-approved clinical trial.[87]

The world in which the child lived was a mother obsessed with gender affirmation, whose only social circle was a service provider, Rainbow Connections, in the district where the child and she lived, 'in a social circle dominated by transgender young people who are older than the child and are undergoing various stages of affirming treatment.'[88] The Family Report, tendered in the case, about the involvement of the mother and the child with Rainbow Connections, explained that the mother's 'acceptance into a marginalised and disempowered subculture probably provided her with [a] sense of belonging.'[89] Further, a doctor who examined the mother reported that she 'is closely aligned to the

84 Re: Devin [2025], par 21

85 Re: Devin [2025], par 70

86 Clayton, A. 2025. What went wrong. *Gender Clinic News | Bernard Lane* 7 May

87 Telfer M M et al, 2020. *Australian Standards of Care and Treatment Guidelines for Trans and Gender Diverse Children and Adolescents*. Melbourne: Royal Children's Hospital version 1.3

88 Re: Devin [2025], par 75

89 Re: Devin [2025], par 202

transgender movement, and is a member of the local gender rainbow group [sic]" and that she "identifies as an abused woman".'[90] The judge found that 'the mother has used the child's fluidity and alleged (but, I have found, unproven) gender dysphoria/incongruence in an endeavour to distance, if not alienate, the child from the father.'[91]

Devastating to the mother's case was the finding of concern, which is 'the reference in [Dr N] February 2023 report to the child having 'dysphoria that results from a lack of affirmation'. However, when this was explored in cross-examination, [Dr N] accepted that, 'throughout her involvement with the child before the end of 2022, there was no evidence of dysphoria that she had directly observed. Thus, it follows that the only dysphoria must have been that reported to her by the mother.'[92] Further, Dr N prepared and filed an opinion that the child met the DSM-5 criteria for gender dysphoria in children, as the trial date approached. The judge found that 'the timing was more than merely coincidental.'[93]

The issue of consent was canvassed. The mother's experts 'contended without explanation that the child would have had the capacity for such self-knowledge by the time of answering the initial questionnaire at the hospital, at the age of merely six years.'[94] The evidence of Dr N was that 'because the child says so, the child is, and must unquestioningly be affirmed as being, female in gender identity.'[95] The judge found that both experts dismissed 'the possible relevance of other factors, such as maternal influence and underlying neurodivergence, playing any part in the child's presentation.'[96]

Professor Telfer criticised the Cass Report in a way that the judge found was 'misleading or omitted findings/material that detracted from her

90 Re: Devin [2025], par 204

91 Re: Devin [2025], par 206

92 Re: Devin [2025], par 81

93 Re: Devin [2025], par 87

94 Re: Devin [2025], par 89

95 Re: Devin [2025], par 74

96 Re: Devin [2025], par 90

opinion' and 'contrary to the obligations as an expert witness.'[97] Telfer would do well to read the 2025 U.S. Department of Health and Human Services review of paediatric gender dysphoria, which, like the Cass Report, was scathing of the affirmation model.

> *Diagnosis of gender dysphoria is based entirely on subjective self-reports and behavioral observations, without any objective physical, imaging, or laboratory markers. The diagnosis centers on attitudes, feelings, and behaviors that are known to fluctuate during adolescence.*[98]

The U.S. review made clear that, in many areas of medicine, treatments are first established as safe and effective in adults before being extended to paediatric populations. The review also found no independent association between gender dysphoria and suicidality, and there is no evidence that paediatric medical transition reduces the incidence of suicide.[99] In this case, however, the opposite occurred. A true public health approach was used: action was taken without giving any serious consideration to causes of the 'condition', unforeseen negative consequences, or other alternatives. Clinician-researchers developed the paediatric medical transition protocol in response to disappointing psychosocial outcomes in adults who underwent medical transition. The review found that the quality of evidence on the effects of intervention on psychological outcomes, quality of life, regret, or long-term health was very low. This suggests that the beneficial effects reported in the literature differ substantially from the interventions' effects. The risks of paediatric medical transition include infertility/sterility, sexual dysfunction, impaired bone density accrual, adverse cognitive impacts, cardiovascular disease and metabolic disorders, psychiatric disorders, surgical complications, and regret.

The review damned WPATH's Standards of Care, Version 8 guidelines, finding that 'in the process of developing SOC-8, WPATH suppressed systematic reviews its leaders believed would undermine its favoured

97 Re: Devin [2025], par 101

98 U.S. Department of Health and Human Services, 2025, 10

99 U.S. Department of Health and Human Services, 2025, 16

treatment approach. SOC-8 developers also violated conflict of interest management requirements and eliminated nearly all recommended age minimums for medical and surgical interventions in response to political pressures.'[100] In addition to condemning WPATH the review found that U.S. medical associations played a role in creating a perception that there was professional consensus in support of paediatric medical transition. The apparent consensus, however, was driven by a small number of specialised committees, influenced by WPATH. It was unclear whether the official views of these associations were shared by their members. There was evidence that some medical and mental health associations had 'suppressed dissent and stifled debate about this issue among their members.'[101] A recent paper by Dr Jillian Spencer and Dr Patrick Clarke has added weight to the demolition of the affirmation model as espoused by the Australian group AusPATH.[102]

See you in court

Public health has long relied on the legal system to get what it wants, but in a small ray of hope, it seems that system may finally turn back on public health. Professor Patrick Parkinson has suggested the many grounds on which doctors and clinics may be sued by children who have suffered from affirming treatment.[103] The first chink in the ideological armour of the affirmation proponents was the insurer, MDA National, which no longer covered General Practitioners-initiating gender-affirming treatment for adolescents.[104] Parkinson outlines seven causes of action:

---

100 U.S. Department of Health and Human Services, 2025, 14

101 U.S. Department of Health and Human Services, 2025, 15

102 Spencer J & Clarke P, 2025. AusPATH: activism influencing health policy. *Australasian Psychiatry* 33(2), 273

103 Parkinson P, 2025. Legal issues in treatment of minors. *Proceedings: The Future of Youth Gender Medicine Seminar*. NSW Parliament House, 78

104 Anastasia Tsirtsakis, 2023. Insurance cut for gender-affirming care 'sends such a negative signal.' 29 May *GP News*

1. Failure to apply the DSM-5 criteria properly

In Australia, the prescription of puberty blockers or cross-sex hormones to a minor is only lawful if there is a diagnosis under the DSM-5 criteria of gender dysphoria. In practice, the only criterion applied is that the child has been insistent about their transgender identification.

2. Failure to consider and rule out other explanations for gender incongruence

In some cases, there is a refusal to consider any alternative explanation for gender incongruence other than that the child or young person has an innate gender identity that is discordant with their natal sex.

3. Failure to take a history from both parents

If one marker of persistent gender incongruence is that it was evident from early childhood, then the history of the child's interests and behaviours in early childhood is essential. As the Strum judgment indicates, children referred to gender clinics are often greatly affected by parental conflict, and it is not uncommon for the parents to be living separately.

4. Failure to consider alternative treatment options

Failure to consider and rule out less drastic treatment options, including psychotherapeutic approaches to manage distress and build resilience as outlined by Professor Kenny, would be grounds for a suit.

5. Unlawful treatment of non-binary adolescents

Treatment that affects fertility and is not for the treatment of an illness or disease of a non-binary adolescent is outside the parents' capacity to consent. It needs court approval. Could a court find that it is clinically necessary and in the best interests of the child to provide body-altering treatments to a non-binary adolescent when the treatment does not have any proven therapeutic benefit and is not intended to help them 'pass' as the opposite sex?

6. Failure to assess Gillick competence properly

Clinics insist that a young person must be 'Gillick competent' before prescribing cross-sex hormones. This concept is poorly understood within the medical profession.

7. Failure to obtain a fully informed consent

To provide fully informed consent, the patient must be able to make an informed judgment about whether the likely benefits of the treatment outweigh the known impacts and risks to physical health, fertility and sexual function. Queensland's chief psychiatrist has been placed on notice that, if they persist in administering affirmation treatment, Queensland Children's Hospital and individual QCGS staff could be held liable for any damage to their patients.[105]

One central idea of the gender-affirming model of care is that children know who they are. This is an ideological assertion that is inconsistent with all existing models of human development. As a result of allowing itself to be swept up in this ideology that hands power to those gripped by 'infantile omnipotence', the profession should make amends in various ways, by establishing specialist health services for detransitioners, a statutory compensation scheme, remedial training for the profession, and, most importantly, a statement of culpability and apology.[106]

Conclusion

Whenever the spectre of suicide and the need to avoid that tragic outcome is raised to justify some unrelated and ideologically-charged course of action, we should be very wary indeed. This is one of public health's favoured tactics to shut down any dissent and gain unquestioning support for its latest fashionable crusade. It is also a wonderful way to encourage good professional people to stray into ways of thinking that undermine the normally cautious scientific method and end up causing harm.

105 Lane B, 2025. Stop this sterilising of children. *Gender Clinic News*. 26 October

106 Spencer J, D'Angelo R & Clarke P, 2025. The Profession that failed. *Gender Clinic News* 29 August. This article was offered to but rejected by the journal *Australasian Psychiatry.*

Believing that you are helping to save somebody's life feels good. And to feel good about the work they do, some practitioners are susceptible to ego-enhancing ideologies; they overreach.

The antidote to public health overreach is contestability and openness within professions. Too many have looked the other way, failed to ask questions of their colleagues, preferring to not rock the boat to avoid professional punishments, ostracism, and ridicule. Too many remain silent when bad ideas creep in, and patients suffer as a result. All in the name of public health.

7

Aboriginal Health: measuring ideology

One string among many of the public health lobby's bow is the claim that Aboriginal community-controlled health services are better for Aboriginal clients. This stretches the idea of social determinants into the realms of who 'owns' and is delivering services. But, is it true, or just another example of public health's latest ideological preoccupation, hiding behind claims of better health outcomes? Public health's rhetoric about Aboriginal controlled services reveals another of its favoured tactics: confounding methods to achieve better health outcomes with measuring outcomes. The preferred methods are intermediaries, such as cultural safety, but not outcomes, such as years of life. Most government programs are subject to evaluation to determine their effectiveness and the worthiness of the investment. Most evaluations will state an explicit theory of change, that is, a specific and measurable description and illustration of how and why a program is supposed to work. What happens, though, when the theory of change for Aboriginal community-controlled organisations is based on the principles of self-determination and cultural integrity?[1] What if the means — self-determination and cultural integrity – defeat the outcomes, for example, in closing the gap in life expectancy? Which does public health choose then? The answer, sadly, is not surprising.

1 Aboriginal Affairs NSW, 2025. *Monitoring, Evaluation and Learning Package: Closing the Gap Grant Program*, 7

The need is great, but is the remedy correct?

There is a great need for effective interventions in Aboriginal health because of the gap in life expectancy between Aboriginal people and other Australians, which is nine years for males and eight years for females. This is, indeed, a matter public health is right to concern itself with. Aborigines living in remote areas have the lowest life expectancy, five years lower than that of Aborigines living in major cities and regional areas. However, location is not the determining factor in Aborigines' life expectancy, as the most significant difference in life expectancy between Aborigines and other Australians occurs in remote areas, where the gap is 12 years. Some people live long lives in remote areas, but this is not the case for Aborigines.

Is socioeconomic disadvantage the determining factor in Aboriginal life expectancy? Aboriginal men living in the most socioeconomically disadvantaged areas have a life expectancy that is about five years lower than that of those living in the least disadvantaged areas. Aboriginal females in the most disadvantaged areas had a life expectancy of around three years lower than those in the least disadvantaged areas.[2] It seems to be part of the answer, as better-off people —not just Aborigines — tend to take better care of their health. That journey may have something to do with behaviour and culture, but not in a way that public health officials would want to hear. Location and class are acceptable lenses to understand public health inequity. What is less acceptable is the way people live, including their culture.

There is no lack of research or spending in this field. Aboriginal health research publications more than doubled between 2010 and 2021.[3] Expenditure by the Australian Government on Aboriginal-specific health programs increased by nearly 30 per cent in real terms between 2010 and

---

2 Australian Institute of Health & Welfare and National Indigenous Australians Agency, 2024. *ATSI Health Performance Framework, 1.19 Life Expectancy at birth*

3 Jennings W et al, 2021. Rapid review of five years of Aboriginal and Torres Strait Islander health research in Australia: persisting under-representation of urban populations. *Australian and New Zealand Journal of Public Health* 45, 53

2020.[4] In 2020, total expenditure per person on admitted patient care, Medicare Benefits Schedule, and Australian Government Department of Health and Aged Care grants to Aboriginal Community Controlled Health Services was $9,374 per person in remote and very remote areas, $5,166 per person in inner and outer regional areas, and $4,797 per person for major cities. In 2020, the average health expenditure per person for Aborigines was $1.50 for every $1 spent per person for other Australians. Funding per person for community health services for Aborigines was 3.5 times the amount for other Australians.[5] There is not a single program or dollar that admits personal habits as a cause of ill health. All causes are externalised. Indeed, public health sets out to disguise inappropriate behaviour as cultural safety, a problem for the majority to adjust to.

Cultural safety is born

The Public Health Association of Australia devotes considerable space to Aboriginal health, particularly to concepts such as cultural safety.[6] Cultural safety is a major recommendation of the Australian Human Rights Commission report on health inequity, as is the co-design of health programs.[7] Indeed, the Royal Australian College of General Practitioners recently reaffirmed its support for the Uluru Statement, a demonstration of how deeply the rot of ideology has infiltrated the medical profession.[8] Flowing from these ideas is the firm policy to hire more Aboriginal health

4 Australian Institute of Health & Welfare and National Indigenous Australians Agency, 2024, 92

5 Australian Institute of Health & Welfare and National Indigenous Australians Agency, 2024, 3.21

6 Williams R, 1999. Cultural safety: what does it mean for our work practice? *Australian and New Zealand Journal of Public Health* 23(2), 213. Mithen V et al, 2021. Aboriginal patient and interpreter perspectives on the delivery of culturally safe hospital-based care. *Health Promotion Journal of Australia* 32(S1), 155

7 Australian Human Rights Commission, 2025. *Health Inequities in Australia: A Scoping Review on the Impact of Racism on Indigenous and Other Negatively Racialised Communities' Health Outcomes and Healthcare Access*

8 Royal Australian College of General Practitioners, 2025. *Reaffirming our Commitment to the Uluru Statement from the Heart.* 13 June

workers to reduce health disparities, promote cultural safety and cultural responsiveness in health organisations,[9] adopt a community-led service model that respects and incorporates Indigenous culture, and, of course, make sure these jobs are well remunerated,[10] plentiful,[11] sensitive to the diversity of Aboriginal cultures and regional variations[12] and Indigenous occupational wellbeing.[13] The policy leap is made that cultural safety is the preserve of Aboriginal community-controlled health services. It is argued to be the key weapon in the fight to close the health gap. In one definition, a culturally safe health system is

> *spiritually, socially and emotionally safe, as well as physically safe for people; where there is no assault, challenge or denial of their identity, of who they are and what they need.*
>
> *This extends beyond cultural 'awareness' and cultural 'sensitivity'. It requires that all human beings receive services that take into account all that makes them unique.*[14]

What makes a person unique is their DNA and response to their environment. Instead, the public health mindset prefers to chase down a rabbit hole. As early as 2007, medical deans were prevailed upon to provide a forum for medical educators in Aboriginal health.[15] In

---

9 Webster E et al, 2022. Building cultural responsiveness in a mainstream health organisation with '8 Aboriginal Ways of Learning': a participatory action research study. *Australian and New Zealand Journal of Public Health* 46, 517

10 Bailey J et al, 2020. 'We Are working for our people': growing and strengthening the Aboriginal and Torres Strait Islander health workforce, *Career Pathways Project Report*, Melbourne: The Lowitja Institute

11 Campbell M A et al. 2018. Contribution of Aboriginal community-controlled health services to improving Aboriginal health: an evidence review. *Australian Health Review* 42(2), 218

12 Scrimgeour M & Scrimgeour D, 2007. Health care access for Aboriginal and Torres Strait Islander people living in urban areas, and related research issues: a review of the literature. *Cooperative Research Centre for Aboriginal Health*, Darwin

13 Raciti M & Gibson C, 2025. A call to indigenise occupational wellbeing. *Medical Journal of Australia* 222 (11)16 June, 534

14 Quoted in Australian Indigenous Doctors' Association, 2017. *Report on the Findings of the 2016 AIDA Member Survey on Bullying, Racism and Lateral Violence in the Workplace*. Canberra, preface

15 Anderson I P S et al, 2009. Indigenous medical workforce development: current status and future directions. *Medical Journal of Australia* 190(10), 580

2015, the Aboriginal Health and Medical Research Council of NSW considered that 'culturally safe health care includes the provision of services underpinned by Indigenous Australians' beliefs and values.'[16] In 2016, the Australian Health Ministers' Advisory Council agreed to the proposition that 'the provision of culturally safe care is essential to meet the health care needs of Indigenous Australians effectively and requires health professionals to have considered power relations, cultural differences and patients' rights.' They also agreed that 'While the Indigenous workforce plays an important role in the provision of culturally appropriate services, it is the responsibility of the health-care system to ensure that mainstream health services are culturally competent through high-quality professional development and training, appropriate management where cultural respect is lacking, and staff developing awareness of their own unconscious bias.'[17] The latest iteration is the Lowitja Institute convening all health ministers of the nation to embed meaningful cultural safety through 'organisational truth-telling'.[18] Is there any basis for these confabulations?

Much of the cheering is promotional

Much of the literature in the field is designed to advocate for Aboriginal health workers. It lacks evidence that the specific intervention would improve the health of Aboriginal people. Each of the following studies has been quoted from the Australian Institute of Health and Welfare, an official government publication. For example, considering the barriers to nursing training in Queensland, the authors assert (emphasis added), 'The provision of a well-trained and *culturally safe* health workforce is critical to the alleviation of health inequities for Australian Indigenous

16 Aboriginal Health and Medical Research Council of NSW, 2015. *Aboriginal Communities Improving Aboriginal Health: An Evidence Review on the Contribution of Aboriginal Controlled Health Services to Improving Aboriginal Health*

17 Australian Health Ministers' Advisory Council, 2016. *Cultural Respect Framework for Aboriginal and Torres Strait Islander Health 2016 –2026: a National Approach to Building a Culturally Respectful Health System*

18 Lowitja Institute, 2024. *2024 Aboriginal and Torres Strait Islander Health Roundtable: Outcomes Report*, 11

peoples.' The reasoning is that 'Indigenous nurses bring a set of *unique skills, knowledge and understanding* to health service delivery. Their contribution has the *potential* to enhance future outcomes for Indigenous people by improving access to health services, ensuring services are *culturally appropriate* and respectful, and assisting non-Indigenous nurses to deliver *culturally appropriate* care.'[19] Others suggest a preference among Aborigines for care by Aboriginal health professionals, and *qualitative* research has shown that Aboriginal health staff *appeared to sustain better connection*, rapport and trust with Aboriginal patients[20] and *reduce their anxiety* and enhance communication.[21]

These various claims are repeated *ad infinitum* in the literature. Scant evidence exists that the claims contribute to closing the gap in health outcomes between Aboriginal and non-Aboriginal people. A culturally safe workforce may produce a culturally appropriate outcome, but does it necessarily lead to fewer instances of ill health? A study using a U.S. 'minority health survey' was lauded for its findings that people preferred a doctor of their race (race concordance). For example, 'people prefer seeing health professionals from the same ethnic background, and that improved health outcomes *can* result.' Delving a little deeper, however, the study concluded it is one thing in 'doctor-patient relationships to perceive a more engaging communication style, to express greater satisfaction with their health care or even perceive that they received better quality care, but it is quite another matter for patients' illness

19 West R, Usher K, & Foster K, 2010. Increased numbers of Australian Indigenous nurses would make a significant contribution to 'closing the gap' in indigenous health: what is getting in the way? *Contemporary Nurse* 36(1–2), 121

20 Hayman N, 1999. The poor health status of Aboriginal and Torres Strait Islander peoples. Can more indigenous doctors make a difference? *New Doctor* Summer, 19. de Witt A et al, 2018. 'It's just presence,' the contributions of Aboriginal and Torres Strait Islander health professionals in cancer care in Queensland. *Frontiers in Public Health* 6(1-8), Article 344

21 Freeman T et al, 2014. Cultural respect strategies in Australian Aboriginal primary health care services: beyond education and training of practitioners. *Australian and New Zealand Journal of Public Health* 38(4), 355

behavior *to be influenced by race concordance.*'[22]

Australian research claims that Aborigines want their health care to include Aboriginal staff and 'affirms the desire to hire and retain more Aboriginal health workers.'[23] Indeed, their absence is seen as a barrier to the accessibility, quality and effectiveness of healthcare. The obstacles to doing so are familiar: work environment, heavy workloads, poorly understood roles and responsibilities, low salary and a perception of salary disparity, and 'the influence of community as both a strong personal motivator and source of stress when work/life boundaries could not be maintained.'[24] This list would be familiar to any trade union representative of a medical workforce, but the latter elements are most intriguing. The 'influence of community' is a source of stress in a humbugging culture where a professional is pressured to look after their own first and foremost, not to mention share their income. Of course, it is stressful, and it is no surprise that those who escape 'community' to complete their studies may not return. None of this is mentioned in government reports, as it would be seen as a threat to the overarching theme of cultural safety. Real cultural safety would entail changing the community, not the profession.

Some studies claim to provide evidence of improved outcomes, but what kind of evidence? For example, Roseby and others suggested that Aboriginal health workers may help improve attendance at appointments.[25] As is often the case in this field, one study quotes another as proof. In this instance, they cited a Gwynne survey on the

---

22 LaVeist T A, Nuru-Jeter A & Jones K E, 2003. The association of doctor-patient race concordance with health services utilization. *Journal of Public Health Policy* 24(3-4), 312

23 Aspin C et al, 2012. Strategic approaches to enhanced health service delivery for Aboriginal and Torres Strait Islander people with chronic illness: a qualitative study. *BMC Health Services Research* 12, 143

24 Lai G C et al, 2018. Factors affecting the retention of Indigenous Australians in the health workforce: a systematic review. *International Journal of Environmental Research and Public Health* 15(5), 1

25 Roseby R et al, 2019. Not just a policy; this is for real. An affirmative action policy to encourage Aboriginal and Torres Strait Islander peoples to seek employment in the health workforce. *Internal Medicine Journal* 49(7), 908

recruitment and retention of Aboriginal health workers; however, the study provided no evidence of improved attendance at appointments.[26] A survey by Jongen and others, undertaken at the Gurriny Yealamucka Health Service in Yarrabah, North Queensland, involved interviews with 17 staff from Aboriginal community-controlled health organisations (ACCHOs).[27] They mapped out strategies such as strong leadership and growing capability, but provided no evidence of effectiveness. Various benefits were proposed, including acceptance of treatment, reduced discharge against medical advice, increased patient contact time, enhanced referrals, and improved follow-up, which would result from Aboriginal control and staffing.[28] To support their claim, they cited a study by Taylor and others aimed at enhancing Aboriginal inpatient care and improving the utilisation of outpatient cardiac rehabilitation at a tertiary hospital in Western Australia. One Aboriginal health worker was recruited. The impact of the recruitment was assessed through interviews with the cardiology Aboriginal health worker, other hospital staff, including another Aboriginal health worker, and recent Aboriginal cardiac patients. The impact of the health worker 'included facilitating culturally appropriate care, bridging communication divides, reducing discharges against medical advice, providing cultural education, increasing inpatient contact time, improving follow-up practices and enhancing patient referral linkages.'[29] The study claimed to demonstrate that Aboriginal health workers 'can have significant impacts on Aboriginal cardiac inpatient experiences and outpatient care.'[30] But no hard evidence was reported.

Another study referenced by the Australian Institute of Health and

26 Gwynne K & Lincoln M, 2017. Developing the rural health workforce to improve Australian Aboriginal and Torres Strait Islander health outcomes: a systematic review. *Australian Health Review* 41(2), 234

27 Jongen C et al, 2019. Working well: strategies to strengthen the workforce of the indigenous primary healthcare sector. *BMC Health Services Research* 19(910), 3

28 Jongen C et al, 2019, 2

29 Taylor K P et al, 2009. Exploring the impact of an Aboriginal health worker on hospitalised Aboriginal experiences: lessons from cardiology. *Australian Health Review* 33(4), 549

30 Taylor K P et al, 2009, 549

Welfare review suggested *preliminary evidence* of the *potential* for Aboriginal health workers to improve diabetes screening. It was preliminary indeed. The study, by Murray and others, found nothing more than that 'Screening for diabetic retinopathy performed locally by Aboriginal health workers and nurses with fundus cameras can be successfully sustained with regional support.'[31] Nothing is reported about better outcomes with Aboriginal health workers compared to other health workers. The literature about the impact of Aboriginal health workers on Aboriginal health outcomes abounds with the phrase *preliminary evidence shows potential for.* Indeed, a study in palliative care of Aboriginal patients at a facility in the Kimberley was typical. Interviews with staff and carers amounted to little more than a plea for more hiring. For example,

> *The other problem we have with our respite is Aboriginal women working in the respite, where they can't get on with that family because the older one [will] tell you [what to do all the time] and they [are] real demanding at that stage, when they get older [and] grumpy. They want a family member working there like from that group, clan group or tribal group ... They like to see their own people looking after them.*[32]

These sentiments are quite understandable, but they could apply to all people in need rather than serving as a rationale for employing a particular group.

Participants in a Brisbane study of government-controlled Aboriginal medical services and Aboriginal community-controlled services reported marked health improvements in their communities due to the establishment of these services, as well as their role in addressing

31 Murray R B et al, 2005. Sustaining remote-area programs: retinal camera use by Aboriginal health workers and nurses in a Kimberley partnership. *Medical Journal of Australia* 182(10), 520

32 McGrath et al, 2007. The case for Aboriginal health workers in palliative care. *Australian Health Review* 31(3), 430

the adverse health effects of discrimination.[33] But there are no actual measurements of improvements. Two focus group discussions were conducted with clients of two health services, involving 11 participants in one service and 10 in the other. There were the usual bromides. 'Participants of this study spoke very highly of the health services they accessed, and how these issues are addressed through the provision of culturally appropriate and evidence-based services.'[34] Would it not be sensible to interview those who were not attending these services as a control group? Regarding measures of outcome, one general practitioner service reported a significant increase in clientele following the successful integration of cultural safety principles. No study was made; it was simply the word of a practitioner — and what practitioner would be brave enough to say that these holy cultural safety principles had done nothing? No evidence was presented to substantiate the claim that recognising the practitioners' cultural biases resulted in dramatic increases in Aboriginal clientele.[35] Were there other factors that drove the increase? Did another clinic in the area close? Were they a service that bulk-billed where others did not? One interviewee praised the clinic for its care of her mother's diabetes because she 'got diagnosed here and they've done everything for her here.' In contrast, the interviewee patient had not received the same care elsewhere. Might that not be a common reason why patients consider moving surgeries? Public health loves to say that the absence of evidence does not mean evidence of absence. It is easy to see why.

Cultural safety is an impossibly high bar to achieve, and there is weak evidence that it improves health outcomes. Cultural safety may serve as an incentive for people not to perform their professional duties, yet the claims for its efficacy are repeated endlessly. These become the measures of success rather than the health outcomes of those who use the health

---

33 Baba J T et al, 2014. Aboriginal medical services cure more than illness: a qualitative study of how Indigenous services address the health impacts of discrimination in Brisbane communities. *International Journal for Equity in Health* 13:56

34 Baba J T et al, 2014, 4

35 Baba J T et al, 2014, 5

facilities run by Aboriginal community-controlled organisations. And so public health champions something ideologically pleasing and virtue signalling, that has no demonstrated impact on actual health. Who cares if health outcomes are not shifting if public health is seen as progressive?

Is there more substantial evidence to prove NACCHO's claims?

The National Aboriginal Community Controlled Health Organisation (NACCHO) is the national peak body representing 146 Aboriginal community-controlled health organisations across Australia. They make many claims to be effective organisations, and that the more of them there are, the better Aboriginal clients would be served. For example, it claims that 16 per cent of Aboriginal and Torres Strait Islander people said they wanted to access an Aboriginal community-controlled service but were unable to do so, where they were living.[36] This claim could not be found in the reference provided. Nevertheless, it may be true, but it must be compared with other reasons for non-attendance. In 2018–19, 30 per cent of Aboriginal people reported that they needed to but did not see a health care provider on at least one occasion in the previous 12 months, about the same as for all patients reported in a later survey.[37] The reasons were that they were too busy (36 per cent) or could not afford it (34 per cent), and this was higher in non-remote areas (36 per cent) than in remote areas (21 per cent). Further, 23 per cent said they disliked the service or were embarrassed or afraid – a higher percentage in non-remote areas (24 per cent) compared with remote areas (15 per cent).[38] The latter figure supports the argument that some patients would prefer to attend a service where they were not embarrassed or afraid. These are important considerations, but of course, they do not discount the possibility that they were embarrassed or scared to attend a particular

36 National Aboriginal Community Controlled Health Organisation, 2025. *Key Facts February 2025,* 6. The figure quoted was 20 per in the 2024 report, same reference cited.

37 Australian Bureau of Statistics, 2025. *Patient Experiences*

38 Australian Institute of Health & Welfare and National Indigenous Australians Agency, 2024.

Aboriginal community-controlled service.

Some Aborigines may prefer a community-controlled service, but is it for the wrong reasons, or under a misapprehension that it will deliver 'traditional' medicine? The anthropologist Peter Sutton reported that healers are still employed by government-funded health services, which entails both the recognition of custom and its denial: healers deny science, while the health service utilises it.[39] Sutton made clear that 'well-meaning whitefellas who support traditional doctors in their quest to peel back the postcolonial power differential have to face the fact that … traditional healers … are likely to constitute a danger to the already disastrous health of their communities.'[40] Dr Patrick Maher of the Northern Rehabilitation Network, Royal Darwin Hospital, has offered an insight into the persistence of traditional practices and passive resistance to Western medicine. He instructed new practitioners to be aware that the Aboriginal model of causation often meant that the priority was not individual health, but the discharge of social obligations. For example, a car accident may create a web of blame quite removed from the actual cause. By contrast, serious illness, especially for those other than the frail aged or infants, may be attributed to supernatural causes or a breach of a taboo.[41] Wanting to attend a community-controlled health service may have nothing to do with improving health.

Numerous claims are made about the economics of Aboriginal community-controlled health services. For example, NACCHO complained that compared to similar-sized general practice clinics, community-controlled clinics received $920,000 less in mainstream funding each year ($0.56 million vs $1.48 million). The reason for this gap, however, is that the Baseline Practice Payment is not intended to replace other forms of block funding that some primary care organisations receive outside the Practice Incentives Program and

39 Sutton P, 2006. Custom not in common: cultural relativism and customary law. *Macquarie Law Bulletin* 6, 162

40 Sutton P, 2006, 163

41 Maher P, 1999. A review of 'traditional' Aboriginal health beliefs. *Australian Journal of Rural Health* 7(4), 229

Workforce Incentive Practice schemes. For example, the community-controlled sector receives block funding through the Indigenous Australians' Health Programme.[42] Additionally, significant costs are associated with specialist services, and since the local GP refers people to these specialists, it is not necessary to fund the centres for these purposes.

It is also claimed that Aboriginal people have a caseload with greater health needs and a 2.3 times higher burden of disease, resulting in higher costs.[43] There is no doubt that health needs, on average, are higher for many Aboriginal people.[44] If crude economics is applied, it is possible to claim a huge gap in funding, suggesting that Aboriginal health should be funded for every ailment.[45] The answer to most Aboriginal ailments, however, relates to lifestyle choices,[46] and the expenditure to change these is not the same as the endpoint medical interventions suggested.

Most important are the claims of cost-effectiveness. 'Our cost benefit per dollar spent is $1.19. In remote areas, our cost benefit can be fourfold. The lifetime health impact of interventions delivered by [Aboriginal community-controlled health services] is 50 per cent greater than that of mainstream health services.'[47] These claims were based on the research by Vos and others. In their study, however, Vos concluded that there was a lack of quantitative evidence on the costs and effectiveness of interventions delivered through community-controlled services, on which to base economic evaluations. Vos and others based their work on the Aboriginal subset on costs, as well as participation and adherence assumptions from Ong (discussed below). The Vos study concentrated

42 Expert Advisory Panel Report to the Australian Government, 2024. *Review of General Practice Incentives*, 20

43 NACCHO, 2025. *Key Facts February 2025*, 7

44 Alford K, 2014. *Investing in Aboriginal Community Controlled Health Makes Economic Sense*. National Aboriginal Community Controlled Health Organisation

45 Equity Economics, 2022. *Measuring the Gap in Health Expenditure: Aboriginal and Torres Strait Islander Australians*. NACCHO, 6

46 Australian Institute of Health and Welfare, 2024. *Determinants of Health for First Nations People*

47 NACCHO, 2025. *Key Facts February 2025*, 7

on the effectiveness of health interventions, most of which recommended tobacco and alcohol taxes. It admitted that these may not be effective in Aboriginal communities.[48] The Vos study had an altogether different purpose than the one NACCHO claimed. None of these explanations accounts for the significantly poorer health of remote and very remote Aborigines compared to those in cities.

The Australian Institute of Health and Welfare is not the only institution to claim that there is growing evidence that Aboriginal community-controlled health services can improve outcomes for Aboriginal and Torres Strait Islander people.[49] The Productivity Commission, in its review of Closing the Gap, has fallen into the same trap, confusing ideological outcomes with health outcomes. It is unclear what evidence the Commission relied on to support the claim of growing evidence. There is no indication of whether the evidence was robust, and — where it was positive — whether it could be applied to all community-controlled services across all Aboriginal communities. The Commission supported a submission by NACCHO in their inquiry, which placed great weight on a 2012 study by Ong and others that found services delivered by Aboriginal community-controlled services increased intervention costs, utilisation, and treatment adherence rates.[50] However, the study provided a mechanism by which intervention data obtained from mainstream sources could be adapted to facilitate its economic evaluation *as if it were* delivered from a community service.[51] This is not definitive proof of superior service outcomes.

The Ong study relied on highly qualified estimates, such as the enhanced rate at which Aboriginal people use Aboriginal community-controlled services.

---

48 Vos T, Carter R & Barendregt J, 2010. *Assessing Cost-effectiveness in Prevention ACE: Prevention Final Report*. Brisbane: University of Queensland

49 Productivity Commission, 2024. *Review of the National Agreement on Closing the Gap Study Report: Supporting Paper Volume 2*, 64

50 Ong K et al, 2012. Differences in primary health care delivery to Australia's indigenous population: a template for use in economic evaluations. *BMC Health Services Research* 12(1), 1

51 Ong K et al, 2012, 5

> *It is impossible to know ... how much of this difference is a reflection of under-identification of Indigenous people... or to what extent it represents lower use of GP services by Indigenous Australians.*[52]

In other words, no weight should be given to the claim of higher utilisation rates by Aboriginal community-controlled services. The study also quoted two sources for estimates of adherence: the rate at which Aboriginal people continue their medication and other health regimes when they use Aboriginal community-controlled services. The first study estimated childhood immunisation rates.[53] This study did not mention Aboriginal community-controlled services. The second study estimated immunisation rates for different social classes and groups, including Aboriginal ones. It did not refer to Aboriginal community-controlled services.[54] It did not identify immunisation rates in remote areas. Instead, it quoted from another study, a North Queensland survey of Aboriginal children and their vaccinations, which concluded that the 'vaccination status of Indigenous children who reside in remote communities is substantially better than that of Indigenous children from either rural towns or urban settings.'[55] The North Queensland study could not explain the better result for the remote setting. By contrast, a later study using the Australian Childhood Immunisation Register concluded a 'clear trend in coverage for Indigenous children by remoteness was not evident.'[56]

Another example the Productivity Commission relied on was a study

---

52 Trewin D & Madden R, 2005. *The Health and Welfare of Australia's Aboriginal and Torres Strait Islander Peoples*. Australian Bureau of Statistics, 105

53 Hull B et al, 2004. Evaluation of immunisation coverage for Aboriginal and Torres Strait Islander children using the Australian Childhood Immunisation Register. *Australian and New Zealand Journal of Public Health* 28(1), 47

54 Haynes K & Stone C, 2004. Predictors of incomplete immunisation in Victorian children. *Australian and New Zealand Journal of Public Health*, 28(1), 78

55 Hanna J, 1998. The vaccination status of Aboriginal and Torres Strait Island children in Far North Queensland. *Australian and New Zealand Journal of Public Health* 22(6), 667

56 Rank C & Menzies R, 2007. How reliable are Australian childhood immunisation register coverage estimates for indigenous children? An assessment of data quality and coverage. *Communicable Diseases Intelligence* 31(3), 286

by Pearson of the health equity ambitions of Aboriginal community-controlled services, which they assert 'provide culturally informed, holistic health services that directly and indirectly address the social determinants of health.'[57] The study consisted of a textual analysis of annual reports of 67 Aboriginal community-controlled services. The social determinants of health methodology was applied; however, as discussed in Chapter 2, this observation does not provide a solution to how the poor can become less poor, which is not a medical issue. In the Aboriginal context, it drifts into the belief that only Aboriginal organisations can help.

The Aboriginal-led Pearson team looked for evidence among the annual reports that activity aimed to influence 'societal values towards greater inclusion of Aboriginal people.' An example of this was an Aboriginal community-controlled service that hosted 'cultural immersions for key external service partners and members of government.' Another was 'a working partnership with students and staff from [a local private school] in painting a mural.' Another, while addressing clinical care 'held a men's painting group ... addressing cultural, spiritual and social wellbeing.' The study concluded that social capital and social cohesion were enhanced, such as when 'regular community meetings and events were introduced so that all members and the broader community can meet with Board and management representatives.'[58] Actual health outcomes were not reported, a prime example of how public health tends to confuse health with an ideological goal that has nothing to do with health. Another consequence of accepting the right of Aboriginal community-controlled services to deliver services is that experienced providers vacate the field and weaken the level of provision to Aboriginal people. For example, Life Without Barriers, Australia's largest out-of-home care provider, has ceded service delivery for Aboriginal children to community control. They hope that the 'commitment to transition children to community

57 Pearson O et al, 2020. Aboriginal community-controlled health organisations address health equity through action on the social determinants of health of Aboriginal and Torres Strait Islander peoples in Australia. *BMC Public Health* 20, 1859

58 Pearson O et al, 2020, 1859

control will ensure they grow up strong in family, kin, and culture.'[59] It is no consolation to Aboriginal people hoping for a better outcome if they receive worse or no services because of this commitment.

The totality of NACCHO's claims does not hold. In any event, could it be argued that these services are the same when they are locally controlled? In addition, Western medicine is delivered by non-Aboriginal staff. Aborigines make up 51 per cent of the workforce in Commonwealth-funded Aboriginal primary health care organisations, with nearly all these employees employed at Aboriginal community-controlled services. Fewer than five per cent were doctors or nurses, and 29 per cent were administrative staff. Thirteen per cent were Aboriginal and Torres Strait Islander health workers, including individuals with a minimum qualification in primary health care work or clinical practice. Eight per cent were Aboriginal and Torres Strait Islander Health practitioners who had completed a Certificate IV in Aboriginal and Torres Strait Islander Primary Health Care (Practice).[60] In other words, the outcome that has been achieved is that most health care workers in Aboriginal services are not Aboriginal, but they get Aboriginal people to do their paperwork for them. Public health's answer to that has been to successfully lobby to lower the entry standards for Aboriginal people entering medical courses and to make it easier to earn those degrees. Why is it right by public health for Aboriginal people to be treated by workers who have had less rigorous standards applied to them than the standards applied to non-Aboriginal health workers? Could it be that, beneath public health's veneer of caring for the less fortunate, the lot of the less fortunate is not the primary concern?

59 Life Without Barriers, 2022. *Elevate Reconciliation Action Plan 2022-2025*, 63

60 Australian Institute of Health & Welfare and National Indigenous Australians Agency, 2024. *Aboriginal and Torres Strait Islander Health Performance Framework, 3.12*

Actual evaluations

A study by Harfield and others provides a comprehensive description of the elements aimed at producing better outcomes for Aboriginal patients in an Aboriginal community-controlled health service (Figure 7.1).[61] Identifying possible factors that contribute to better outcomes is the first step, but is each element necessary, and can we distinguish the impact of each component? Are all these required for the magic to occur? For example, the Katherine West Coordinated Care Trial evaluation sought to test whether funds managed by the newly established Katherine West Health Board Aboriginal Corporation in 1997 would lead to Aboriginal control over the provision of services, whether fund pooling would increase resources, improve care co-ordination, improve administration and in turn whether these would lead to improved health screening and greater adherence to plans by diabetes sufferers. The difficulty in evaluating the improvement was that several factors coincided, and none alone could account for the change in health outcomes. More funds, pooling, better coordination, the appointment of administrative officers to assist nurses, and the establishment of the Board were not distinguishable. Did the Aboriginalisation of the Board make any difference, were their skills superior to others, would their or other services have been better utilised under other arrangements, would anything different have happened but for the extra funds, or the agreement to coordinate? Unless each contributing element can be determined, it is impossible to determine what creates a service that yields the best outcomes. No results were recorded for improved screening or greater adherence.

61 Harfield S G et al, 2018. Characteristics of indigenous primary health care service delivery models: a systematic scoping review. *Globalization and Health* 14(1), 12

Figure 7.1 Characteristics of Indigenous Primary Health Care Service Delivery Model

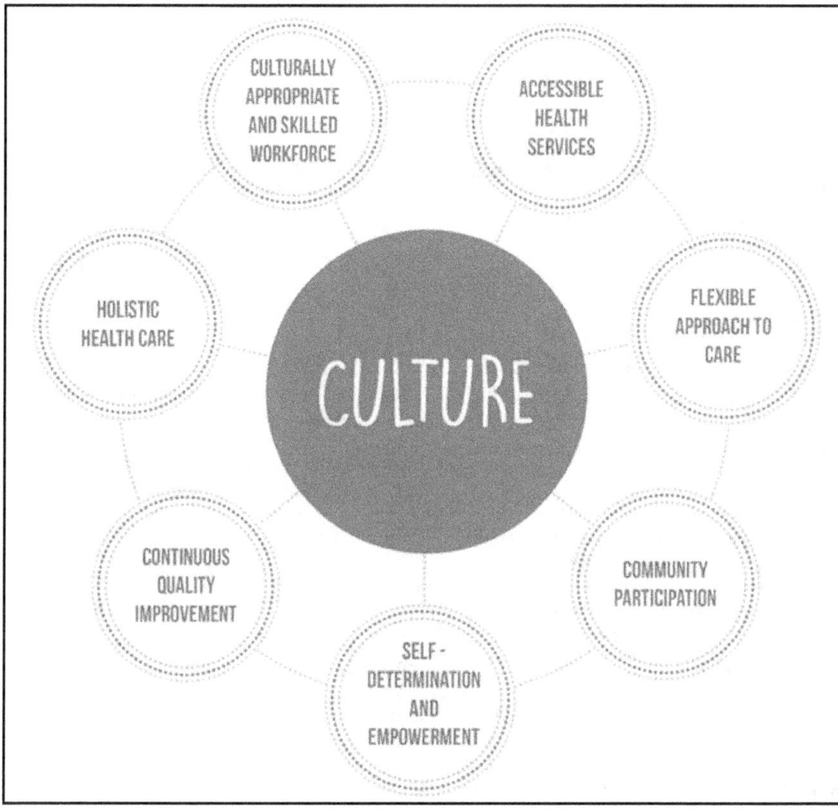

Source: Harfield S G et al, 2018. Characteristics of indigenous primary health care service delivery models: a systematic scoping review. *Globalization and Health* 14(1), 6

Birthing on Country (in Our Community (BiOC)) is a case study of a best-practice Aboriginal maternity service in Brisbane. Birthing on Country is used as a metaphor for the best start in life for Aboriginal and Torres Strait Islander babies.[62] The evaluation of the Birthing on Country, at Mater Mothers' Public Hospital, Brisbane, and the BiOC Community Hub located in Salisbury, Brisbane, aimed to answer the research question: for women pregnant with an Aboriginal baby, does

62 Kildea S, 2018. Birthing on Country (in Our Community): a case study of engaging stakeholders and developing a best-practice Indigenous maternity service in an urban setting. *Australian Health Review* 42, 230

an Aboriginal-led maternity BiOC decrease the likelihood of babies being removed by Child Protection Services (CPS) at birth, compared to women who received standard care?[63]

Table 7.1 Compare Birthing in Our Community to standard care, Brisbane 2013 to 2019

Birthing in Our Community service	Standard care
Aboriginal steering committee.	No Aboriginal governance.
Dedicated manager, community based hub, operated by the Institute for Urban Indigenous Health.	The service operates from the hospital, electronic correspondence between agencies.
Midwifery Group Practice, primary midwife providing 24/7 continuity of carer by a midwife throughout pregnancy, birth and up to six weeks postnatally.	Birthing support likely to be by a midwife the woman has never met. Can call hospital birthing suite in emergency. Postnatal visit or phone call from a rostered community midwife usually for <2weeks.
Aboriginal Family Support Worker through pregnancy and postnatal period.	None
Aboriginal governance, leadership and workforce all support a strong framework of cultural safety.	Frontline staff may seek out their own cultural training or clinical supervision, not routinely provided.
Transport services provided by Aboriginal staff employed through the BiOC	None
Women and infants can access the majority of specialist and allied health services at the BiOC Hub.	Women may be referred to allied health services.

Source: O'Dea B et al, 2024. Breaking the cycle: effect of a multi-agency maternity service redesign on reducing the over-representation of Aboriginal and Torres Strait Islander newborns in out-of-home care: a prospective, non-randomised, intervention study in urban Australia. *Child Abuse & Neglect* 149(106664), 3

The evaluation was not based on a random or controlled selection of cases; however, the researchers took great care to ensure that the two cohorts, those in the hospital and those in the community centre, had similar propensities for a child to be removed. For example, mothers who were more likely to have their baby removed were more likely to be Aboriginal, have lower educational attainment, be without a partner,

63 O'Dea B et al, 2024, 2

report use of illicit drugs in pregnancy, smoke in pregnancy, have major worries or stressors in the previous 12 months, have prior involvement with child protection services (CPS), have children living in the care of other people, have experienced domestic violence, or have pre-existing mental health issues.

Between 2013 and 2019, 1988 women gave birth to 2044 Aboriginal babies, with 40 women having babies removed at birth, nine from BiOC and 31 from standard care. This is an excellent and statistically valid result, and if replicated, it would give hope that the cycle of despair among too many Aboriginal families can be broken. Was the success achieved because of Aboriginal control, or was it the extra resources and attention brought to bear on what was a cohort of mothers with enormous problems, as shown in Table 7.1 (where differences are underlined)? Unfortunately, no control group was included to test that possibility. The researchers describe the BiOC as an Aboriginal-owned community hub providing 'continuity of midwifery care with First Nations governance, supported by a First Nations workforce under a First Nations cultural safety framework, providing holistic and coordinated wrap-around services.'[64] Family Support Workers are community women employed in the model to work closely with families and midwives to improve access to safe housing and financial, legal, and other supports when needed (e.g., transport, food vouchers).

Women accessing BiOC services were less likely to have their babies removed. Still, was it because of 'access to an Indigenous-led model of comprehensive community-based maternity care, supported by continuity of midwifery care and underpinned by Indigenous cultural governance, safety, and workforce was protective', or was it due to more resources? Was it Aboriginal 'ways of knowing, being and doing' that created an opportunity to deliver 'culturally appropriate, strengths-based, respectful care, responsive to the specific needs of the community it aims to serve', or was it more money? Was it the belief in 'holistic health and wellbeing, which requires more considered responses inclusive of

64 O'Dea B et al, 2024, 3

culturally appropriate programs and wrap-around supports', or was it more money, time and effort?

Would any mothers at risk respond more favourably when showered with such attention? Should every community or identity group be similarly showered with resources of an appropriate type of care? At the same time, the rest of the Brisbane mothers had only the attention of the Mater Hospital staff. A possible further hole in the analysis is that children removed from their mothers sometime after birth were not reported.

The official evaluation

A systematic review on the scope and quality of economic evaluations of Aboriginal and Torres Strait Islander health programs undertaken by Doran and others concluded that 'despite significant investment in strategies to close the gap in health outcomes for Aboriginal and Torres Strait Islander people, there is limited evidence about what constitutes a cost-effective investment in Aboriginal and Torres Strait Islander health care.'[65] The same appears to be true of official evaluations, such as the Australian Government Department of Health's Indigenous Australians' Health Programme (IAHP) Economic Evaluation Phase One, which was published in mid-2018. It focused on the return on investment of the IAHP, as measured by potentially preventable hospitalisations, and on the relative costs of Aboriginal-specific compared with non-Aboriginal-specific primary health care services.[66] The report showed that higher attendance at Aboriginal community-controlled health services reduced the likelihood of hospital admission, while also providing health benefits. It concluded that, while the provision of care through mainstream services may be cheaper, 'it is likely to be associated with worse health outcomes due to less comprehensive and integrated care that may not be culturally

65 Doran C M et al, 2022. Scope and quality of economic evaluations of Aboriginal and Torres Strait Islander health programs: a systematic review. *Australian and New Zealand Journal of Public Health* 46, 361

66 See also, Australian Institute of Health and Welfare, 2025. *Aboriginal and Torres Strait Islander Specific Primary Health Care: Results from the Online Service Reports and National Key Performance Indicators Collections*

competent and may not meet patients' needs and expectations.'[67] These findings were used to demonstrate the cost-effectiveness of Aboriginal community-controlled health services, but methodological constraints limited them. For example, the Dalton paper relied on Ong's methodology to assess the cost savings from preventing hospitalisations following care in Aboriginal community-controlled health services. It accepted much higher costs for primary care in Aboriginal remote settings, not only because of remote expenses, but also due to the holistic nature of Aboriginal community-controlled health services care. So, was there a payoff in terms of keeping people out of the hospital?

The analysis revealed that a modest reduction in hospitalisation rates was associated with Aboriginal community-controlled health services; however, the methodological approach had significant limitations.[68] Notably, the evaluation was concerned that a mere conventional economic evaluation was used, which reflected 'a biomedical model approach to quantifying health gains'. The evaluation pleaded the case that these 'should ideally be a social model of health that reflects the holistic approach to health most valued by Aboriginal and Torres Strait Islander peoples.' Indeed, a challenge for the development of IAHP funding policy was to 'resolve the tension between the conventional approach of governments that analyses the performance of non-Aboriginal programs through … financial efficiency and effectiveness, and the needs and preferences of the Aboriginal and Torres Strait Islander communities.'[69] In other words, governments are stuck in a world of their own making, following an ideology that eschews valid evaluation, incurs significant costs and results in greater ownership of medical approaches, property, and organisations, but does not necessarily lead to better health outcomes. Public health officials should be briefing their ministers about this, but instead, they are actively facilitating more of the same.

---

67 Dalton A, 2018. *Economic Evaluation of the Indigenous Australians' Health Programme Phase I.* Deakin Health Economics Centre for Population Health Research, Faculty of Health Deakin University

68 Dalton A, 2018, 5

69 Dalton A, 2018, 5

The Phase One evaluation was announced in 2017, but apart from the tentative report of mid-2018, there has been no further update. The answer to this excessive delay probably lies in the fact that the evaluation drew on the 'perspectives' of Aboriginal and Torres Strait Islander stakeholders, so that as of 2024, the Department of Health and Aged Care was working with the IAHP Yarnes Health Sector Co-design Group on finalising the evaluation. At present, the Department of Health, Disability and Ageing has stated on its website that it is 'evaluating investments in Aboriginal and Torres Strait Islander primary health care through the Indigenous Australians' Health Programme which funds Aboriginal Community Controlled Health Services and that they expected the evaluation to speed up progress towards Closing the Gap'[70] While the evaluation was completed by a consultancy in 2023,[71] the Department has not publicly acknowledged this nor responded to or acted on the report.[72]

Conclusion

The public health lobby is very concerned about Aboriginal health – or so they like everybody to know. Unfortunately, they, along with government departments, have promoted the ruse that culture is a substitute for health, working through magical pathways of social determinants. Of course, there are Aboriginal people whose behaviour and understanding of the causes of their ills are so minimal that they need special attention. Still, the game of catering to special needs and handing over ownership of taxpayer resources to Aboriginal community-controlled agencies has not closed the gap. Nor is it likely that the gap will close until and unless the public health industry decides that actual health outcomes are more important than being seen to be progressive.

70 https://www.health.gov.au/topics/aboriginal-and-torres-strait-islander-health/primary-care/evaluations#iahp-primary-health-care-system-evaluation as of 5 June 2025

71 Confirmed to the author by the consultant.

72 https://allenandclarke.com.au/project/evaluation-of-the-indigenous-australians-health-program/ as of 5 June 2025

8

Mental Health and NDIS: diagnostic inflation

Patrick McGorrie[1] and Ian Hickie[2] argue that the mental health of young Australians represents a public health crisis. McGorrie argues that despite the 'scale and urgency of the crisis', the political will is yet to emerge to solve it.[3] Is it accurate to say that a response is yet to emerge? If the bottom line is that every young Australian should receive the medical care that they and clinicians desire, then McGorrie is correct. But do young people need what McGorrie, Hickie, and their fellows are promoting? The real world of limited resources and competing priorities, such as the crises in public hospitals,[4] aged care[5], the rise in disability and the NDIS response,[6] in health care alone threaten Australia's public finances. An ageing population may account for inadequacies in hospitals and aged care. More visits to doctors have also placed resources under pressure; since Medicare was introduced in 1984, visits to general

1 Patrick McGorrie is Professor of Youth Mental Health at the University of Melbourne and founding editor of the journal Early Intervention in Psychiatry.

2 Ian Hickie is a Professor of Psychiatry and the Co-Director of Health and Policy, Brain and Mind Centre, University of Sydney. See Hickie I B et al, 2025. Novel youth mental health services in Australia: what differences are being reported about the clinical needs of those who attend and the outcomes achieved? *Australian & New Zealand Journal of Psychiatry* 59(2), 99

3 McGorry P D et al, 2024. The Lancet Psychiatry Commission on youth mental health. *The Lancet Psychiatry* 11(9), 731

4 Australian Medical Association, 2025. *Public Hospital Report Card*

5 Committee for the Economic Development of Australia, 2022. *Duty Of Care: Aged Care Sector in Crisis*

6 National Disability Insurance Agency, 2024. *Annual Report 2023–24*

practitioners have increased from 3.8 to 6.8 per person per year,[7] and visits to other medical professionals have also ballooned.[8] Public health sees it as a win that people want more medical attention and continue to promote new illnesses. Given the budget deficit and the ongoing demands for service, is there room for further investment in health at the current standard of living? And has public health contributed to creating the very crises it seeks to fix, to maintain its seat at the table?

Mental health

Political leaders addressing disability and mental health, especially psychiatric disability, must consider all other demands on the public purse. The relatively latecomers to this discussion – disability and mental health, particularly youth mental health – confront significant questions. To what extent does diagnostic and prevalence inflation influence their claims to public resources? The Diagnostic and Statistical Manual of Mental Disorders (DSM), published by the American Psychiatric Association,[9] has long been viewed as the authoritative reference for diagnosis. Allen Frances dedicated twenty years to periodically updating the DSM. In 2013, as work on DSM-V was set to begin, he concluded that the DSM 'had become too powerful for its own good and for society's.'[10] He was concerned that it cast an overly broad diagnostic net, potentially creating false epidemics and generating millions of new patients. He described this phenomenon as diagnostic inflation and argued that excessive treatment is given to the worried well, who ultimately suffer from it.

> *[D]espite our efforts to tame excessive diagnostic exuberance, DSM-IV had since been misused to blow up the diagnostic bubble. Even though we had been boringly modest in our goals, obsessively meticulous*

---

7 Australian Institute of Health and Welfare, 2024. *General Practice, Allied Health and other Primary Care Services*

8 Australian Institute of Health and Welfare, *General Practice*, 2024.

9 Other manuals exist, for example, the *World Health Organization International Classification of Diseases*, Tenth Revision

10 Frances A, 2013, 83

> *in our methods, and rigidly conservative in our product, we failed to predict or prevent three new false epidemics of mental disorder in children—autism, attention deficit, and childhood bipolar disorder. And we did nothing to contain the rampant diagnostic inflation that was already expanding.*[11]

Lucy Foulkes and Jack Andrews have suggested that 'mental health problems and awareness efforts are affecting each other in a cyclical, intensifying manner.'[12] Increased rates of mental health problems drive more awareness efforts, but the awareness efforts might lead to increased reporting and symptoms. They coined the term prevalence inflation to describe this cycle. If people are repeatedly told that mental health problems are common and that they might experience them – and this is especially true for young people who frequently receive mental health information in schools and through their peers – then it makes sense that they might start to interpret any negative thoughts and feelings through this lens.[13]

Whatever the credibility of the proposed causes of an increase in the prevalence of mental health disorders, for example, technology and social media,[14] inequality[15] and climate change,[16] the very act of making others more aware of these disorders through improved recognition and overinterpretation may be driving a propensity to seek a diagnosis. Improved recognition may be legitimate, but awareness arguably encourages overinterpretation. Where there is overinterpretation, the

---

11 Frances A, 2013, 85

12 Foulkes L & Andrews J L, 2023. Are mental health awareness efforts contributing to the rise in reported mental health problems? A call to test the prevalence inflation hypothesis. *New Ideas in Psychology* 69(10110)

13 Foulkes L & Andrews J L, 2023, 3

14 Twenge J M, 2025. *Generations: The Real Differences Between Gen Z, Millennials, Gen X, Boomers, and Silents—and What They Mean for America's Future*. Atria Paperback

15 Kirkbride J B et al, 2024. The social determinants of mental health and disorder: evidence, prevention and recommendations. *World Psychiatry* 23(1), 58

16 Hickman, C et al, 2021. Climate anxiety in children and young people and their beliefs about government responses to climate change: a global survey. *The Lancet Planetary Health* 5(12), e863

result is serious mental health problems competing with lesser mental health problems (or the 'worried well' as many psychologists privately term them).

A stunning illustration of diagnosis and prevalence inflation is the advocacy of Suicide Prevention Australia (SPA), which advocates for a National Suicide Prevention Act, to ensure that 'every government department and official, whether in housing, education, social security, or health, must consider suicide prevention when conducting their work.'[17] SPA backs up its claims with an online survey suggesting that 19 per cent of Australians (18-34) have experienced suicidal distress in the last 12 months, including 'having serious thoughts of suicide, making a suicide plan, or attempting to take their life.'[18] Deaths by suicide are statistically rare events, but suicide is the invincible bogeyman that public health relies on, and arriving at big numbers is the key to the advocacy game. In 2023, 298 Australian young people (aged 18–24 years) died by suicide. Suicide is the leading cause of death among Australians aged 15–24 years because people in these age groups do not tend to die from other causes.[19] The SPA took a sample of adults, online, from which they derived a subset for 18-24 year olds, which contains an undefined concept of suicidal distress, which includes serious thoughts of suicide. These very small numbers and poorly defined concepts may well suit the definition of inflationary prevalence, not to mention that people who complete online surveys are frequently not representative of the general population, and tend to take part in specific surveys because they have some form of experience or perspective that makes that survey seem relevant to them.

SPA makes clear, quite correctly, that many people who lose their

17 Suicide Prevention Australia, 2025. *National Policy Platform*, 10

18 Suicide Prevention Australia, Young Australians demand political action on suicide prevention. *Media Release* 6 March 2025. A nationally representative sample of 1,516 Australian Citizens/Voters aged 18 years and older was undertaken by YouGov Australia between 3–10 of February 2025.

19 Australian Institute of Health and Welfare, 2023. *Deaths By Suicide Among Young People*

lives to suicide do not have a mental health condition. The non-mental health factors that increase the risk of suicide include childhood abuse, addiction, bereavement, financial crisis, insecure housing, low education, unemployment, stressful life events in general, and social isolation. Suicide prevention is important, but the contributors to suicide are so diverse, and also experienced by so many people who do not become suicidal, that passing an Act that is meant to force all government departments to think about suicide prevention seems a meaningless way to tackle the problem. However, such an Act would give public health even greater authority to comment on, and meddle in, any aspect of daily life – not to mention government decision making — that it wishes to. It would, of course, also lend itself to significant social engineering in the name of suicide prevention.

The Australian Bureau of Statistics (ABS) reported in 2020-22 that 43 per cent of adults had experienced a mental disorder, 29 per cent had experienced an anxiety disorder such as social phobia or post-traumatic stress disorder, 16 per cent had experienced an affective disorder such as a depressive episode, and 20 per cent had experienced a substance use disorder. Furthermore, 18 per cent of adults consulted a health professional for their mental health in the 12 months preceding the survey. While 22 per cent had a 12-month mental disorder, anxiety was the most common group. Disturbingly, 39 per cent of 16–24-year-olds had a 12-month mental disorder. The ABS report comes with the usual apologia and a list of crisis support services.

> *The ABS recognises people who have a lived experience of mental health concerns and that having – or not having – mental health concerns does not define a person. We acknowledge that people are living productive, purposeful and meaningful lives with mental health concerns. We acknowledge their unique experiences, and those of carers, families and supporters of people living with mental health concerns.*[20]

As the prevalence of mental health problems increases, organisations such as public health bodies, charities and schools understandably

---

20 Australian Bureau of Statistics, 2023. *National Study of Health and Wellbeing*

respond by disseminating more awareness-raising information to help individuals identify difficulties and access support. However, these efforts themselves might increase prevalence rates.[21] Is this the excessively broad diagnostic net, potentially creating false epidemics and generating millions of new patients with relatively minor concerns or low level conditions that Frances predicts? Is this a result of prevalence inflation due to improved recognition and overinterpretation, as Foulkes and Andrews propose? An impressive counter to diagnosis and prevalence inflation is risk assessment. Most at-risk people will not develop a mental disorder. For example, suppose the incidence of a mental disorder in the next year is one per cent of the population, and the relative risk of a high-risk group is four per cent. In that case, this means that almost all people with this risk factor (96 per cent) will not develop the disorder. Suppose that a preventive intervention can reduce this risk from four per cent to two per cent. That means that, of the 100 high-risk participants in the intervention, 96 would not have developed the disorder anyway, and of the four who would, only two would benefit from the preventive effect. This is neither cost-effective nor ethical.[22] However, to counter this, public health advocates the precautionary principle, which treats any risk as excessive, thereby making it far easier to justify costly interventions. We also see 'risk creep' – where something that would once have been considered low risk, becomes treated as higher and higher risk over time.

Governments are suckers for lobbies. As SPA and myriad other health groups, including lived experience groups,[23] infect their bureaucracies, pressure builds. Sure enough, the Commonwealth has announced a National Suicide Prevention Strategy which incorporates a suicide prevention in all policies mindset.[24] No doubt, a 'Suicide Prevention Act' will arrive, and more public health dollars will follow.

---

21 Foulkes L & Andrews J L, 2023, 4

22 Cuijpers P, Smit F & Furukawa T A, 2021, 224

23 National Suicide Prevention Office. National suicide prevention office lived experience partnership group appointed. *Announcement* 21 December 2022

24 National Suicide Prevention Office, 2025. *National Suicide Prevention Strategy 2025–2035*, 68

NDIS—the leviathan

In a mental health saturated society, it is unsurprising that the source of disability in Australia has changed. For example, while the workers' compensation claims rate declined from 11 (per million hours worked) in 2008-09 to five in 2022-23 for all claims (although the rate for serious claims remained steady at 6.6), workers' compensation claims for mental health conditions (disease-related claims) increased from 6,104 in 2008-09 to 14,585 in 2022-23. Claims for mental stress conditions rose from 5,839 in 2008-09 to 13,866 in 2022-23.[25] Has work become more hazardous, or are Australians gaining a diagnosis previously not available? The age-standardised disability rate was 19 per cent in 2022, an increase from 16 per cent in 2018.[26] The ABS attributes the growth to a growing awareness of disability in Australia, a general increase in the prevalence of some long-term health conditions and an online self-completion questionnaire being offered as an option for the first time in 2022. In the ABS Survey of Disability, a person is considered to have a disability if they have any limitation, restriction, or impairment that restricts everyday activities and has lasted, or is likely to last, for six months or more. In 2022, of the 5.5 million Australians who had a disability, almost 4.8 million people (87 per cent) had a limitation with at least one of the core activities of communication, mobility or self-care, a schooling or employment restriction.

As a proportion of the Australian population, four per cent had a profound limitation, four per cent had a severe limitation, three per cent had a moderate limitation, six per cent had a mild limitation, and 10 per cent had a schooling or employment restriction. Who would have thought there were so many disabled people in Australia and so many with mental health problems? The UK Labour government has begun to tackle the problem of what they term overdiagnosis of mental

25 SafeWork Australia https://data.safeworkaustralia.gov.au/interactive-data/topic/workers-compensation

26 Australian Bureau of Statistics, 2024. *Disability, Ageing and Carers, Australia: Summary of Findings*

health problems.[27] For example, the UK Institute for Fiscal Studies said that 1.3 million people of working age were claiming disability benefits for conditions such as depression and anxiety, nearly twice as many as a decade ago. This accounts for 44 per cent of disability benefit claimants.[28] Where there is an incentive to seek a diagnosis, such as a disability payment, and where a patient in distress wants something tangible from their doctor, prevalence inflation seems assured. The much-touted but unaffordable universal basic income,[29] whereby every citizen receives a regular payment for being a citizen, is becoming a reality. No surprise that an ideological goal has slipped through under the guise of public health.

The NDIS was established in 2013. It replaced the previous, primarily state-based welfare system of disability care and provides a single, national insurance-based approach to fund support for people with disability. It provides funding to 'eligible people with disability' to access 'reasonable and necessary' supports and services. This is a wonderful idea in theory, because just about everybody would want people with profound or serious disability to receive support and care. But, who is eligible, and what is reasonable and necessary? Of the many definitions of disability above, who decides who gains access to NDIS and who misses out? It supports more than 661,000 participants.[30] The cost was $41.8 billion in 2024, approximately $30 billion from the Commonwealth and the remainder from the states. The scheme experienced 19 per cent growth over the 12 months ending 30 June 2024, down from 23 per cent over the previous year. The *National Disability Insurance Scheme Amendment (Getting the NDIS Back on Track No. 1) Act 2024* commenced in August 2024. The name alone is cause for embarrassment. The cost of getting the scheme 'back on track' was another $ 0.5 billion.

27 Steven Swinford, UK labour to cut back welfare for a million. 18 March 2025 *The Australian*

28 Latimer E, Ray-Chaudhuri S & Waters T, 2025. *The Role of Changing Health in Rising Health-related Benefit Claims*. Institute of Fiscal Studies, 2

29 Bidadanure J U, 2019. The political theory of universal basic income. *Annual Review of Political Science* 22, 481

30 National Disability Insurance Agency, 2024. *Annual Report 2023–24*

Projected Scheme expenses on an accrual basis are $58.4 billion in 2027–28. The number of people joining the NDIS continues to grow (Figure 8.1), as does the average payment received by participants.[31] Recent and proposed reforms are expected to stabilise the growth in scheme expenses, in other words, to stabilise a sinking ship. Total Scheme expenses are estimated at $47 billion in 2024–25, rising to $58 billion in 2027–28, and $93 billion in 2033–34 (on an accrual basis). Scheme expenses are estimated at 1.7 per cent of GDP in 2024–25, rising to 2.1 per cent in 2033–34.

Figure 8.1 NDIS actual and projected participants, 2019 to 2034

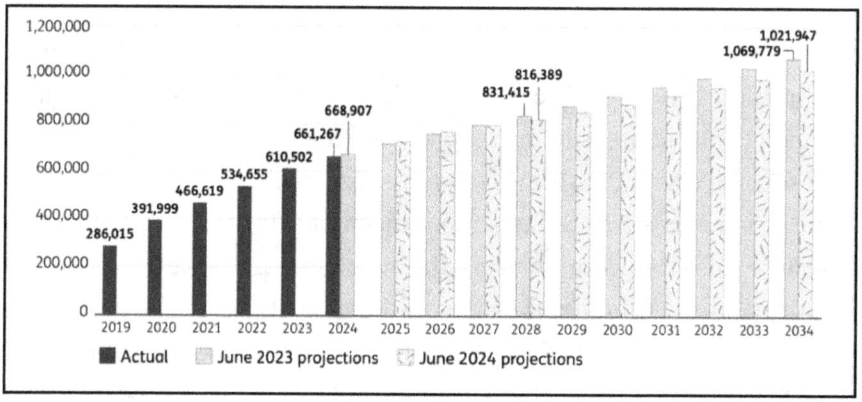

Source: National Disability Insurance Scheme, 2024. *Quarterly Report.* December, 88

In its 2011 report on disability, the Productivity Commission made some heroic claims for NDIS: that benefits would exceed the costs, that costs would be monitored rigorously, that voluntary links between the community and people with disabilities would be stronger, that people with 'enduring and significant psychiatric disabilities' who would comprise 15 per cent of the group, and the disability workforce pressures would rise as aged care expanded.[32]

The Commission asserted that the benefits would outweigh the costs, depending on a specific definition of cost. It stated that the net economic

31 National Disability Insurance Scheme, 2024. *Quarterly Report.* December, 12

32 Productivity Commission, 2011. *Disability Care and Support*

cost of the NDIS was not the budgetary cost of around $6.5 billion (which is a transfer), but rather the distortionary impacts of raising the revenue, approximately $1.6 billion. Thus, the NDIS would only need to generate a gain of $3,800 per participant to satisfy a cost-benefit analysis. The reforms would yield the equivalent of a $2.7 billion (in constant prices) annuity. This figure appears to be based on the costs associated with running the scheme.[33] The dismissive attitude to the overall costs of the scheme, by calling these monies merely transfers, assumes there were no other uses for such monies. This transfer is a gain to some paid by others, and the gains would not be permanent, except for the minority who may become self-supporting.

The factors driving scheme costs were always going to be the number and profile of those granted access, the scope and amount of support provided to participants in the scheme, and their associated costs. By the 2017 scheme review, multiple cost pressures emerged from the trial sites as the scheme was rolled out across Australia.[34] It was already apparent that more children were entering the scheme than expected,[35] and that the prevalence was higher than that of the modelling. As shown in Table 8.1, by the end of 2024, there were 159,354 children under nine years old with an NDIS plan, and a further 23,679 children accessed early connections throughout the last quarter of 2024. While forty-two per cent of participants are aged 0-14, the number of children entering the NDIS continued to grow faster than that of older participants. Of the 43,065 participants who entered and received a plan in the 2024–25 financial year to date, 67 per cent were children under 15. NDIS participants are, on average, younger than the Australian population and are becoming younger over time.

33 Productivity Commission, 2017. *NDIS Costs*, 78

34 Productivity Commission, 2017. *NDIS Costs*, 122

35 Productivity Commission, 2017. *NDIS Costs*, 87

Table 8.1 Participant profile per quarter by age group – national

Age Group	Prior Quarters - Count	Prior Quarters - Percentage	2024-25 Q2 - Count	2024-25 Q2 - Percentage	Total - Count	Total - Percentage
0 to 8	149,449	22%	9,905	51%	159,354	23%
9 to 14	131,885	20%	3,041	16%	134,926	19%
15 to 18	65,819	10%	1,405	7%	67,224	10%
19 to 24	58,748	9%	748	4%	59,496	9%
25 to 34	59,825	9%	927	5%	60,752	9%
35 to 44	49,803	7%	897	5%	50,700	7%
45 to 54	55,725	8%	928	5%	56,653	8%
55 to 64	66,147	10%	1,351	7%	67,498	10%
65+	36,023	5%	196	1%	36,219	5%
Total	**673,425**	**100%**	**19,398**	**100%**	**692,823**	**100%**

Source: National Disability Insurance Scheme, 2024. *Quarterly Report. December, Supplement E:* National, 8

Table 8.2 shows the profile of disabilities, with 73 per cent of disabilities categorised as psychosocial or allied. Autism accounts for 38 per cent of the NDIS participants, and the Minister recognises that catering for the autistic is a big problem,[36] which is going to get bigger. Autism Aspergers Advocacy Australia, quoting the full description of Autism Spectrum Disorder from the Diagnostic and Statistical Manual of Mental Disorders, 2022, is unhappy with the Commonwealth government that 'funding [above and beyond NDIS] is yet to be secured.'[37] There is more to come. A meta-analysis of numerous studies on neurodevelopmental conditions revealed that many share similar executive functions and a range of cognitive processes, including planning, working memory, attention, inhibition, self-monitoring, self-regulation, and initiation. Neurological developmental conditions allied to autism include attention-deficit/hyperactivity disorder, specific learning disorders, and developmental coordination disorders.[38] The more science understands these conditions, the more hope for better management, but the greater public health lobby pressure to have each disorder added to the NDIS list of approved disorders.

36 The Hon Amanda Rishworth MP, Launch of National Autism Strategy. *Speeches* 14 January 2025

37 *A4* Autism Aspergers Advocacy Australia, *Media Release* 25 February 2025

38 Guastella A J, 2024. Executive function in children with neurodevelopmental conditions: a systematic review and meta-analysis. *Nature Human Behaviour* (8) December, 2357

Table 8.2 Participant profile per quarter by primary disability group - national

Primary disability group	Prior Quarters - Count	Prior Quarters - Percentage	2024-25 Q2 - Count	2024-25 Q2 - Percentage	Total - Count	Total - Percentage
Autism	254,044	38%	7,573	39%	261,617	38%
Intellectual disability	93,003	14%	832	4%	93,835	14%
Developmental delay	75,910	11%	6,198	32%	82,108	12%
Psychosocial disability	63,917	9%	599	3%	64,516	9%
Hearing impairment	27,847	4%	441	2%	28,288	4%
Other neurological	23,323	3%	622	3%	23,945	3%
Other physical	19,881	3%	173	1%	20,054	3%
Acquired brain injury	18,781	3%	331	2%	19,112	3%
Cerebral palsy	17,965	3%	101	1%	18,066	3%
Global developmental delay	16,483	2%	1,078	6%	17,561	3%
Other	11381	2%	606	3%	11,987	2%
Down syndrome	<11,630	n/a	<60	n/a	11,682	2%
Multiple sclerosis	11,078	2%	241	1%	11,319	2%
Visual impairment	10,392	2%	158	1%	10,550	2%
Stroke	9,728	1%	294	2%	10,022	1%
Spinal cord Injury	6,097	1%	87	0%	6,184	1%
Other sensory/speech	<1,970	n/a	<11	n/a	1,977	0%
Total	**673,425**	**100%**	**19,398**	**100%**	**692,823**	**100%**

Source: National Disability Insurance Scheme, 2024. *Quarterly Report. December, Supplement E:* National, 6

Furthermore, there were increased package costs beyond the impacts of inflation and ageing, and a mismatch existed between the benchmark package costs and the actual package costs.[39] As it has evolved, the percentage of NDIS participants receiving PBS prescriptions increased steadily over the years. There was also the hope that early investment in some disabilities would reduce costs by 0.35 per cent per year.[40] Unfortunately, the number of exits from the scheme due to successful early intervention is lower than expected, 'as it can take some years for the benefits of early intervention to accrue.'[41] Indeed, the latest report shows only five per cent of children who have benefited from the Scheme and no longer need support.[42] Those are not encouraging figures – unless you want to argue for more money, forever, in which

39 Productivity Commission, 2017. *NDIS Costs*, 123

40 Productivity Commission, 2017. *NDIS Costs*, 99

41 Productivity Commission, 2017. *NDIS Costs*, 106

42 The 2022-23 year reported in National Disability Insurance Agency, 2024. *Annual Report 2023–24*, 35

case they are a godsend.

The worry has been that if the NDIS agency were to use the assessment criterion for access to the scheme loosely, for example, broad or vague assessment criteria for funded support, or if there were exaggerated claims for support, or the increasingly generous use of assessment tools by assessors, public funding would threaten the scheme's sustainability. The hope was that people making assessments would be independent of the client (unlike general practitioners), properly trained in the use of the tools, and approved or appointed by the National Disability Insurance Agency to conduct NDIS assessments. The level of independence required may not have been achieved. Laughably, the original Productivity Commission report mused that 'an additional safeguard would be the reluctance by many people to receive more than the necessary personal care by non-family members.'[43] The 2023 NDIS Review, in essence a lobby for the scheme, was happy to report one disabled person's observation 'that some participants are reluctant to use their allocated funding, due to being considered as a "burden to society", means that they might leave things until they escalate into a crisis situation.'[44]

As for the expected increase in voluntary links between the community and the disabled, many former providers, often charities, exited the field, leaving it flooded with 16,000 registered providers, over 154,000 unregistered providers, and more than 325,000 workers.[45] Despite legislating pay rises for staff in the sector, finding staff is still a problem.[46] Most regions require a 50 to 150 per cent increase in the workforce.[47]

One of the key claims for the NDIS was the hope that many people with disabilities would be able to enter the workforce. For participants of

43 Productivity Commission, 2011. *Disability Care and Support,* 21

44 Department of the Prime Minister and Cabinet, 2023. *Working together to deliver the NDIS - Independent Review into the National Disability Insurance Scheme: Final Report*, 99

45 Department of the Prime Minister and Cabinet, 2023, 227

46 The Hon Amanda Rishworth MP, Launch of the What's My Future national disability support worker recruitment campaign. *Speeches* 19 February 2025

47 Productivity Commission, 2017. *NDIS Costs*, 37

working age (15 to 64) who have been in the NDIS for two years, the employment rate has increased slightly, from 19 per cent to 21 per cent. Those in the NDIS for three to five years also experienced similar increases of up to two percentage points. For participants who have been in the NDIS for six years or more, there has been little change in the percentage of participants in work, which remains at 26 per cent (Figure 8.2).

Figure 8.2 Change in the percentage of participants in work

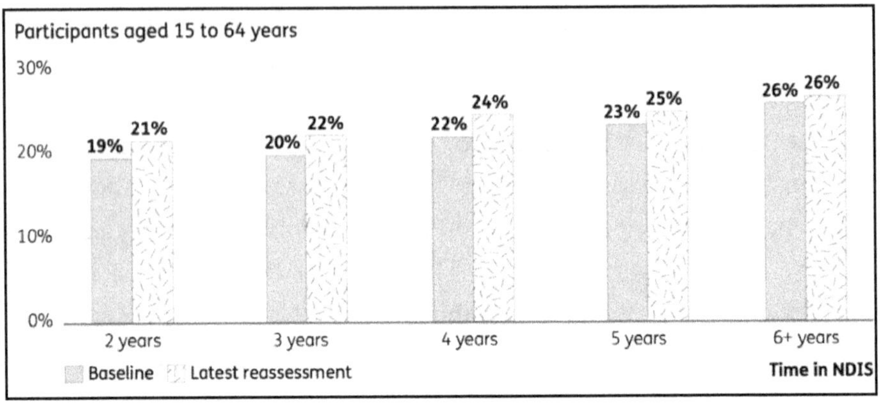

Source: National Disability Insurance Scheme, 2024. *Quarterly Report. December, 40*

The second line of hope was that employment opportunities for families and carers would increase, thereby reducing their responsibilities for caring for their disabled family member. The percentage of families and carers in paid employment among participants who have been in the NDIS for at least two years has improved over time. Comparing responses at the most recent plan reassessment (between two and eight years after entry) with responses at entry to the NDIS, the changes were an eight percentage point increase from 46 per cent to 54 per cent for families and carers of participants aged 0 to 14 years and a two percentage point increase from 48 per cent to 50 per cent for families and carers of participants aged 15 years and over. Overall, for families and carers of all participants, there has been a five percentage point increase, from 47 per cent to 52 per cent. These are modest improvements, and the NDIS cost does not account for the price of supported employment, which may be a substantial part of the employment story for people with disabilities.

A further weakness in the public health approach is to praise any measure of success, no matter how benign. For example, 'less specific outcomes' are improving for participants aged 0 to 14. A growing proportion of parents and carers of young children reported that their child used specialist services, which helped their child develop life skills and assisted them in supporting their child. Children who participate in community activities tend to feel welcome and actively included. School-aged children are becoming more independent, and they are increasingly likely to manage the demands of their world effectively, integrate into family life, and form friendships with people outside their family. More participants formed friendships with people outside their family while also fitting well into family life.[48] The measures used could not test whether these things would have happened anyway, especially in an era when disability is thankfully less subject to exclusion and social distance.

For older participants, aged 15 and over, it seemed that there was more to be done. Participants wanted more choice and control; a higher percentage than in previous surveys said they could not do something they wanted to in the last 12 months. This is a magnificent illustration of the inflation of expectations that comes with free services. Ultimately, they disappoint because they assume a participant can have whatever they desire. Most disturbing is that labour force participation, which includes those who are neither working nor actively looking for work, has shown little change over time. The percentage of participants in the labour force, which consists of those employed and/or actively seeking employment, has declined over time. Of the 23 per cent of participants who have a paid job,[49] many of these are government jobs, and probably not otherwise made available except to people with a disability, which means there are extra costs associated with the program.

48 National Disability Insurance Scheme, 2024. *Quarterly Report*. December, 31

49 National Disability Insurance Agency, 2024. *Annual Report 2023–24*, 34

Most disappointing of all is the general deterioration in self-rated health over time across all age groups and duration cohorts. Older participants are typically less likely to rate their health as Excellent, Very Good or Good. There is an increasing desire among participants to see friends and family more often, and a decreasing percentage have friends other than family or paid staff (e.g. paid support workers).[50] The same is true for the self-rated health of families and carers, which has deteriorated over time. These are feeble measures and results and should be sufficient to have the entire program torn down, but once ideas get a head of steam and institutions built and public health officials in place and recipients funded, it is almost impossible to stop. Once more, public health path dependency takes over.

But wait, there's more …

Bruce Bonyhady, perhaps the most important person in the establishment of the inaccurately named National Disability Insurance Scheme, commented in 2021 that while 500,000 people were able to access support under the scheme, those outside the scheme, referred to as tier 2 disabled, received very little.[51] He wanted more. And he got more. In 2024, following Bonyhady's review of the NDIS, the Australian government announced the tier 2 program, relabeled Information, Linkages and Capacity Building (ILC) to avoid creating a hierarchy of disability.[52] ILC is the NDIS component that provides information, linkages, and referrals to connect people with mainstream support. It is intended to ensure that the NDIS establishes and facilitates capacity-building supports for any person with a disability who is not directly linked to a person through an individually funded package. This was not news, as the Productivity Commission's 2017 review acknowledged

50 National Disability Insurance Scheme, 2024. *Quarterly Report.* December, 32

51 Jewel Topsfield. 'You're either in or you're out': NDIS architects say scheme is inequitable. *The Sydney Morning Herald* 22 July 2021

52 National Disability Insurance Scheme, undated. *A Framework for Information, Linkages and Capacity Building*

that four million Australians had a disability and that funds had been allocated to these programs since 2016.[53] Nevertheless, while the Minister's speech to update the disability strategy through to 2031 seems more like a reannouncement than a new program,[54] there is no doubt that the pressure remains to ensure that every Australian with any disability has access to the care they believe they deserve.

The 2023 review, packed with lobbyists and bureaucrats, followed public health's well-worn strategic path: find more problems in order to create more bureaucracy. The review's demands were comprehensive. There were no fewer than 26 recommendations and 139 actions consequent upon them. These are in addition to the 12-volume report of the 2023 Royal Commission into Violence, Abuse, Neglect and Exploitation of People with Disability, with 222 recommendations.[55] The review sought answers to five questions:

- Why is the NDIS an oasis in a desert?
- What does reasonable and necessary mean?
- Why are there many more children in the NDIS than expected?
- Why aren't NDIS markets working?
- How do we ensure the NDIS is sustainable?

The report argued that in trying to correct for the underfunded, inconsistent and unfair arrangements that existed before the NDIS, governments have come to rely on the NDIS as the dominant, and in some cases only, source of support for people with disability — the oasis in the desert. This is a reflection on the contribution by state and local governments to disability services, which, in some circumstances, have declined but have otherwise not kept pace with the significant new contributions from the Commonwealth. There is no suggestion that funds from all sources have declined.

The reasonable and necessary complaint is two-fold. That which is

53 https://www.ndis.gov.au/community/information-linkages-and-capacity-building-ilc/funded-projects

54 The Hon Amanda Rishworth MP Speeches Updated Australia's Disability Strategy 2021-2031, building a more inclusive Australia 29 January 2025

55 Royal Commission into Violence, Abuse, Neglect and Exploitation of People with a Disability, 2023. *Final Report*

reasonable and necessary is applied to every part of a support package, not the needs of the whole person. Claimants do not know what evidence to provide to show their support is reasonable and necessary, or how the evidence will be used. Consequently, applicants present their most vulnerable versions to gain support. The Report considers that the authority is adopting an adversarial approach, which is naïve. Almost 22,000 participants have taken disputes to the Administrative Review Tribunal since 2021.[56] If someone wants something from the taxpayer, the authority must uphold the taxpayer's trust by being cautious with the funds. If the disabled person wants more, of course, there is conflict.

Why are there many more children in the NDIS than expected? With so few supports outside the NDIS, it is not surprising that parents are fighting to get their children with developmental concerns or disability into the NDIS. After receiving early intervention support, they are reluctant to leave the scheme, fearing they will be left without support. The prevalence of disability and developmental concerns in children, currently 20 per cent of all Australian children, makes this a mainstream issue requiring a mainstream response. With children making up half of all NDIS participants, it is clear mainstream supports are not meeting the needs of children and families, who are turning to the NDIS as the only source of support. There is no recognition in this line of reasoning that services create demand for services, nor is there any hint that medical interventions create demand.

The report notes that the NDIS markets differ from other markets. This is sensible. The current fee-for-service model rewards providers for the volume of support they deliver, with little incentive to improve quality, innovate, or respond to the needs of all participants. Price caps have become price floors. The Authority sets service prices and determines access to them. The only market is in providers who bid for clients. The pricing arrangements are complex, as any centrally controlled market

56 NDIS, 2024. *Report to Disability Ministers Quarter 2 2024-25, Supplement*, 30

for complex services must be.[57] The participants' perception of choice and control for selected providers is only 53 per cent.[58]

The definition of the financial sustainability of the NDIS (as defined in the 2016 Insurance Principles and Financial Sustainability Manual) is a wonder to behold. The NDIS is held to be successful 'on participants' views that they are getting enough money to buy enough goods and services to allow them reasonable access to life opportunities, that is, reasonable and necessary support contributors think that the cost is and will continue to be affordable, under control, represents value for money and, therefore, remain willing to contribute.'[59] The assumption is made that, if contributors to the NDIS agree to the budget and the forecast, the 'state of financial sustainability' has been met for the reporting period.[60] More guff has not been written in a long time. It would be easier to answer, 'how long is a piece of string?', except that the answer can be finite by cutting the string. The so-called contributors who are to decide these matters are taxpayers, but they have no direct interest; they do not pay an insurance premium as such.

The review brazenly aligned with the United Nations Convention on the Rights of Persons with Disabilities. It argued that the NDIS was one of the most important global innovations in disability rights and was 'essential to Australia meeting its obligations under the UNCRPD.' Their recommendations sought to uphold a rights-based approach.[61] This thinking is conceited and beggars society. As with the Productivity Commission's original sin of suggesting that the bulk of funds to NDIS were merely transfers, as opposed to economic costs, economics can never be abolished. Only so much can be afforded, and when government power is used to take monies from some citizens to give to

57 NDIS Pricing Arrangements. https://www.ndis.gov.au/providers/pricing-arrangements#ndis-pricing-arrangements-and-price-limits

58 National Disability Insurance Agency, 2024. *Annual Report 2023–24*, 30

59 National Disability Insurance Agency, 2024. *Annual Report 2023–24*, 27

60 National Disability Insurance Agency, 2024. *Annual Report 2023–24*, 28

61 NDIS Review, 2023. *Our Final Report: A Guide for People with Disability and their Families*, 2

others, citizens should never lose their right to resist. Only those citizens can decide what is right, not a politician who glories in a speech at the United Nations, hoping to be retired when the bills fall due.

The befuddled and deliberate obscurity of the sustainability formula is too much for the disability lobby, which, as a favourite and increasingly powerful instrument of public health, retreats to the hoary notion of human rights. The review's solution to the question of how to ensure the NDIS is sustainable was to invoke the principle that 'A human right which cannot be sustained is a human right denied.' This is very woolly thinking. Human rights are a battering ram to squeeze as much as possible from others. If the sector is concerned about the taxpayer's forbearance, they should stop asserting a human right to others' money. 'As a standard setter within the disability service system, the NDIS should ensure people with disability are at the centre of service delivery and empowered to exercise their rights.'[62] There is no suggestion by these advocates that there are limits to support, no insight or acknowledgement that there are other, equally essential calls on public funds. As the 2017 Productivity Commission review of costs noted, 'the scheme is only uncapped to the extent that taxpayers are willing to pay for it.'[63]

The Australian Federation of Disability Organisations were highly critical of Prime Minister Anthony Albanese's moving the NDIS to Mark Butler and the broader health portfolio, warning the decision 'risks medicalising disability and undermines the scheme's social model foundations.' The lobby wanted a dedicated minister for disability – someone accountable not only for the NDIS but for the 5.5 million Australians with disability, including the 690,000 NDIS participants. There was more,

> *Placing the NDIS with the health portfolio potentially risks medicalising disability and undermines the scheme's social model foundations, which are based on choice, control, and inclusion.*[64]

62 National Disability Insurance Scheme Review, 2023. *Our Final Report: A Guide for People with Disability and their Families*, 36

63 Productivity Commission, 2017. *NDIS Costs,* 462

64 Sarah Ison, Passing the buck to Mark Butler and health 'risks undermining NDIS'. *The Australian* 14 May 2025

This claim is precisely the opposite of reality. Disability has been medicalised to receive benefits. The concept of the social model amounts to assuming that taxpayers are willing to transfer their or someone else's money to pay for a better life for a disabled person. How much and what level of impairment qualify are moral questions, based on medical assessments that, in turn, are affected by social circumstances such as an ever-broadening definition of disability. Invoking human rights does not relieve the essentially economic constraints of who is willing to pay for whom.

Foreshadowing the difficulty of fighting the public health lobby

The Grattan Institute analysis of the NDIS has some valuable insights, the main one being that 'an unsustainable NDIS risks upending … essential coverage for Australians with permanent and profound disability.'[65] Parents and charities seeking help for the profoundly disabled were the driving forces behind the disability sector, and few would want to see the profoundly disabled robbed of care. However, under a public health approach that seeks to expand its remit, mental health diagnoses have soared continually. A vast array of mental health conditions – not just those that can reasonably be considered profound or serious – have found their way into the scheme, which has now morphed into rights-based justifications and a vastly expanded opportunity for less disabled people to access taxpayer support beyond the wildest hopes of the pioneers in the struggle for the disabled.

The most essential thing in reining in the NDIS is for politicians not to cave into the disability lobby, which includes the disabled and their advocates, but also the providers, who have experienced a boom market for many years.[66] 'The disability community … does not support the government's timeline for NDIS reforms; however, the Agency must

65 Bennett S, Jessurun M & Orban H, 2025. *Saving The NDIS: How To Rebalance Disability Services To Get Better Results*. Grattan Institute, 21

66 Sarah Ison, Don't cave: 'critical' NDIS decree bureaucrats' warning to ministers. *The Australian* 17 July 2025

remain on the timeline if we are to achieve the national cabinet's annual 8 per cent growth target,' the NDIA brief said. Governments have created a rod for their back, and the taxpayer, by paying the lobby handsomely to 'co-design the system.[67] It is astounding how public health – usually so shrill in demanding that perceived lobbyists for something it does not like should have zero say — is happy for lobbyists to design systems when it suits their ideological bent.

A theme that will be explored in the final chapter is the difficulty of fighting an entrenched lobby that enjoys public health support. For example, a typical criticism by the sector of the feeble ability and intentions by the government to rein in costs is Children and Young People with Disability Australia chief executive Skye Kakoschke-Moore, who stated, 'it's being justified by a need to meet a financial target rather than the needs of people with disability.' The Australian Federation of Disability Organisations said it was 'deeply concerned by the NDIA's assertion that, despite acknowledging the disability community does not support the current reform timeline, the Agency intends to proceed regardless to meet an arbitrary financial target set by national cabinet.'[68] All financial targets are arbitrary; indeed, the scheme itself is arbitrary because the funds are not endless. Someone must miss out. Although there is parliamentary scrutiny of the scheme, it is yet another forum in which pressure is applied to the government to keep money rolling in. There is a lack of appetite for restraint, especially as many members of the parliamentary committee are non-governmental, indeed independent, and will never have to be responsible for Budgets.[69]

The Grattan suggestions, which include strengthening eligibility criteria for when an impairment should be considered permanent and reallocating NDIS funds to 'foundational supports for children with developmental

67 The Hon Bill Shorten MP, Minister for the National Disability Insurance Scheme, NDIS reforms boosted by greater investment in co-design with disability representative organisations. 6 June 2024

68 Sarah Ison, *The Australian* 17 July 2025

69 Joint Standing Committee on the National Disability Insurance Scheme, 2024. *General Issues: Annual Report No. 2 of the 47th Parliament*

delay or disability' to reduce the number of claimants in that category, have a frighteningly small payoff.[70] The recommended reforms were estimated to bring the growth rate of the NDIS down from eight per cent, which is the Commonwealth government's hoped-for reduction in the rate of growth, to 7.5 per cent per year by 2033-34.'[71] Under those changes, the behemoth remains. Australia is not paying its way at present, and future taxpayers may not appreciate the public health and rights-based approach that has driven the behemoth.

Bold medicine is necessary, if not always easy to achieve. If the behemoth of the NDIS is to be reined in, its growth path must be understood. The first step is to recognise an earlier public health putsch, for the de-institutionalisation of the mentally ill, was an experiment that has failed.[72] Further, part of the reining in of the extravagant claims of the lobby is that a better allocation of funds to the seriously mentally ill is needed.[73] There may be a shortfall in Australian adult psychiatric care. Still, the burden has fallen on those whose needs are greatest, those with severe mental illnesses such as schizophrenia, bipolar disorder, and severe major depression. Patients languish in emergency departments, are cared for in brief hospital stays, and/or are discharged to under-resourced public mental health services in the community. Prioritising care for those with severe mental illness is essential, yet public health continues to push mental health awareness and education that results in overdiagnosis and overtreatment of the worried well at the expense of the seriously unwell.

At the same time, broad access schemes have not improved the health of the less mentally ill. The suggestion is that there is no detectable benefit to the mental health of Australians from the introduction of the Better Access scheme. Under Better Access, patients can be referred to a clinical psychologist, another psychologist, or an allied health practitioner (such

70 Bennett S, Jessurun M & Orban H, 2025, 4

71 Bennett S, Jessurun M & Orban H, 2025, 80

72 Australian Medical Network, 2023. *Deinstitutionalisation of Mental Health*

73 Looi J C L et al, 2024. The corrosion of adult mental healthcare in Australia: can we meet the needs of those who need the most? *Australasian Psychiatry* 32(4), 285

as an occupational therapist or social worker) by a medical practitioner as part of a GP Mental Health Treatment Plan or referred by a psychiatrist or paediatrician.[74] The findings are consistent with previous reports from both Australia and other countries that significant increases in treatment do not appear to reduce the prevalence of mental disorders.[75]

The sugar on the table is so great that parents will chase an ADHD or Autism diagnosis and allied conditions for their child. This sector alone is destroying the system's financial viability. Several changes will be needed to counter this cohort. First, is to tighten the diagnosis for such conditions, and second, is to ensure that a Commonwealth medical officer makes those diagnoses. A private, fee-paying medical practitioner is not in a position of responsibility to make a diagnosis that has significant financial implications for the parents and the taxpayer. It may be necessary to grandfather the scheme, to create a new scheme that has much tighter eligibility criteria, and, because the young are a large proportion of the NDIS clientele, ensure that those on the existing scheme undergo an annual review and, in any event, must exit the scheme at age 15, which corresponds to the compulsory years of schooling.

Conclusion

The NDIS is not an insurance scheme. No one pays a premium. There are good reasons why such a scheme would not be viable when profound disability is considered or life-changing accidents are considered. Nevertheless, the essence of an insurance scheme is that the pool of premiums is the pool of money from which claims must be paid. In other words, there should be a cap on payouts. A reserve is essential to even out claim payouts over time and to avoid disturbing support for long-

74 Looi J C L et al, 2024, 286

75 Jorm A F, 2018. Australia's 'Better Access' scheme: has it had an impact on population mental health? *Australian & New Zealand Journal of Psychiatry* 52(11), 1061

term clients.[76] Without a cap, the scheme is nothing more than an open cheque for future politicians to buy votes. The public health lobby, with its endless promotion of more and more ills that people will find they have if they just look hard enough, should have been restrained by those who knew better but failed to speak up.

---

76 National Disability Insurance Agency, 2024. *Annual Report 2023–24*, 18. See also, Productivity Commission, 2017. *NDIS Costs,* 464 and Bennett S, Jessurun M & Orban H, 2025, 83

Tackling the public health lobby

The public health lobby has to learn about the costs and benefits of any proposed scheme. They also have to learn to conduct these honestly.

In lieu of such honesty, there are many ways in which those involved in or concerned for health policy should fight the lobby.

9

Costs and Benefits: honest evaluation

Perhaps the greatest weapon in rational public health policy is the application of rigorous cost-benefit analysis. Politicians and public officials should ensure that such analyses assist them in their deliberations, if only as a defence against any lobby that seeks to have others pay for their real or claimed misfortune. Unfortunately, as with techniques of control and influence such as statistics, regulation and taxation, cost-benefit analysis can hide as much as it reveals. Hence, the pleas for an honest evaluation that takes into account all relevant factors across a lifetime.

The Commonwealth Department of Health's national alcohol strategy warns that the risks associated with alcohol are often underestimated.[1] Perhaps not. Professor Steven Schwartz, a former professor of psychology and former vice-chancellor at Macquarie University, commented on the U.S. Surgeon General's proposal to place cancer warnings on wine bottles. He explained a typical statistical sleight of hand in such warnings—the distinction between relative and absolute risk. Alcohol consumption is linked to certain cancers, but should the alarm stemming from the Surgeon General's policy proposal be taken seriously, especially when most drinkers consume in moderation? Setting aside the

1 Commonwealth of Australia Department of Health, 2019. *National Alcohol Strategy 2019–2028*, 6

problematic predictive strength of risk factors in medical conditions,[2] relative risk describes how much something increases (or decreases) the likelihood of an outcome. For instance, consuming alcohol may raise the relative risk of breast cancer by about 10 per cent per standard drink per day. That figure sounds significant until the absolute risk is considered. Absolute risk assesses the actual likelihood of developing a disease. For a woman in her 40s, the absolute risk of developing breast cancer over the next decade is roughly 1.5 per cent. If she has one glass of wine daily, a 10 per cent rise in relative risk results in her absolute risk climbing to 1.65 per cent. Comparing 1000 women who do not drink with 1000 who enjoy one glass of wine each day, among the non-drinkers, about 15 will develop breast cancer over the next decade. That number rises to 16.5 among the wine drinkers – a difference of 1.5 cases. The power that public health feels when it convinces legislators to make big alcohol quite literally label itself as harmful, outweighs any such analysis.

Another factor is whether the labels affect the target audience. Warnings may be effective for drinkers who are unlikely to develop breast cancer or for those whose breast cancer is linked to their consumption of alcohol. Alcohol can be appealing to those dealing with anxieties that might affect their health and who have become desensitised to the warnings. Additionally, moderate drinking might merely shift the risk of death. If a glass of wine raises the risk of breast cancer but lowers the risk of heart disease, one health risk is traded for another. Public health messaging seldom addresses this trade-off, instead focusing on worst-case scenarios.[3] If the health warnings were genuinely effective, the estimated 1.5 lives saved would be overstated. Incidentally, this figure does not consider the loss of enjoyment or the various social and psychological benefits. If we are being generous, we could say that is the precautionary principle at work again. If we are being realistic, we could say that the more worst-case scenarios there are, the more relevant

2 Cuijpers P, Smit F & Furukawa T A, 2021. Most at-risk individuals will not develop a mental disorder: the limited predictive strength of risk factors. *World Psychiatry* 20(2), 224

3 Schwartz S, 2025. Cancer warning labels on wine? Put a cork in it. *The Australian* 4 January

public health remains.

Dr Steve Robson, a surgeon specialising in breast cancer, strongly opposed Schwartz's advice: 'Some male commentators have publicly attempted to downplay the role that alcohol consumption plays in breast cancer. This does women a disservice and puts them at risk.'[4] The surgeon viewed society and its individuals as if they were a hospital ward. While there is undeniable suffering associated with cancer, it remains uncertain whether labels will change the behaviours of those whose drinking habits could be improved by completely abstaining or drinking less. No evidence was provided. Instead, in true public health fashion, yet another constraint on the lives of all alcohol consumers was suggested.

A decade ago, St Vincent's Health Australia urged political parties to commit to a target of reducing alcohol-related illness by 20 per cent by 2025.[5] St Vincent's has been working with alcoholics and others since 1964, so, understandably, they might be frustrated. This may explain their desire to push for a national policy. They pursued this goal, knowing that only 3.4 per cent of drinkers fall into the 'harmful' category.[6] They also acknowledged that there has been a decline in per capita alcohol consumption in Australia since 1960.[7] Some of their policies are specific and traditional, such as providing treatment services for people with alcohol dependence, but most aspects are designed to apply to nearly everyone. Echoing tobacco regulation, St Vincent's calls for a ban on all alcohol advertising and sponsorship, alcohol taxation based on its content and level of harm (a volumetric tax), pictorial health warnings, and various restrictions on trading hours.[8]

---

4 Robson S, 2025. Drinking risks are real – women should know them. *The Australian* 5 January

5 St Vincent's Health Australia, 2016. *Restoring the Balance: A New Approach to lcohol in Australia*. Melbourne: St. Vincent's Health Australia

6 Six standard drinks per day. Marsden Jacob 2015, 13

7 Australian Bureau of Statistics, 2015. *Apparent Consumption of Alcohol, Australia, 2013-14*

8 St Vincent's Health Australia, 2016, 15

Poorly targeted

Politicians need to address two significant issues before they do St Vincent's bidding. If it is not possible to recover the costs of alcohol-related harm caused by drinkers that spill over to others, who else must pay, and how much? Is it feasible to reduce the amount of harm without hindering others' enjoyment? As Joshua Byrnes eloquently stated, 'How much pleasure should be foregone among those who drink moderately to dissuade those who over-indulge?'[9] This is the essence of all harm regulation, played out in painstaking detail, particularly in alcohol taxation.

If the tax on alcohol could be aimed at that one drink too many, it might help to curb harmful consumption or, at the very least, generate funds to cover the damage caused by those who overindulge. However, imposing a charge on every drink that exceeds what someone considers one drink too many is not feasible. Consequently, taxes on alcohol are applied to all products, which ultimately increases the cost of drinking for everyone. This makes tax a blunt tool for alleviating the external costs of alcohol use. It means that consumers who enjoy alcohol responsibly end up paying an unjustifiably high price. While the tax on alcohol generates revenue for the government, it is not a cost-free method of tackling alcohol misuse. As with any policy intervention, the advantages of taxation must be weighed against its costs.[10]

A study based on the Australian National Drug Strategy Household Surveys aimed to determine who altered their drinking habits and by how much following price (tax) increases.[11] The results indicate that Australian drinkers reduced their overall alcohol consumption primarily by increasing the number of occasions on which they abstained altogether and by decreasing the instances of low-intensity drinking. They did not significantly reduce their frequency of moderate- and high-

9 Byrnes J et al, 2013. Can harms associated with high-intensity drinking be reduced by increasing the price of alcohol? *Drug and Alcohol Review* 32(1), 27

10 Australia's Future Tax System, 2009, E5–1

11 Self-reported patterns of alcohol consumption and demographic data, Australian National Drug Strategy Household Surveys, conducted in 2001, 2004 and 2007, comprising a total of 79 545 respondents. Byrnes J et al, 2013, 27

intensity drinking. In other words, price increases appear unlikely to have significantly reduced the number of occasions on which people consume at higher intensities (5-9 and 10 or more standard drinks). Thus, those for whom drinking is a pleasure and poses little harm were compelled to alter their habits, while those who drank excessively and posed a higher risk of harm changed little. Another public health failure.

The authors noted that price rises were ineffective in reducing problem drinking and that survey respondents may have under-reported their drinking levels, potentially undermining the accuracy of the impact price had on demand at various intensity levels. Additionally, price increases may have been ineffective because retailers might respond with short-term discounts, or drinkers might shift their consumption from pubs to takeaways. To emphasise this point, the study's authors recommend 'complementary legislation, such as earlier closing times for venues that sell alcohol,' to reduce the frequency of high-intensity consumption.[12] State governments have been grappling with this aspect of alcohol policy for generations.[13]

Optimal rate for the social benefit of alcohol taxation

The Foundation for Alcohol Research and Education commissioned economists Marsden Jacobs to estimate the optimal rate for the social benefits of alcohol taxation in Australia. To achieve this, they needed to assess the costs and benefits associated with alcohol consumption. Estimates of Australia's annual social costs vary widely, ranging from \$3.8 billion to \$36 billion.[14] St Vincent's used a figure of \$20 billion. The discrepancies in calculated social costs reflect differing opinions on which costs should be included and how they should be measured.

12 Byrnes J et al, 2013, 30

13 New South Wales Auditor-General, 2013, 2

14 Laslett A-M et al, 2025. *Alcohol's Harm to Others in Australia: Patterns, Costs, Disparities and Precipitants*. Melbourne: Centre for Alcohol Policy Research, La Trobe University, 7

When calculating the costs and benefits of alcohol consumption at a specific price, careful judgments must be made regarding the rationality of drinkers. Marsden Jacobs sensibly employed two scenarios: one where heavy drinkers gained benefits from excessive consumption and another where they received only a portion of those benefits. Assuming there was no loss of benefits for heavy drinkers due to increased excise rates, the excise increase estimated to maximise net benefits to society was 145 per cent. This adjustment would generate $688 million in net benefits annually. Such a policy would lead to an annual increase in excise and tax revenue to the Commonwealth government of $6.6 billion. When they relaxed the assumption that harmful levels of alcohol consumption had no benefit to consumers, the rate of excise increase that would maximise net benefits to society was 74 per cent, yielding $207 million per year in net benefits. This policy change would result in an annual increase in excise and tax revenue to the Commonwealth government of $4.3 billion.

These figures appear impressive, providing overall net benefits by considering the loss of satisfaction among moderate drinkers and the reduction in specific harms associated with alcohol. However, was it realistic? The economists' answer was a startling no. In careful terms, they concluded, 'the percentage increases in excise rates that are found to maximise net benefits to society are well above any changes that have been observed in practice.'[15] In other words, these excise rate increases are implausible. Public health frequently relies on implausible, unrealistic models of human behaviour.

The authors readily acknowledged several limitations and weaknesses in the analysis. First, it does not model the possibility that alcohol consumers might switch to other substances, such as illicit drugs, in response to a price change in alcohol. This means the actual costs of higher excise rates could be understated. The largest figure in the two scenarios was revenue, not benefits. Naturally, its gathering would have a price, and the funds might not be used sensibly.

15 Marsden Jacob, 2015, 20

In Jonathan Pincus's terms, the momentous numbers favoured by public health advocates to justify controlling individual consumption choices are derived through various methods. The most recent tack is to survey at a population level those who believe others' use of alcohol has harmed them. A 2021 survey in Australia generated a huge number – '48 per cent of all Australians reported experiencing harm (negative effects or specific harms) from others' drinking in the previous 12 months.'[16] There is contention regarding how to measure the costs associated with the use and misuse of alcohol and about which costs are private versus those that are spillover (non-private). Some researchers have identified and quantified community expenses and losses correlated with alcohol misuse, including certain costs incurred by the drinker. This method has generally led to a comparatively large estimate of social costs. Conversely, other researchers have disregarded costs borne by private individuals. This alternative approach has tended to classify numerous costs as private, resulting in a smaller estimate of social costs.

A further distinction between private and spillover costs is the differentiation between tangible and intangible costs associated with alcohol misuse. The variation in cost estimates across studies is due mainly to whether intangible costs are factored in.[17] Tangible costs arising from alcohol misuse and its consequences include medical services and hospital-related expenses. Intangible costs, conversely, encompass the effects on health and quality of life for both the drinker and their family members. The Marsden Jacob study expressly excluded intangible costs from the overall cost of alcohol misuse due to the uncertainty surrounding these estimates. In such cases, the resulting cost estimate has been deemed a minimal cost to society attributable to alcohol misuse.

To conclude the debate about the costs associated with alcohol's effects, the issues of what should be included and how costs are allocated

16 Laslett A-M et al, 2025. *Alcohol's Harm to Others in Australia: Patterns, Costs, Disparities and Precipitants*. Melbourne: Centre for Alcohol Policy Research, La Trobe University, 2

17 Laslett A-M et al, 2025

represent a common error made by the public health lobby: neglecting to account for consumer surpluses.

> *So it is a mystery how the researchers felt able to draw their conclusions about the effects of a minimum alcohol price on health, crime, absentee rates and so on. If they do not know by how much a minimum alcohol price will increase the consumption of DIY alcohol, illegal drugs, glue fumes and the rest, they cannot know its effects on public health, crime and employment.*[18]

Creating significant numbers is a crucial part of the lobby's toolkit. Another aspect is rushing to solutions without understanding their costs and impacts.

In assessing economic evaluations for health interventions, spillover costs can be defined very broadly, for instance, as 'all impacts from an intervention on all parties or entities other than the users of the intervention being evaluated.'[19] An ACIL Allen discussion paper examined the extent to which public policy measures can alleviate the spillover costs of alcohol. It emphasised the significance of understanding the extent to which various public policy measures can mitigate costs, a point that the debate regarding the magnitude of different cost estimates has somewhat overshadowed.[20]

While spillover costs encompass all expenses imposed on individuals external to a drinker due to alcohol consumption (externalities) and the costs not accounted for by the drinker, policy-relevant spillover costs only include those that public policy measures can influence. Policy-relevant spillover costs exclude private costs to the individual resulting from alcohol misuse. ACIL Allen argues that policy-relevant spillover costs should be defined in a manner that helps address the following questions:

18 Whyte J, 2013. *Quack Policy Abusing Science in the Cause of Paternalism.* The Institute of Economic Affairs, 25

19 Mendoza-Jiménez M J, van Exel J & Brouwer W, 2024. On spillovers in economic evaluations: definition, mapping review and research agenda. *European Journal of Health Economics* 25(7), 1239

20 ACIL Allen, 2014, 4

- What impacts should be considered as a basis for potential government intervention in alcohol consumption decisions?
- What are the relevant policy costs, and how do they vary with the severity of alcohol misuse?
- What avoidable costs can public policy initiatives and behaviour change address?
- Which costs can be addressed through public policy measures?
- What public policy interventions effectively reduce the policy-relevant costs associated with alcohol misuse?[21]

These are sensible questions, and their answers may prompt public health advocates to be cautious about generating significant figures that might preempt a rush towards taxation and regulation as the solution for alcohol-related issues affecting a small group. Given public health's history of interfering in people's lives using any means it can, we should not hold our breath.

What is the aim?

Public health advocates must be clear about their goals and actions. For instance, regarding alcohol, is the aim to change culture, such as reducing violence linked to alcohol, or simply to decrease overall alcohol consumption? What if weak self-control is a common underlying factor in the clustering of heavy drinking, violence, and other deviant behaviours among young people?[22] Some researchers, such as anthropologist Anne Fox, have faced criticism as alleged supporters of the alcohol industry.[23] Still, others have raised similar questions about the connection between alcohol and violence. For example, what if the link between adolescent drinking and aggression is 'non-causal because the same set of individual

21 ACIL Allen, 2014, 27

22 Gottfredson M R & Hirschi T, 1990. *A General Theory of Crime*. Stanford University Press

23 Bartlett A & McCambridge, J, 2021. Doing violence to evidence on violence? How the alcohol industry created doubt in order to influence policy. *Drug and Alcohol Review*. 41

and environmental factors predicts both behaviours'?[24] Or, what if the effect of drinking is limited to those who tend to suppress their angry feelings?[25]

What if drunken behaviour is culturally determined? Like the decline in smoking, governments can help shape our understanding, but individuals ultimately make their own choices. As Fox has noted, 'It is unlikely that we will achieve real and positive change in the drinking culture until we have a better understanding of what is driving it.'[26] Fox observed that as long as alcohol exists, no amount of regulation, education, propaganda, restriction, or taxation will deter the hard core of dedicated abusers from periodically (or regularly) exceeding the official maximum safe allowance. The social significance of the substance needs to be understood before solutions are devised.[27] In a drinking culture such as the Irish, for instance, and in a relatively uniform group like students, a 2013 study found a strong family history of drinking habits. Parental and sibling drinking influenced both actual alcohol consumption and standards for what is considered normal or acceptable drinking behaviour. Additionally, the culture also functioned at regional and national levels, combining to create 'complex deep-rooted cultural and historical factors that facilitate alcohol consumption.'[28]

Drunkenness and drunken behaviour are often considered directly proportional to the amount of alcohol consumed. However, the same person on the same alcohol dose can react differently on various occasions and in different settings. This variation would not occur if the responses were purely physiological. Morphologically similar humans in

24 White H R, 1997. Longitudinal perspective on alcohol use and aggression during adolescence. *Recent Developments in Alcohol* 13, 81

25 Norstrom T & Pape H, 2010. Alcohol, suppressed anger and violence. *Addiction* 105 (9), 1580

26 Fox A, 2015. Understanding behaviour in the Australian and New Zealand night-time economies: an anthropological study. *Unpublished,* 5

27 Room R & Mäkelä K, 2000. Typologies of the cultural position of drinking. *Journal of the Study of Alcohol* 61(3), 475

28 Delaney L et al, 2013. Why do some Irish drink so much? Family, historical and regional effects on students' alcohol consumption and subjective normative thresholds. *Review of Economics of the Household* 11(1), 25

other cultures respond quite differently to being under the influence. Some cultures experience very little violence and anti-social behaviour despite having comparable levels and patterns of consumption compared to other nations with high levels of such harm. A recent analysis of all current statistics on both reported and estimated unreported alcohol-related assaults in Australia, along with the estimated number of 'nights out', revealed that only 0.11 per cent of nights out result in alcohol-related violence.[29] In other words, 99.89 per cent of drinking occasions remain violence-free. If alcohol were a prescribed medication, a side effect reported in just 0.11 per cent of cases would not be considered caused by the drug. Fox reported that a policewoman confirmed this with an insightful observation based on several years of weekend patrols in a major Australian city: 'I have never met a violent drunk who was not also violent when sober.'[30] In other words – alcohol may facilitate, but it is not a cause.

The regional Australian city of Newcastle was the site of an experiment aimed at reducing weekend violence and chaos. In 2008, a range of measures was implemented for licensed venues, including earlier closing times, lockouts starting at 1 am, restrictions on the sale of certain drinks, and other regulations governing the management of drinking establishments. The Newcastle police adopted a zero-tolerance approach to misconduct in the nightlife economy and imposed heavy, on-the-spot fines for all misdemeanours. While the results of the Newcastle experiment seem impressive, showing a reduction in violent incidents from 99 per quarter in the Newcastle CBD before the changes to 68 per quarter afterwards, they have not been replicated as successfully in other areas, such as Geelong. One reason may be that Newcastle police employed another strategy: a significant increase in bail compliance checks. As Newcastle police Superintendent John Gralton explained, 'five per cent of the population causes 90 per cent of the problem ... Our bail compliance checks have gone from 40 to 400 a month.'[31] Each night, the police in Newcastle

29 Data Analysis Australia Pty Ltd, 2014. How often does a night out lead to an assault. *Unpublished,* 4

30 Fox A, 2015, 51

31 Fox A, 2015, 53

systematically verify that offenders out on bail or probation, who are subject to curfew, are not on the streets.

Believing that the benefits of drinking outweigh the harms, Fox argued that alcohol education should focus on the perceived benefits and assist individuals in achieving these essentially social goals without causing damage. Young people are concerned with being attractive, desirable, socially accepted, and confident. They seek pleasure, fun, novelty, and excitement in their lives, and for many, alcohol serves to that end. Fox suggested that changing a culture of drunken 'disinhibition' requires questioning what is so strongly inhibited in society that a chemical agent is needed to 'loosen' it. In drinking cultures, the message to children is that they cannot relax, be friendly, sociable, loving, helpful, or tolerant without a drink. The entire ritual, not just the alcohol, binds the group. However, in societies where alcohol is a routine, mundane, everyday, and unexciting part of life, adolescents generally do not use it as a form of rebellion or stolen pleasure. Fox is not implying that the solution is to provide 'toddlers booze and flame throwers'. Instead, she believes that the Australian risk-averse culture should be examined.[32] The only compelling message to control negative or extremely antisocial or violent drinking behaviour is, 'You are in control of your behaviour at all times. Drunkenness is no excuse.'[33]

Healthcare costs may not fall if unhealthy lifestyles are eliminated

It is fair to suggest that obesity is on the rise and that this is not occurring in a vacuum. For example, in 2022, of Australian adults:

- 11 per cent smoked daily
- 20 per cent drank too much
- 57 per cent did not eat enough fruit
- 77 per cent were not sufficiently active
- 94 per cent did not eat enough vegetables.[34]

As a result, while acknowledging that some Australians have biomedical

32 Fox A, 2015, 35

33 Fox A, 2015, 96

34 Australian Bureau of Statistics, 2023. *National Health Survey 2022,* Table 1.3

predispositions, in 2022, 66 per cent of adults were classified as overweight or obese, an increase from 56 per cent in 1995, predominantly driven by the rise in obese adults (19 per cent in 1995 to 32 per cent in 2022). Furthermore, 26 per cent of children aged 2-17 were overweight or obese. The proportion of children and adolescents aged 5-17 who were overweight or obese in 2022 was 28 per cent, up from 20 per cent in 1995.[35] An overweight child is likely to grow into, and remain, an obese adult. While obesity can be harmful, is it, as Obesity Australia argues, no longer merely a personal issue but 'overwhelmingly a societal issue, given its prevalence and costs'?[36] But, for obesity to be deemed a societal issue, there must be some problems that obese individuals create for non-obese individuals. Additionally, the causes of obesity are varied and are not as easily addressed as the issues of tobacco and alcohol. More importantly, there may be no public savings in a 'cure' for all consumption-related concerns.

It is true that medical costs are shared through public medical insurance and that any illness caused by obesity shifts these costs onto non-obese individuals. However, there are two solutions to this issue. One option is for obese individuals to bear a greater share of the expenses, thereby relieving the burden on others. The other, more intriguingly, is to compare the lifestyle costs of health to the lifetime costs of health. Such comparison reveals that healthy lifestyles, rather than unhealthy ones, are more likely to drive up health costs.[37] So, the obese have less to apologise for than is generally claimed.

What if it turns out that obese people, excluding those with genuine underlying medical conditions, are merely those who demonstrate a lack of restraint in a time when food is cheaper and more accessible than

35 Australian Institute of Health and Welfare, 2024. *Overweight and Obesity*

36 Obesity Australia, 2013, 2. See also, Obesity Evidence Hub www.obesityevidencehub.org.au

37 Snowdon C, 2015, 7. See also, Alemayehu B & Warner K E, 2004. The lifetime distribution of health care costs. *Health Services Research* 39(3), 627

ever before or are less inclined to exercise?[38] This is where the fun and games begin. The annual cost of obesity in Australia has been estimated to be between $37 billion and $58 billion a year.[39] But much of the so-called cost of obesity relates to loss of well-being. These losses are not a cost to society but to individuals. That aspect, shared because of public health insurance, is of concern.

The harsh reality of public harm-prevention or health-promotion programs for various consumption issues is that they yield no public savings. The reason is that healthy, rather than unhealthy, lifestyles escalate health costs. While preventive measures like immunising children can save costs, 'hundreds of economic studies have shown that prevention in chronic diseases [like those associated with obesity] typically increases medical costs.'[40] Improving health by preventing obesity is a valuable goal, but it does not necessarily mean that preventing obesity lowers national medical spending.

Medical science and healthier living delay the costs associated with disability and disease while paving the way for more costly non-fatal conditions among the elderly. Non-smokers have lower annual healthcare costs but incur higher lifetime costs due to their longer lifespans. Their additional pension years also contribute to significantly higher social security expenses. Consequently, the general taxpayer effectively saves money when others smoke.[41] The short-term healthcare costs of unhealthy individuals are lower than the long-term healthcare costs of healthy individuals.

Though public health advocates minimise the financial costs associated with healthy living and longer lives, these costs must be considered in

---

38 To the extent that exercise can reduce weight. See Sarma S et al, 2014. The effect of physical activity on adult obesity: evidence from the Canadian NPHS panel. *Economics & Human Biology* 14, 1

39 Colagiuri S, 2016. Is obesity a disease?: economic implications. *Obesity Australia Summit Papers*

40 Russell L, 2009. Preventing chronic disease: an important investment, but don't count on cost savings. *Health Affairs* 28(1), 42

41 Snowdon C, 2015, 23

the policy mix. If the benefits are limited, the public receives less return on its investment in health promotion or harm prevention policies than anticipated. Governments may tax, regulate, and punish wrongdoers, but such actions may not reduce taxpayers' burden. More importantly, the discovery that the lifetime health costs of unhealthy lifestyles are lower than those of healthy lifestyles suggests that the argument for controlling the lives of those who indulge in unhealthy lifestyles carries much less weight than previously claimed. It appears that destructive lifestyles are not public property. But, of course, public health depends on the argument that they are, and that the burden to the taxpayer justifies any number of intrusive measures.

Typical studies on the cost of obesity (and other vices) often generate substantial figures. For instance, the accounting firm PricewaterhouseCoopers estimated that the total costs of obesity in Australia for 2011-12 reached \$8.6 billion (in 2014-15 dollars). This total comprises \$3.8 billion in direct costs and \$4.8 billion in indirect costs. Projections yield even more significant figures; for example, 'there will be 2.4 million more obese individuals by 2025 compared to 2011-12, resulting in an additional \$87.7 billion in costs to society due to obesity over the ten years (from 2015-16 to 2024-25).'[42] The PwC study overlooked any associated benefits.

A study by Buchmueller, which examined the link between obesity and healthcare expenditure in Australia, noted that 'to the extent that obesity leads to premature mortality, savings from a policy that successfully reduces obesity at younger ages may be partially offset by higher lifetime expenditures caused by increased longevity.' This study, however, estimated that 'interventions that are successful in reducing obesity rates may also result in reduced health expenditures.'[43] The PwC study accounted for costs but not the benefits of obesity, while the

42 Price Waterhouse Coopers, 2015. *Weighing the Cost of Obesity: A Case for Action*, iv and v

43 Buchmueller T & Meliyanni J, 2015. Obesity and health expenditures: evidence from Australia. *Economics and Human Biology* 17, 54. See also, Black N, Hughes R & Jones A M, 2018. The health care costs of childhood obesity in Australia: an instrumental variables approach. *Economics & Human Biology* 31, 1

Buchmueller study assessed health expenditure costs but did not formally include other lifetime non-medical costs. Neither has the whole picture.

Whether interventions produce a dividend depends on measuring the costs and benefits of the activity. In any study, it is essential to verify that all costs and benefits are factored in. For example, Crampton's critique of a report by the Department of Health Victoria (featured in Text Box 9.1) on the costs of smoking points out multiple errors. The errors apply to all 'sin' products.

Text Box 9.1 Vic Health's wrong estimates of smoking benefits and costs

- Massively and inappropriately discounted the benefits of smoking while including as a cost of smoking the resources involved in tobacco production. A gross measure of consumer surplus would suffice, but it was not considered.
- It compares the health care costs of a smoker who dies at 63 from lung cancer with those of a non-smoker at the same age. It overlooks the fact that the smoker does not, for example, incur additional health care costs while dying from congestive heart failure at 76. Essentially, it assumes that the smoker could have lived indefinitely without any health care costs had they not smoked.
- Recognises that smoking is linked to other risk-taking behaviours but overlooks the possibility that the costs of smoking might be confused with the costs of other risk-taking activities.
- Ignoring the fact that smokers, by dying earlier, cost the superannuation and pension system significantly less—they contribute to the system but take out much less.
- Ignores that cigarette excise taxes are paid upfront, whereas health care costs arise much later. Essentially, the young smoker pays an annuity to the government to cover excess health costs that won't occur for another 30 or 40 years in the future.

Sources: Crampton E, 2008. Cost-benefit analysis when the conclusion drives the method: a review of 'Report on Tobacco Taxation in New Zealand'. *The New Zealand Medical Journal* 121(1269), 91. Crampton E, 2010. Excess costs of smoking. *Offsetting Behaviour* 16 June

Norman Temple provides a compelling illustration of how to consider all costs associated with interventions designed to persuade people to quit smoking. He points out that many estimates of the costs to encourage people to stop smoking are significantly flawed.[44] Consider a man, aged 40, who has smoked half a pack a day for the past 20 years. If he continues smoking, he will die of coronary heart disease (CHD) at age 65. However, if he quits, he is likely to live until 75 and then die of CHD. Temple poses the question: How does quitting impact healthcare spending? What are the other financial implications of a person stopping smoking? There are three ways to address these questions. The narrow view considers the next 25 years. Quitting reduces health care spending, as preventing death from CHD avoids the costs of treating the man for terminal CHD. Additionally, the man will likely be healthier during those 25 years, thus requiring less medical treatment.

The long-term view encompasses the next 35 years. The man dies at the age of 75 from terminal CHD, so the cost of treatment has not been avoided but merely postponed. Additionally, the savings from improved health before age 65 are likely to be offset, perhaps even surpassed, by the increase in healthcare spending that typically occurs among individuals over 65. The savings in health-care spending are illusory. The big picture considers non-medical expenditures. Since the man in the above example did not smoke between the ages of 40 and 65, he paid no tobacco taxes during that period. As a result, taxpayers lose a considerable amount of revenue. Moreover, he almost certainly receives an age pension, meaning taxpayers, through the government, must provide additional funds for the 10 extra years he lives after turning 65.

From a taxpayer's perspective, the effect of this man quitting smoking at the age of 40 is twofold. Each dollar in savings before age 65 leads to a dollar or more in spending after that. The combined effect of lost tax revenues and increased spending on pension payments has a significant negative impact on government finances. Temple cautions that in various scenarios at older ages, prevention may lead to a longer life with less disability and no increase in healthcare costs. Additionally, prevention can often be more cost-effective than medical treatments. However,

44 Temple N, 2012. Why prevention can increase health-care spending. *European Journal of Public Health* 22(5), 618

over the past 40 years, numerous economic studies have indicated that prevention of chronic diseases such as heart disease, stroke, and diabetes, along with screenings for various cancers and management of chronic conditions, typically results in increased medical spending.[45]

Obesity prevention, for instance, may not lead to cost savings. While effective obesity prevention reduces the costs associated with obesity-related diseases, these savings are offset by increased costs from diseases not linked to obesity when considering life years gained. The study conducted by van Baal in the Netherlands compared the lifetime health costs of obese individuals, smokers, and those who maintain a healthy lifestyle. It predicted that up to the age of 56, yearly health costs are highest for the obese population and lowest for the healthy individuals. In older age groups, the smoking demographic incurred the highest annual costs. However, due to differences in life expectancy (life expectancy at age 20 was five years lower in the obese group and eight years lower in the smoking group than in the healthy-living group), total lifetime health expenditure was most significant for healthy individuals, lowest for smokers, and intermediate for obese individuals.[46] Although public health advocates downplay the financial costs associated with healthy living and longer lives, it is essential to consider these costs in the policy mix. If gains are few, the public will receive less than the expected return on its investment in health promotion or harm prevention policies. So why is public health silent on these nuances? Do economic arguments only matter in public health when they support public health ideology?

Morbidity: compression or expansion?

An essential consideration in these lifetime health cost calculations is the cost of care in later life. Public health theoreticians and practitioners must be honest in informing the public and politicians,

45 Russell L, 2009, 42

46 van Baal et al, 2008. Lifetime medical costs of obesity: prevention no cure for increasing health expenditure. *PLOS Medicine*, 0242

indeed, arming them with facts that will allow them to explain to a baying public and media that a whole-of-life-cycle appreciation of costs is part of any cost-benefit analysis. An important part of such analyses is morbidity.

The compression of morbidity occurs when the age at which aging manifestations and chronic disease symptoms first appear can increase more rapidly than life expectancy. The question of whether the duration of morbidity can be reduced hinges on whether the average onset age of a marker of morbidity (the first heart attack, initial dyspnea from emphysema, first disability from osteoarthritis, or first memory loss) can rise more quickly than life expectancy from the same age. If it does, the interval between that marker and the end of life is shortened.

Absolute compression of morbidity occurs when age-specific morbidity rates decrease more rapidly than age-specific mortality rates. Relative compression of morbidity occurs if the time lived after the onset of the first chronic morbidity diminishes as a percentage of life expectancy.[47] Three broad health scenarios have been proposed to outline the evolution of mortality, morbidity, and disability as well as the health consequences of increasing life expectancy in older age groups (detailed in Text Box 9.2).

47 Fries J, 2005. The compression of morbidity. *The Milbank Quarterly* 83(4), 810

Text Box 9.2 Three scenarios of morbidity

Compression of morbidity

- The period living with ill-health and disability before death is shortened because of a delay in onset of chronic disease or disability and a slowdown in the rate of increase in life expectancy
- If the number of expected years of life with disability falls, there is an absolute compression of morbidity
- If the proportion of expected years of life with disability falls without the number of expected years of disability decreasing (it could even rise), there is a relative compression of morbidity.

Expansion of morbidity

- Increasing longevity is accompanied by more survivors who are frail and suffer from chronic conditions, resulting in a longer period living with disability before death
- If the number of expected years of life free of disability falls, there is an absolute expansion of morbidity
- If the proportion of expected years free of disability falls without the number of expected disability-free years decreasing (it could even rise) there is a relative expansion of morbidity.

Dynamic equilibrium

- The overall level of diseases or disability increases largely due to the increase of less severe diseases or disability, while the prevalence of severe diseases or disability falls or remains stable, due to the rate of progression of disease or disability slowing down
- If the ratio of disability-free life expectancy to total life expectancy is constant, there is equilibrium
- For the severity of disability, if the number of years with disabilities – all levels combined – increases, while the number of years with severe disability remains constant or even falls within life expectancy, there is said to be 'dynamic equilibrium'.

Source: The Australian Institute for Health and Welfare, 2014. Healthy life expectancy in Australia: patterns and trends 1998 to 2012. *Bulletin 126*, 19

Health-adjusted life expectancy extends the concept of life expectancy (the number of years a person can expect to live) by considering the number of years a person of a particular age could expect to live in full health (without disease and/or injury) and in ill health (with disease and/or injury). Life expectancy and health-adjusted life expectancy can be measured at any age, but are typically reported from birth (which represents the average life expectancy in years for a baby born that year) and at age 65, describing health in an ageing population.

Figure 9.1 Life expectancy and life-adjusted life expectancy over time by sex at birth

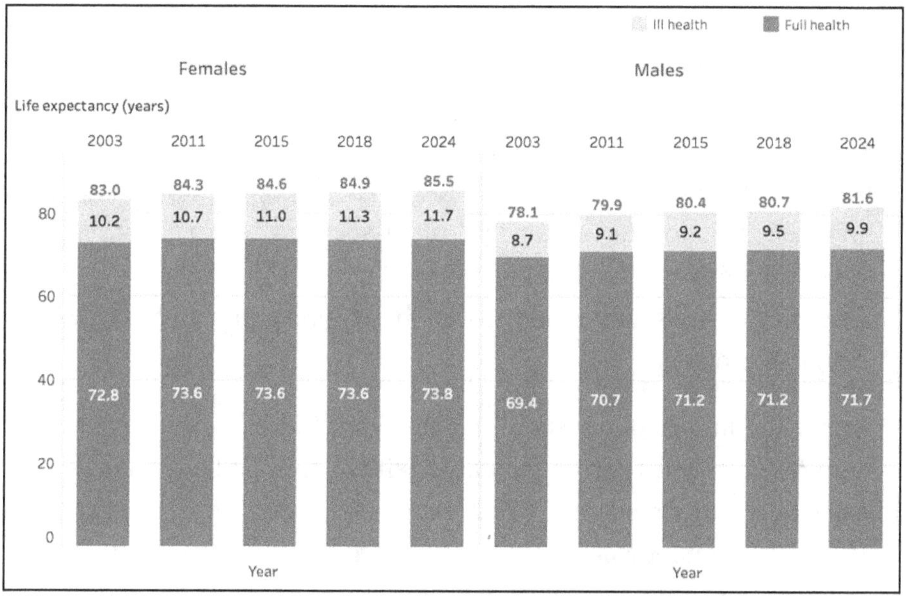

Source: Australian Institute of Health and Welfare, 2024. *Australian Burden of Disease Study 2024*

An analysis by the Australian Institute of Health and Welfare found improvements in life expectancy at birth and at age 65 were accompanied by a rise in expected years both with and without disability or severe or profound core activity limitation (Figure 9.1 shows life expectancy at birth). The results for age 65 cohort were shown in Figure I.2. Life expectancy in both scenarios is rising, life free from disability is rising and years of life with disability is rising.

The increase in expected years of living free from disability is linked to a combination of increasing longevity and declining prevalence rates of disability. Additionally, there is no reliable evidence supporting the dynamic equilibrium scenario for older Australians, as the expected years with severe or profound core activity limitation have continued to rise slightly alongside a rise in years with disability. There is also no evidence of an absolute compression of disability among older Australians, regardless of the disability level. At age 65, the gains in expected years free of disability and severe or profound core activity limitation have not exceeded those in life expectancy. Increases in anticipated years of disability and in severe or profound limitations in core activities have accompanied improvements in longevity. These findings confirm that no single scenario applies in Australia during the study period; instead, a combination of positive and negative changes is evident, aligning with recent international experience.[48] This suggests that there is no imminent solution to the rising costs associated with ageing, such as the lower smoking and drinking rates observed in Australia over several decades. Given its numerous causes, obesity prevention may prove to be even less promising.

As for the non-health costs of ageing, James Fries, a leader in ageing research, advocates that to maintain health in old age 'there should be no mandatory retirement age.'[49] But, the fact is that there is, or at least an age at which retirement benefits become available, and it is inconceivable that a pension will not be available at an age relatively young compared to the rising rate of longevity.[50] Men aged 65 in 2021–2023 could expect to live another 20.1 years, and women aged 65 in 2021–2023 could expect to live another 22.7 years. In 1960, for example, the life expectancy at age 65 was 77.5 for men and 80.7 for women. The pension age was 65 and 60, respectively. In 1960, a man could expect to receive the aged pension for 11.5 years, and a woman for 20.7 years. In 2021, aged pension eligibility was 67, a man could expect to be on the aged

48 The Australian Institute for Health and Welfare, 2014. *Bulletin 126*, 19

49 Fries J, 2005, 819

50 The age at which the aged pension is available in Australia has been lifted in the last few years, but 67 is the new standard for men and women.

pension for 18.1 years, and a woman for 20.7 years.[51] The non-health lifetime costs of ageing are increasing.

Any study that claims to demonstrate savings in harm prevention or health promotion should be treated with caution. While these may be beneficial, they often come with a price tag. Snowdon provides a handy checklist of the ways public health advocates downplay the financial costs of healthy, longer lives, where they,

- Focus on end-of-life health costs while overlooking the health costs of additional years of life
- Give little thought to long-term care costs, which surpass the acute healthcare expenses linked to ageing
- Disregard welfare payments
- Concentrate on per capita expenses instead of the ratio of employed taxpayers to pensioners
- Argue that promoting healthy ageing will lower healthcare costs.[52]

Conclusion

The relationship between prevention and public spending is complex and multifaceted. Some preventive activities can be cost-saving, particularly those that are relatively inexpensive to implement and prevent a condition that is generally non-fatal but costly to treat. A good example is the immunisation of children. However, preventing fatal diseases may increase healthcare spending. This occurs because the extra years of life inevitably lead to a greater need for treating chronic conditions and long-term nursing care. Overall, most medical interventions aimed at preventing disease or improving health increase healthcare spending. This does not argue against treatment, but instead suggests that the cost savings claimed by various advocates may not be accurate.

The costs and benefits of health prevention and other health strategies trumpeted by public health advocates must be subject to honest, whole-of-life-cycle analysis. The rationale for gouging taxes, as seen with tobacco

51 Australian Bureau of Statistics, 2025. *Deaths in Australia.*

52 Snowdon C, 2015, 30

excise taxes, or restricting access, as with alcohol, or implementing highly interventionist programs, such as food labelling, is much shakier when public health interventions do not provide public savings.

Governments may tax, regulate, and bemoan those who indulge, but these actions will not reduce the taxpayers' burden. The justification for controlling the lives of those who choose to indulge holds significantly less weight than previously argued. It appears that when subject to calm analysis rather than public health hyperbole, lifestyles are not public property.

10

Things to do

The public health lobby, or that part that eschews science and embraces ideology, is driven by ego and harms society. Public health types who want to save the world will use all means necessary, particularly taxpayers' money and government fiat, to achieve what they define as population health outcomes. The overriding value in public health, according to one of its young enthusiasts, is that of equity,[1] a highly freighted concept that drives a never-ending search for 'optimal' outcomes for all. No stone is to be left unturned to help even those who did not ask for it. At its centre, it is, as Jessica Flanigan observed, progressive and statist.[2] Public health, in conjunction with more conventional patient point-of-entry medical interventions, is driving nations into debt. The result will be a very unappealing equity, a highly prescribed environment where health is valued above all else and health practitioners rule the polity. Society is not a hospital ward or a medical clinic. Public health needs to be reined in. To counter public health tyranny, various measures require debate.

This book has illustrated some of public health's most prominent strategies and tactics. Collectively, these fall under three broad banners: power, life, and death. Public health craves power over others, meaning that it must always find new problems and groups of people who, according to

---

1 Dr Lauren Richardson, Director, Evidence Based Medicine and Health Policy, Guidelines and Economists Network International. *Public Health Insiders Podcast* Monash University 25 September 2024. She was a member of the COVID-19 Public Health Policy team in Victoria.

2 Flanigan J, 2024, 508

its own righteous judgement, require saving from themselves or from whom society more broadly requires saving. Public health is also obsessed with its narrow view of what 'living' means; it endlessly promotes the idea that long lives are necessarily better lives, even as it takes away the things that make life pleasurable. Apparently, a long, miserable life subject to the straitjacketed social norms that public health deems acceptable, beats a shorter but happier life in which people can indulge in enjoyments and freedoms that public health finds deeply offensive. And finally, public health is about death — or, more precisely, an insistence that the only type of death that is tolerable is one at an advanced age. Public health attempts to persuade that illness, injury, and 'premature' death are in some way abnormal, rather than just part of life, and that it is worth trading off parts of our lives in the attempt to delay death. And it uses our growing unfamiliarity with death to generate monumental fear — not only for our own lives, but for those of the people we love. After all, a fearful population is an easy one to control.

Being able to identify public health's modus operandi means calling it out, which is a first and essential step towards ending public health's conceited control over our lives and societies. We encourage readers to apply the points raised in this book whenever possible. However, we provide below some immediate actions that relate to the specific case studies and examples we have given.

1. Stop insidious ideology: let people do their job

The Trojan Horse used to undermine the medical profession in pursuit of public health progressive ideology is the various codes of ethics. For example, since 2018, the International Council of Nurses' Code of Ethics for Nurses and Midwives has been in effect for all nurses in Australia, replacing the 2008 Australian codes. The International Council code expanded the meaning and reach of ethics in the profession considerably. For example, (emphasis added),

> *1.6 Nurses share with society the responsibility for initiating and supporting action to meet the health and social needs of all people.*
>
> *1.7 Nurses advocate for equity and social justice in resource allocation, access to health care and other social and economic services.*
>
> *1.8 Nurses demonstrate professional values such as respect, justice, responsiveness, caring, compassion, empathy, trustworthiness and integrity. They support and respect the dignity and universal rights of all people, including patients, colleagues and families.*

Nurses and other medical professionals should not sign up to be political actors. Supporting action to meet social needs, whatever they are, or advocating for equity and social justice, or the universal rights of all people, should not be the subject of a profession's code of ethics. These are a political call to arms, both progressive and statist, or, in old-fashioned terms, socialist. Further,

> *4.4 Nurses contribute to population health and work towards the achievement of the United Nations Sustainable Development Goals.*
>
> *4.5 Nurses recognise the significance of the social determinants of health. They contribute to, and advocate for, policies and programmes that address them.*
>
> *4.6 Nurses collaborate and practise to preserve, sustain and protect the natural environment and are aware of the health consequences of environmental degradation, e.g. climate change. They advocate for initiatives that reduce environmentally harmful practices to promote health and well-being.*
>
> *4.7 Nurses collaborate with other health and social care professions and the public to uphold principles of justice by promoting responsibility in human rights, equity and fairness and by promoting the public good and a healthy planet.*

Nurses should not sign up for, especially under threat of registration, the achievement of UN sustainable development goals, all of which are political and contestable, and incidentally, frequently at cross-purposes. They should not have to agree to protect the natural environment, which has nothing to do with their profession, or promote the public good, a meaningless concept, or a healthy planet, an equally useless concept.

Figure 10.1 ICN Code of ethics for nurses professional values

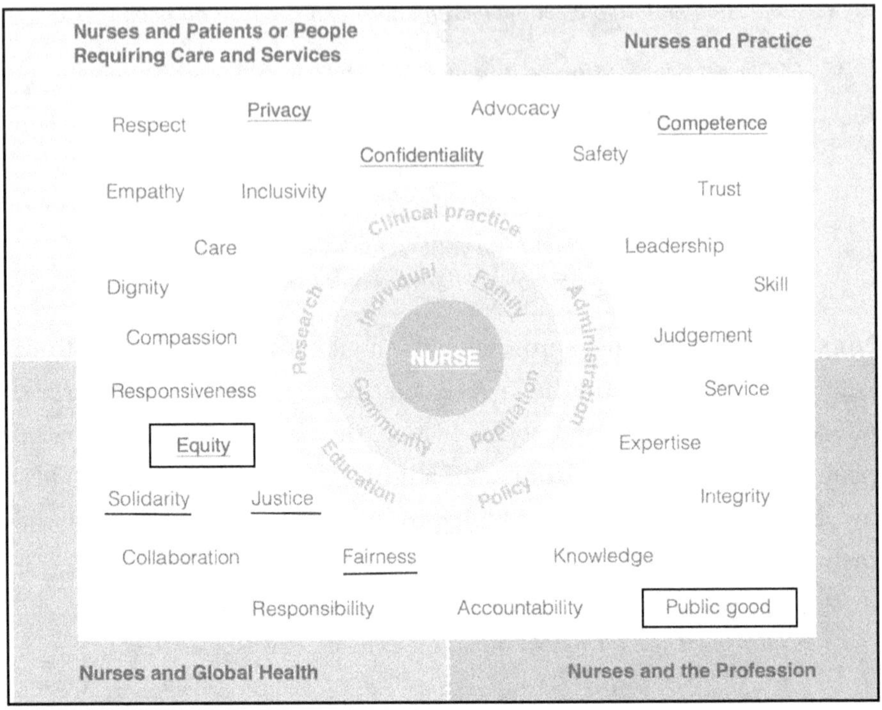

Source: International Council of Nurses, 2021. *The ICN Code of Ethics for Nurses,* 21

The international code of ethics is set out in Figure 10.1. Those parts of the code that relate to practice, care, and services are reasonable and closely aligned to the profession of nursing. Still, those relating to nurses, the profession, and the public good are outside a sensible remit. Those related to nurses and global health are extreme and should never be a condition of a nurse's registration.

2. Push back on the use of legislation: amend Public Health Acts

As Forbes argued to the Commonwealth Inquiry, Chief Health Officers 'must never again be afforded the unchecked powers applicable during the COVID-19 pandemic.'[3] An essential value must be that compulsion to restrict the daily lives of its citizens during a pandemic, including the

3 Forbes G, 2024. *Submission to the Commonwealth Government COVID-19 Pandemic Response Inquiry*

right to peaceful protest, must never be used unless there is overwhelming evidence of significant risk to many individuals without such measures and, crucially, that each intervention will be effective and time-limited.[4] The issue is to find feasible ways to do this.

The Commonwealth government and some State governments closed their borders as a response to the pandemic.[5] The result of Clive Palmer's challenge to the West Australian government's closure of borders under its emergency powers was unsuccessful. In *Palmer v. Western Australia*, the High Court of Australia unanimously determined that the Western Australian Government's pandemic border restrictions were not invalid under section 92 of the Australian Constitution. Their powers are unassailable. There is also no joy in challenging the authority of the Commonwealth government to close the national border.[6] Several federal court cases have sought to challenge the validity of both the Governor-General's declaration of a human biosecurity emergency and the Minister for Health's invocation of human biosecurity emergency powers to implement measures such as a travel ban. So far, every challenge has failed.[7] The discussion around border closures, primarily state borders, should occur within the framework of authority granted by emergency legislation.

A recent review of emergency powers exercised under public health legislation across all Australian jurisdictions found that inadequate accountability mechanisms are entrenched in the statutes and insufficient transparency regarding decisions made by the Executive under public

4 Appleby G, O'Sullivan M & Partlett W, 2021. *The Public Health and Wellbeing Amendment (Pandemic Management) Bill 2021* (Vic) The Centre for Public Integrity. See also, Law Institute of Victoria submission on the Bill, 10 November 2021

5 Suraweera A, 2022. *Palmer v Western Australia*: pandemic border closures and section 92 of the Australian Constitution. *Sydney Law Review* 13 44(2)

6 Commonwealth Government, 2024. *COVID-19 Response Inquiry,* 171

7 Commonwealth Government, 2024. *COVID-19 Response Inquiry,* 107 and see *Athavle & Ors v NSW Minister for Health, Vic Minister for Health, State of NSW, State of Vic and Commonwealth of Australia*, Federal Court of Australia, NSD 894/2021; *Knowles & Ors v Commonwealth of Australia & Ors*, Federal Court of Australia, VID 579/2021; *Gary Newman v Minister for Health and Aged Care*, Federal Court of Australia, NSD 388/2021; *LibertyWorks Inc v Commonwealth*, Federal Court of Australia, NSD 1312/2020

health emergency powers. There are few options within the public health emergency legislation for reviewing executive actions concerning legality, merit, and fairness.[8] More concerning is that the state fails to provide regular accounts or justifications for its use. Although public health powers are subject to administrative review and, in some jurisdictions, forms of judicial oversight, violations of administrative justice concerning coercive public health powers can lead to irreversible consequences.[9]

Far from ensuring restraint on emergency powers, some members of the public health fraternity argue that these Acts could be used to advance their broader health objectives, particularly in addressing the commercial determinants of health, which they allege contribute to non-communicable diseases. For example,

> *Modernised public health acts may enable governments to develop and implement regulatory strategies that sit under the act, without facing the complexities that are often associated in passing new legislation. Careful wording of provisions could also avoid attention and reduce unwanted pushback from unhealthy commodity industries and lobby groups.*[10]

It is wise to always beware of the term 'modernised'. The proponents of the surreptitious use of public health legislation to expand their remit praise the *South Australian Public Health Act* 2011, particularly where the Minister may declare a medical condition to be a non-communicable condition if they consider that the disease or medical condition poses a significant public health concern. The active principles that give effect to the Act are precautionary, proportionate, sustainable, population-focused, and equitable.

---

8 O'Brien P & Waters E, 2021. COVID-19: public health emergency powers and accountability mechanisms in Australia. *Journal of Law and Medicine* 28(2), 346

9 Carter D J, 2020. The use of coercive public health and human biosecurity law in Australia: an empirical analysis. *University of New South Wales Law Journal* 43(1), 150 and Rajan R & Topp S M, 2022. Accountability mechanisms of inquiries and investigations into Australian Governments' responses to the COVID-19 pandemic. *Australian and New Zealand Journal of Public Health* 46(4), 488

10 Heenan M, Ralph M & Shantosh J, 2024, 2

The chameleon-like precautionary principle cannot assist decision-making without a value system; for example, it does not specify whom to protect from what. What happens when the facts change during a pandemic response? This is the point made by Coatsworth in his submission to the Commonwealth COVID-19 Inquiry. The facts changed, but the response remained the same. At its simplest, the precautionary principle advises that a proponent should proceed with caution before undertaking an action where there is a risk of potential harm. But this principle is not so simple.[11] Although widely invoked, the principle does not necessarily aid in risk management. For example, a widely accepted definition of the principle is as follows: 'When an activity raises threats of harm to … human health, precautionary measures should be taken, even if some cause-and-effect relationships are not fully established.'[12] This formulation is value-laden in what might be called a health direction: 'A principle that is presented by its proponents in the guise of a value-neutral guide to policy-making in the face of uncertainty is nothing of the kind.'[13] Taking precautionary action such as lockdowns is a perversion of the precautionary principle—an analogue of the Hippocratic do no harm concept — which is designed to maintain the *status quo* in the presence of scientific uncertainty.'[14]

The difficulty with the statement lies in the absence of a definition for three crucial elements: the threat of harm, uncertainty about risks and causal relationships, and the level of precaution in response to the threat. If the threat of harm is taken to mean the actual risk of an activity, then the principle says too little: stay safe. If, on the other hand, the threat of harm refers to the public perception of hazard, then the precautionary principle may be applied too broadly; it can be invoked to halt benefits such as everyday life, the economy, and other medical procedures. If,

11 Beloin V, 2009. *Public Policies Guided by The Precautionary Principle.* National Collaborating Centre for Healthy Public Policy

12 Cussen K, 2009. Handle with care: assessing the risks of the precautionary principle. *Australasian Journal of Environmental Management* 16(2), 67

13 Cussen K, 2009, 69

14 Annas G J, 2007. Your liberty or your life. Talking point on public health versus civil liberties. *EMBO Reports* 8(12), 1093

in response to harm, human health is the fundamental value, all other values — the health and prosperity of the non-vulnerable on whom the vulnerable rely — are given little or no weight.

The South Australian Act article 6(1) states that 'If there is a perceived material risk to public health, lack of full scientific certainty should not be used as a reason for postponing measures to prevent, control or abate that risk.' During the COVID-19 response, it seems that this part of Article was invoked, but the remainder, (2)(b) and (c), were not, that is, 'decision-making and action should be proportionate to the degree of public health risk' following an 'assessment of the risk-weighted consequences of options' and 'an aim to ensure minimum disruption to an individual's activities, a community's functioning and commercial activity.'[15]

Every part of the responses to the risk of the virus — lockdowns, masks, testing and tracing, vaccines and so on — should have been assessed for harm and cost. If the precautionary principle is to be invoked, it must apply to both the interventions and the original threat to health. Other fine-sounding principles — proportionate regulation, sustainability and population focus — are similarly biased when applied through the lens of a single threat to health.[16] They sound fine but are of no practical use, although they can be invoked to cause significant harm to the public in all of life's dimensions other than the specific threat to a particular cohort.

By contrast, the equity principle (13), 'consideration should be given to health disparities between population groups', has become an obsession among policy makers. For example, the Commonwealth COVID-19 Inquiry provided a rote recitation of 'vulnerable' communities, beginning with Aboriginal people and the usual list of others. Only those people at heightened risk of infection should have been vaccinated. The notion of equity was abused. The SA Act also has Specific principles that

15 *South Australian Public Health Act 2011*, part 2

16 *South Australian Public Health Act 2011*, part 2

restrictions should be 'proportionate to any risks presented to others', and that 'any requirement restricting the liberty of a person should not be imposed unless it is the only effective way remaining to ensure that the health of the public is not endangered.'[17] The equitable response was to assess the vulnerable cohort and then assess the response for both the vulnerable cohort and all others. If the response had taken notice of 14(4)(e) and (6), it may have been balanced. These many principles give the appearance of rational evaluation, but operate to cover values hidden in the minds of advisers.

3. Challenge coercive control: restrict mandatory vaccination

During the pandemic, State and Territory governments made public health orders and enforceable government directions requiring certain workers to be vaccinated against COVID-19. The Fair Work Ombudsman confirmed that employers could require their employees to be vaccinated where a public health order or enforceable government direction required it, or they give their employees a lawful and reasonable direction to be vaccinated.[18]

Using NSW as an example, COVID-19 was managed in the same way as any workplace health and safety hazard, by applying a risk management approach to eliminate and/or minimise COVID-19 exposure and transmission risks in the workplace.[19] An employer may still be able to give their employee a lawful and reasonable direction to get vaccinated, even if no public health order, agreement or contract with terms about COVID-19 vaccination applies. A key consideration included the effectiveness of vaccines in reducing the risk of transmission or serious illness.[20] The leading case was heard in the NSW Supreme Court on

17 *South Australian Public Health Act 2011*, part 2

18 Fair Work Ombudsman, COVID-19 vaccinations https://www.fairwork.gov.au/find-help-for/covid-19-and-workplace-laws/covid-19-vaccinations

19 NSW Safe Work, 2025. *COVID-19 Vaccination*

20 Fair Work Ombudsman, COVID-19 vaccinations https://www.fairwork.gov.au/find-help-for/covid-19-and-workplace-laws/covid-19-vaccinations

appeal from a decision of the Fair Work Commission and relying on a dissenting decision of a deputy president.[21] The primary challenge raised in the cases concerned the effect of the impugned public health orders on the rights and freedoms of those persons who chose not to be vaccinated, particularly their freedom and right to their bodily integrity.

The NSW Supreme Court held that 'So far as the right to bodily integrity is concerned, it is not violated as the impugned orders do not authorise the involuntary vaccination of anyone.' The plaintiffs submitted, however, that the practical effect of such an interpretation was that a person's consent is essentially weakened because of being threatened with the loss of their capacity to work. The argument was that employees could not have exercised a free choice to consent and that any such vaccinations amounted to battery. The NSW Supreme Court categorically rejected this in saying that 'while none of the plaintiffs have been so overborne', so far as 'the consent necessary to negative the offence of battery [this] is satisfied by the patient being advised in broad terms of the nature of the procedure to be performed.' But the patients could not have been well informed; the adverse effects of the vaccines were unknown. It would be helpful for the court to practice the recommendation that, in receiving scientific evidence, they have a compliance checklist as recommended by Armstrong and Green.[22]

The Chief Justice stated that assertions about the efficacy and safety of COVID-19 vaccines and other aspects of the public health response to COVID-19 were not reflected in the evidence.[23] The Chief Justice was unaware that the Australian Health Practitioner Regulation Agency and National Boards' statement on 21 March 2021, that 'There is no place for anti-vaccination messages in professional health practice'[24], was part of

21 *Kassam v Hazzard; Henry v Hazzard* [2021] NSWSC 1320

22 Armstrong J S & Green K C, 2022, 169

23 *Kassam v Hazzard; Henry v Hazzard* [2021] NSWSC 1320, 69

24 Australian Health Practitioner Regulation Agency and National Boards, 2021, 21 March. AHPRA's failure to warn vaccinators not to collaborate with COVID-19 vaccination mandates is subject of complaint to the National Health Practitioner Ombudsman.

a regimen to suppress dissent. It became clear very early, however, that the COVID-19 vaccines did not prevent transmission and may not have reduced the likelihood of serious illnesses among a working-age cohort in otherwise good health. And yet, the compulsion continued.

The law should not license an overly protective mindset. It penalises workers. A future case against an employer may not be so trusting of the evidence on the efficacy of vaccines or the potential loss of employment in a mandatory vaccination regime.

4. Oppose the WHO pandemic Agreement

The WHO panicked during the COVID-19 pandemic and abandoned its trusted responses on lockdowns and masks.[25] It was lured into a false sense of control in the authoritarian Chinese state.[26] The Chinese government's suppression of information and delayed disclosure of critical data, not to mention silencing Chinese medical staff, damaged its credibility.[27] Lack of transparency hindered the investigation into the virus's origin and fueled the spread of the lab-leak or intentional manipulation hypotheses.[28] Why the UN changed its mind on aspects of the response, and indeed, many governments followed a Chinese-style suppression, is a mystery born of conspiracy and panic.[29]

Controversy has not deterred the UN's intentions to be better prepared for the next pandemic. In December 2021, the World Health Assembly established an intergovernmental negotiating body to draft and negotiate a convention, agreement or other international instrument under the Constitution of the WHO 'to strengthen pandemic prevention,

---

25 United Nations, 2019. *Non-pharmaceutical Public Health Measures for Mitigating the Risk and Impact of Epidemic and Pandemic Influenza*

26 World Health Organization, WHO Director-General's Opening Remarks. *Media Briefing on COVID-19*, 11 March 2020

27 United Nations, 2020. *Report of the WHO-China Joint Mission*, 16

28 Yoo J H, 2025, e153

29 Macedo S & Lee F, 2025, 300 quoting emails among members of the Joint Mission when drafting and editing their report, February 22–24, 2020

preparedness and response.' WHO Member States have adopted two other global, legally binding agreements to protect and promote people's health: the WHO Framework Convention on Tobacco Control and the International Health Regulations, which provide a public health response to the international spread of disease. Of course, how this new agreement fits with the myriad other priorities is anyone's guess. Bjorn Lomborg has pointed out that the long list of UN priorities amounts to no priorities.[30]

Undeterred, the agreement was obsessed with 'inequities at national and international levels that hindered timely and equitable access to health products to address coronavirus disease (COVID-19).' Worryingly, the agreement states that an adequate pandemic response is part of a 'continuum to combat other health emergencies and achieve greater health equity through resolute action on the social, environmental, cultural, political and economic determinants of health', and 'the importance and public health impact of growing threats such as climate change.'[31] Other worrying elements are the One Health approach for pandemic prevention, which recognises 'that the health of humans is closely linked and interdependent with the health of domestic and wild animals, as well as plants and the wider environment (including ecosystems), aiming for a sustainable balance … which contributes to sustainable development in an equitable manner.'[32] Whatever this means is almost certainly expensive and bound to slow progress and wealth creation.

Notably, the Agreement demands the 'best available science and evidence as the basis for public health decisions for pandemic prevention, preparedness and response'[33], but it failed to do so during COVID-19, severely weakening trust in medical responses to pandemics. The Agreement refers to zoonotic diseases jumping from animals to humans

---

30 Lomborg B, 2023

31 World Health Organization, 2025. *14 May*, 5

32 World Health Organization, 2025, 7

33 World Health Organization, 2025, 9

and 'laboratory biological risk management, which is a relief for those who worried the UN would be too afraid to raise the prospect in light of accusations against the Chinese Wuhan laboratory.[34] Wrapped in the language of health equity,[35] the bottom line is, as always, the bottom line, with the proposal for additional financial resources to support 'developing country Parties implement the Agreement.'[36]

Given the propensity for the Albanese government to do whatever is fashionable at the UN, it is likely to be an enthusiastic adopter.[37] The Agreement is one more pillar in the edifice of top-down decision-making, enhancing the appearance of unity in medical responses—one false move at the UN, as occurred during COVID-19, and the world panics. There will be a conference of the parties to maintain the conversation, no doubt with a rolling message of crisis and the need for regulation and funding. Better that each nation takes its account of risks, albeit understanding that its actions are not alone in halting the spread of a disease or, more appropriately, preparing a response to manage those who will likely suffer.

5. No more bureaucracy: oppose the Centre for Disease Control

The Commonwealth Inquiry recommended establishing an Australian Centre for Disease Control, to which the government has agreed. Coatsworth observed,

> *The creation of a separate institution risks ... institutional group think and single-minded pursuit of disease-control over all other priorities ... There is no evidence at all to suggest that nations with CDC's performed any better during the pandemic.*[38]

The future will present a contest between cabinet government, where

34 World Health Organization, 2025, 10

35 World Health Organization, 2025, 5

36 World Health Organization, 2025, 25

37 Commonwealth of Australia Department of Foreign Affairs and Trade, 2025. *Global Health Reform*

38 Coatsworth N, 2023, 9

ministers and departments advise and deliberate, and a CDC that supports a chief medical officer and medical committee. Evidence must be explicit to justify chief medical officers or their delegates implementing lockdowns, closing borders, mandating masks and vaccines, denying employment to the unvaccinated, shutting down schools, and indeed any measures associated with a pandemic. Above all, the doctor-patient relationship must be preserved despite the existence of the interim CDC,[39] based on existing institutions such as the Doherty and Burnet Institutes and the University of Melbourne.[40] These institutions' recommendations for COVID-19 included lockdowns, border closures, masks, testing, tracing, isolation, quarantine, and vaccines. They also advocate ongoing vaccinations, testing, tracing, and isolation efforts. An Australian CDC will ensure a comparable response in future pandemics unless alternative sources of advice emerge.

The Centre for Disease Control, with the likelihood of a Chief Paediatrician and the National Children's Commissioner on the Australian Health Protection Committee, will not readily loosen the regulatory noose during a pandemic.[41] The fact that children not at risk from COVID-19 suffered due to the pandemic response, particularly school closures, does not justify the need for more Commissioners. Instead, it reflects a public service mentality of creating more jobs for public servants. Establishing a disease-first bureaucracy, followed by other bureaucrats addressing unintended consequences, is unwise. It is crucial to have alternative sources of advice to complement the CDC. Whether it adopts a red team/blue team model, as suggested by Peter Ridd[42] or James McCaw[43] or the Alberta Inquiry[44], it must act as

39 Commonwealth of Australia Department of Health, Disability and Ageing, 2025. *The Interim Australian Centre for Disease Control*

40 Burnet Institute, 2023

41 Commonwealth Government, 2024. *COVID-19 Response Inquiry*, 13

42 Ridd P, 2024. Trump's revolution is coming for the health technocrats. *The Australian* 5 December

43 McCaw J, 2024. *Submission to the Commonwealth Government Covid-19 Response Inquiry*

44 Alberta COVID-19 Pandemic Data Review Task Force, 2025, ch 4

a significant counterbalance not only to medical officials but also to prominent politicians who may seek approval from frightened voters for harmful actions that lead to lockdowns, mandated masks, and vaccinations where the costs outweigh the benefits.

6. Real-time evaluations of non-pharmaceutical interventions

Unlike vaccines, non-pharmaceutical interventions (NPI), such as quarantining healthy individuals, mass testing, and contact tracing, do not require formal approval. This area operates as a free-for-all, with each chief health officer enforcing their remedies. A significant change would be to require all non-pharmaceutical interventions to undergo real-time evaluation, including risk-benefit analyses. Sabhlok believes that drug regulators are best placed to compile the scientific evidence needed to evaluate non-pharmaceutical interventions. He suggests a role for a CDC to prepare a scientific proposal on NPIs for submission to a relevant authority, such as the Therapeutic Goods Administration, which would conduct a cost-benefit analysis.[45] He further suggests that empirical evidence is essential, while non-empirical methods, like mathematical models based on assumptions about implementation and efficacy, would not suffice. 'Blanket claims that the "validity" of a model should be viewed with suspicion.'[46] Meaningless mathematics can create a false sense of control over complex phenomena. 'Undue acceptance of modelling results is a common consequence of an "interpretation pitfall," where the model's users – decision-makers lack distance from the model's shortcomings.'[47] Simulation model results of infection spread should not be released to the public.

Although the cost-benefit analysis methodology may not suit the TGA's

45 Sabhlok S, 2024. Non-pharmaceutical interventions should be approved by the drugs regulator – Parts 1 and 2. *The Times of India* December 24

46 James L P et al, 2021. The use and misuse of mathematical modeling for infectious disease policymaking: lessons for the COVID-19 pandemic. *Medical Decision Making* 41(4), 383

47 Alberta COVID-19 Pandemic Data Review Task Force, 2025, ch 3

skills, it is crucial to educate the public health community on how to assess human health and well-being using cost-benefit analysis to ensure that regulators never again treat society like a hospital ward. Whether a CDC proceeds without a proper correction process, authorities may overreach, leading to a false sense of consensus. This situation can solidify the trajectory of a public health emergency response in a flawed direction. Alberta raised several questions that Coatsworth referred to, including the need for an agreed-upon ethical framework that is not focused solely on the risks posed by a single source —specifically, the disease. The balance between essential public health measures and the preservation of professional autonomy and judgment must be clarified early in a pandemic response.

7. Oppose social justice ideological contagion in AHPRA

The Australian Health Practitioner Regulation Agency (incorporating Medical Boards) exercises power over the doctor-patient relationship by being able to deregister practitioners. It exercises this power, however, often in the context of the Australian Medical Association's code of conduct, and more narrowly, its code of ethics, which affirms professional autonomy and clinical independence and advocates for the freedom to exercise professional judgment in the care and treatment of patients without undue influence from individuals, governments, or third parties.[48] While malpractice is a concern, a wide range of medical practices are disputed by expert opinion. If patients are informed of all potential risks and benefits, the decision on whether to use therapies (whether for pandemics or gender dysphoria) should remain between the patient and the doctor.

A case, still in train, provides an excellent illustration of risks in the suspension of a medical practitioner's licence for reasons not immediately related to professional competence but for the political views held and

48 Australian Medical Association, 2024. *Member Consultation Draft, Revised Code of Ethics*

publicly expressed. The Medical Board commenced an investigation of Dr Kok for his social media post in 2018 and suspended his registration as a medical practitioner in 2019. In 2020, the Victorian Civil and Administrative Tribunal confirmed the suspension of registration. Dr Kok sought to respond and did so in 2024, and the reasons were published in July 2025, with proceedings to continue in March 2026.

The tribunal found that Dr Kok, a conservative Christian, engaged in professional misconduct by posting on social media words that denigrated, demeaned and slurred medical practitioners who provided abortion treatment, and those who recognised and treated gender dysphoria.[49] Further, he expressed views that denigrated, demeaned and were disrespectful of and derogatory to LGBTQI+ persons and community, and denigrated, demeaned and slurred persons that accepted and considered it right to follow COVID-19 public health orders, and about COVID-19. He also drew on and legitimised antivaccination and vaccine hesitancy rhetoric and contained misleading information regarding vaccines.[50]

The Medical Board of Australia relied on the Good Medical Practice: A Code of Conduct for Doctors in Australia to provide the context for evidence of misconduct.[51] For example, the code describes, but does not define, concepts such as 'culturally safe and sensitive practice', for instance, by 'Acknowledging the social, economic, cultural and behavioural factors influencing health, both at individual and population levels.' These concepts can be weaponised to silence or suspend doctors who some in the profession believe do not fit the mould. The Code also states that 'all doctors have a right to have and express their personal views and values.' However, as a doctor, 'you need to consider the effect of your public comments … online, … and how they reflect on your role

49 Conduct that is substantially below the standard reasonably expected, whether occurring in connection with the practice of the health practitioner's profession or not. *Health Practitioner Regulation National Law Act 2009*, 76

50 *Medical Board of Australia v Kok (Review & Regulation)* [2025] VCAT 650

51 *Medical Board of Australia v Kok (Review & Regulation)* [2025] VCAT 650, par 34

as a doctor and on the reputation of the profession.'[52] His barrister has set out the story in a recent speech to the Medico Legal Society of Victoria.[53]

The Australian Doctors Federation and the Australian Medical Professionals Society regard the doctor-patient relationship as sacrosanct and disagree that a doctor should be suspended from registration for their political views, however expressed, so long as these do not interfere with the practice of their profession. However, when a public health academic took issue with opinion articles written by the Secretary of the Australian Medical Professionals, the secretary was formally referred to the regulator, the Australian Health Practitioner Regulation Agency, via the Office of the Health Ombudsman.[54]

The regulator should never interfere with the doctor-patient relationship unless there is improper conduct, that is, conduct relating to the work of a medical practitioner, not their opinions on any matter. More broadly, where were the medical colleges and societies querying the COVID-19 medical responses? Without robust debate and curiosity from medical and scientific experts, it is difficult for politicians to overcome a wall of opinions. Legislation can guard against panic, but ultimately, the public is in the hands of those responsible for advice. The Alberta Inquiry was very strong on the issue of independence of medical colleges, maintaining that regulatory bodies should not override professional bodies or doctor-patient trust.[55]

---

52 https://www.medicalboard.gov.au/Codes-Guidelines-Policies/Code-of-conduct.aspx

53 Moloney S, 2025. You can't say that! The Medical Board of Australia and other governors – whither freedom of speech and political communication for doctors, lawyers and the public? *Address to the Medico Legal Society of Victoria.* Melbourne Club 6 September

54 Thomas K & Mcintyre A, 2025. Controlled by confidence: the unchecked power of AHPRA and the state. *The Spectator* 12 August

55 Alberta COVID-19 Pandemic Data Review Task Force, 2025, ch 9

8. Stick with matters directly related to health

Writing in the Medical Journal of Australia, an author suggested a fossil fuel non-proliferation treaty as a solution to — what?[56] Doctors for the Environment Australia were adamant, 'We, the undersigned health professionals, call on our government to ban all new coal, oil and gas projects.'[57] Hundreds of their members signed a full-page advertisement in the press, announcing that 'coal, oil, and gas are hazardous to our health and well-being ... we must prioritize the health of people over the interests of the fossil fuel industry.' Dr Monique Ryan MP wants to name killer heatwaves, claiming that 'heatwaves are Australia's most deadly climate hazard.' Doctors adhere to the principle of first, do no harm. Banning coal, gas, and oil would harm their patients by depriving them of medicines and medical devices that alleviate suffering. Without a substantial infrastructure to support renewables, the likely scenario under the doctors' prescription is intermittent electricity, which is inadequate for running hospitals. Should these doctors be suspended? Their prescription would cause enormous harm to society.

If climate change is such a pressing medical issue, why not forgo medical research grants funded by coal, oil, and gas taxation? Green medical researchers are not particularly enthusiastic about that idea. What is their solution for producing ammonia to maintain the same level of medical care with lower CO2 emissions? Without ammonia, there would be no inorganic fertilisers, and nearly half the world could face hunger. Ammonia is also essential for pharmaceuticals. Unfortunately, ammonia production has a significant carbon footprint because it is energy-intensive. The industrial production of ammonia emits more CO2 than any other chemical production process. Why not direct medical research funds towards industrial chemistry to create less CO2-intensive ammonia?

---

56 Colagiuri P et al, 2025. The Fossil Fuel Non-Proliferation Treaty: what it is, its importance for health, and why Australia should endorse it. *Medical Journal of Australia* 222 (6)

57 https://www.dea.org.au/fossil_fuels_are_a_health_hazard

Wind turbines and solar panels can only be constructed on a large scale using fossil fuels during both the mining and industrial production phases. Green doctors should recognise that steel is an essential material for building hospitals.[58] Much of the medical equipment used today is made from oil. Oil products are widely used in health care as transport fuel and feedstock for pharmaceuticals, plastics, and medical supplies. Heart valves and artificial limbs are created from petroleum, as are many of the cleaning and safety products employed by medical personnel. Aspirin and other pharmaceuticals also contain petroleum. Few substitutes are available. Nearly 99 per cent of pharmaceutical feedstocks and reagents are derived from petrochemicals.

Each of these products has a very high melting point, requiring significant industrial-level energy to produce. Boron is used in eye drops, cobalt is used in medical tracers, lithium is used in mental health treatments and pacemakers, niobium is employed in MRI scanners, platinum is used in surgical tools and dentistry, tantalum is used in surgical implants, and titanium is used for medical implants. The enormous energy required to manufacture titanium should be compulsory viewing for virtue-signalling doctors. Viable energy substitutes for industrial processes must be found before they are banned. The consequences for medicine are enormous.

Medical doctors are not particularly well-equipped to assess risk in public policy. Indeed, they may be among the least qualified, as, except in emergencies, their focus is on helping everyone. While doctors possess skills in medical triage and can prioritise based on short-term medical risks, as evidenced by the response to COVID-19, policy triage operates in a different realm. Medical qualifications can just as easily mislead as they can guide policy decisions. They are, of course, always welcome as citizens to engage in these discussions, but that is not how they typically present.

58 https://worldsteel.org/wp-content/uploads/Fact-sheet-Energy-use-in-the-steel-industry.pdf

9. Enough with the social determinants: challenge public health centres

Coercion is a technique common in public health. A prime example is the Rainbow Health tick of approval. The Victorian government funds Rainbow Health Australia (RHA).[59] Rainbow Health Australia is a program that supports lesbian, gay, bisexual, transgender, intersex and queer health and wellbeing through research and knowledge translation, training, resources, policy advice and service accreditation through the Rainbow Tick.

The Rainbow Tick Accreditation Program was established to support health and community organisations in understanding and implementing LGBTIQ-safe, inclusive service delivery. It provides national recognition for those who meet the Rainbow Tick Standards. The handbook emphasises cultural safety, a concept initially developed to apply to health service delivery for Mãori communities, with the hope it would create *a more equal society*. Over time, the concept has been expanded to apply to *inclusive and affirmative health* and community service delivery for other groups, including LGBTIQ communities.[60] The affirmative health reference is, of course, the very heart of the attempt to undermine medical ethics.

The language is very forceful. For example, providing culturally safe services for LGBTIQ people means delivering 'affirmative, responsive, trauma-informed and person-centred care'. It requires acknowledging the unique strengths and vulnerabilities of LGBTIQ people and having structures and processes in place that proactively identify and address potential risks to safety and wellbeing. It means 'challenging heteronormative and cisnormative ideas and assumptions about bodies, genders and sexualities within systems, workplace culture and service delivery.' In short, these people are not to be regarded as people but as identities and treated specially, not as employees, but fragile vessels

59 https://www.latrobe.edu.au/arcshs/health-and-wellbeing

60 Jones J et al, 2020. *Rainbow Tick Standards: A Framework for LGBTIQ Cultural Safety*. Third Edition, 6

to be celebrated and appreciated, not as co-workers or for their talent. Because they are in a minority who live in a liberal society, they are free to express their difference from the heteronormative, but beyond that, they should have no claim to special treatment as employees.

A typical strategy to gain the tick of approval is, for example, to create 'an organisational culture that celebrates diversity of sex, gender and sexuality'. Why celebrate these essentially private matters? Celebration becomes a performance in which all are expected to contribute, lest they be deemed not inclusive. Banners, posters, pronouns and lanyards displayed with the implication that the non-wearer is not a good person. The Rainbow Tick creates an oppressive regime. What if such designated people do not want to celebrate, but rather be appreciated for their skills and contribution to the purpose of their employment?

Cultural safety, if it was ever a sensible idea, has become a highly weaponised concept to press ideologies – society-wide equality and affirmation — on mostly unsuspecting employers. It is a very loose and dangerous concept that 'empowers' individuals to complain about their workplace and indeed not to work at the direction of employers. It is nevertheless lapped up by 'people and culture' employees whose remit, power and prestige it expands.

Not to be outdone, the University of Queensland Mental Health and Climate Change Research Network[61] seeks to answer the question, 'How do we protect and nurture social and emotional wellbeing in a rapidly changing climate?' In parallel with gender-affirming practice, the question should be, 'Is there an illness that requires medical intervention?' Instead, the study is of eco-anxiety among young Australians, who, allegedly, are experiencing high rates of 'distressing emotions and perceptions about climate change'. The study will investigate how a 'guided journal could assist young people' to understand and manage these thoughts and feelings. Could such anxiety be the result of professors burying sensible responses to the possibility of climate change by providing a sense of

61 https://public-health.uq.edu.au/mental-health-and-climate-change-research-network

perspective, as recommended by Bjorn Lomborg, rather than fuelling scenarios in ignorance, as Greta Thunberg does?[62]

The most galling is an examination of the relationship between health and engagement in climate advocacy behaviour. Apparently, 'individuals who engage in climate advocacy experience high rates of burnout.' The study will examine climate activists' and advocates' perceptions of the impacts of their activities on their physical and mental health. This nonsense is funded by The Sunrise Project, which sources most of its $77 million in annual funds from overseas.[63]

10. Remove taxation privileges from public health organisations

If charity incentives cost the taxpayer money via foregone revenue, 'the point of charity law had better be a good one'.[64] So argued a staunch supporter of the charity sector. Taxpayers should not subsidise politically contestable actions or subsidise free speech, and yet, this is precisely what happens in the public health arena. Good policy is judged over long periods through democratic means. When governments support one reasonable conception of 'the good' over any other by subsidising charities that spruik controversial public policy, it brings the sector down and it dishonours at least some taxpayers. The many arguments outlined above should indicate to any government and any donor that, in the health arena, and with seemingly straightforward wrongs to right, public health lobby policy prescriptions are sometimes harmful.

A prime example of political aims fulfilled by a charity is the decision by the Assistant Minister for Charities to lobby to include Equality

62 https://public-health.uq.edu.au/mental-health-and-climate-change-research-network/projects

63 https://www.acnc.gov.au/charity/charities/fd27e06b-38af-e811-a962-000d3ad24a0dprofile

64 McCormack S W, 2010. Taking the good with the bad: recognizing the negative externalities created by charities and their implications for the charitable deduction. *Arizona Law Review* 52, 1025

Australia (which advocates for the LGBTIQ+ community) in the Tax Act and secure DGR status despite this being denied by the Charities Commissioner,[65] whose decision was affirmed by the Full Court of the Federal Court.[66] Equality Australia, courtesy of its tax-deductible status, is raising funds to stop women from excluding transgender women from entering their spaces or joining their group meetings, as a gay woman. In a further example of political advocacy, Project 491 is an initiative led by the Australian Professional Association for Trans Health (AusPATH), a health promotion charity, in response to the Queensland Government's restrictions on gender-affirming care for trans and gender-diverse children.[67] A formal complaint has been lodged with the Australian Charities and Not-for-profits Commission regarding AusPATH, as it is promoting and advocating the Australian Informed Consent Standards of Care for Gender Affirming Hormone Therapy. In doing so, the complaint alleged that AusPATH fails the public benefit requirement imposed on Australian charities because the proven detriment to the public in carrying out its objects outweighs any of its benefits.[68]

The move to limit the charity voice in political fields took a decisive step towards publicly subsidised free speech in a High Court of Australia case. Because of a 2010 decision of the High Court in *Aid/Watch Incorporated v. Commissioner of Taxation*,[69] charities are free to lobby the government and do little, if any, charity work. When charities lobby the government on controversial matters, using the privilege of charity status, should the taxpayer have a right of veto? Charities in Australia have always been free to lobby, so long as charity work remains their dominant purpose. The High Court decided that a charity engaged in 'lawful means of

---

65 Yoni Bashan, Some more equal than others? Equality Australia's free ride to tax free. *The Australian* 29 July 2025

66 https://www.acnc.gov.au/tools/guidance/decision-impact-statements/acnc-decision-impact-statement-equality-australia-ltd

67 https://auspath.org.au/project-491/

68 Complaint lodged by Gary Johns, Duncan Syme, President of the Australian Medical Professionals Society and Kara Thomas, President of the Nurses Professional Association of Australia on 21 August 2025

69 *Aid/Watch Incorporated v Commissioner of Taxation* [2010] HCA 42 (1 December 2010)

public debate concerning the efficiency of foreign aid directed to the relief of poverty is a purpose beneficial to the community.'[70] Justice Heydon, in the minority judgment, found that 'Aid/Watch did not have the goal of relieving poverty. It provided no funds, goods or services to the poor.'[71] Justice Kiefel, in the minority, decided that Aid/Watch's pursuit of a freedom to communicate its views 'does not qualify as being for the public benefit.'[72] If the Australian Taxation Office had challenged a charity set up to cut foreign aid, arguably a public benefit, the High Court would have run a mile.

The Australian Government has written the substance of the High Court decision into law to legitimise 'promoting or opposing a change to any matter established by law, policy or practice in the Commonwealth, a state, a territory or another country.'[73] Advocacy and lobbying have become charitable purposes. Charities will be less constrained in lobbying and will do less charity. How much lobbying charities can undertake, that is, how much charitable resources they devote to politics, is a moot point. Historically, a 'trust for the attainment of political objects' was invalid because courts had 'no means of judging whether a proposed change in the law would or would not be for the public benefit.'[74] The High Court overlooked this matter in Aid/Watch and decided that an association engaged in researching, monitoring and campaigning on the delivery of overseas aid should maintain charitable status.

Charities lobby the government because they reckon it pays dividends. The results of a U. S. study of not-for-profits (charities) indicate that a 10 per cent increase in lobbying expenditures produces a 0.5 per cent increase in contributions.[75] But contributions are not the only gains from

70 *Aid/Watch*, 47

71 *Aid/Watch*, 60

72 *Aid/Watch*, 86

73 The Parliament of the Commonwealth of Australia, *Charities Act 2013* (Cth), Part 3 Division 1(12)

74 Halsbury's, 2013. *Laws of Australia.* LexisNexis Butterworths 75, 290

75 Heckelman J C & Wilson B, 2013. Institutions, lobbying, and economic performance. *Economics and Politics* 25(3), 360

lobbying; they can bring money and favourable rule changes to the cause. That does not necessarily hold for every other cause. Lobbying, just as every other activity, has an opportunity cost. It requires resources that otherwise could have been put to productive use. It may hurt economic activity. For example, 'the higher the quality of economic institutions, the more costly is lobbying with respect to growth.' It depends on 'whether pressure enhances or inhibits institutions that foster economic freedom.'[76]

A standard pro-NGO academic view is that governments view charities and other NGOs as necessary actors that provide access to information, serve as a vehicle for aggregating preferences, and help coordinate the political process, rather than as threats to the status quo. They might argue that governments are likely to remove barriers and facilitate access to resources to encourage NGO formation.[77] The trouble is, public health charities make the same mistakes as every other lobby. Why the taxpayer would favour them is a mystery. If public health charities want to be civil regulators, the presumption of righteousness must be tested. They should have a social license to operate.[78] At the very least, taxpayers should never subsidise campaigning charities. The AID/Watch decision and the amendments to the Charities Act to allow an unspecified amount of lobbying should be scrapped.

In 2010, the Productivity Commission argued that donor tax relief should be extended to all charities. In 2013, a Treasury paper recommended extending that status to all charities with some carve-outs.[79] While it is permissible for a charity to do no more than lobby the government, as many have observed, 'There is something unsatisfactory about taxpayers' money being used to fund charities that are campaigning for

76 Heckelman J C & Wilson B, 2013, 360

77 Bloodgood E et al, 2013. National styles of NGO regulation. *Nonprofit and Voluntary Sector Quarterly* 43(4), 719

78 Morrison J, 2014. *Social Licence: How To Keep Your Organisation Legitimate*. London: Palgrave McMillan

79 Australian Government the Treasury, 2013. *Fairer, simpler and more effective tax concessions for the not-for-profit sector*. Not-for-Profit Sector Tax Concession Working Group. Final Report, rec 6

things that we may disagree with.'[80] A proposal worth considering is that registered charities should be eligible for donor tax relief, as per the Treasury recommendation, and in return, charities must have a means of delivering on their purpose. Charities should not be allowed to spend funds raised in the name of charity on political advertising, partisan or not. Political advertising is not a good use of charitable funds.

These modest changes would strengthen the distinctive contribution charities make to Australian society. They would also help justify the support of Australians through taxation and the opportunity costs implicit in charity work. Charities that think this is burdensome are free not to seek taxpayer support and can focus on their mission. Public health organisations are narrowly focused on one, albeit significant value: health. Still, they can distort public policy to ends that either harm health or other values, such as the environment or the standard of living, or, in the case of trans ideology, the very base of science.

Conclusion

In any field of endeavour, those who profess expertise are liable to want to be heard and often to acquire power and prestige in the name of that expertise. When these experts want to exert power over public policy the issue for elected officials, is to recognise whether the expertise is applicable to the professed public purpose. Climate change experts grew in proportion to the perception that climate change was a public concern. Too many jumped aboard and perverted science to chase research money and prestige, no doubt believing in the cause of saving the world. Public health aficionados are not alone in these regards, but they have the added power, an aura of untouchability, that a medical background brings.

80 Seddon N, 2007. *Who Cares? How State Funding and Political Activism Change Charity*. Civitas: Institute for the Study of Civil Society London, 62

Bibliography

Acts

Births, Deaths and Marriages Registration Act 2023 (Qld)

Charities Act 2013 (Cth)

Health Practitioner Regulation National Law Act 2009

Public And Environmental Health Act 2011 (NT)

Public Health Act 1997 (ACT)

Public Health Act 2010 (NSW)

Public Health Act 2005 (Qld)

Public Health Act 1997 (Tas)

Public Health Act 2016 (WA)

Public Health and Wellbeing Act 2008 (Vic)

Sex Discrimination Act 1984 (Cth)

South Australian Public Health Act 2011(SA)

Cases

Athavle & Ors v NSW Minister for Health, Vic Minister for Health, State of NSW, State of Vic and Commonwealth of Australia, Federal Court of Australia, NSD 894/2021

Bay v Australian Health Practitioner Regulation Agency [2024] QSC 315

Bell and another v The Tavistock and Portman NHS Foundation Trust [2021] EWCA Civ 1363

Davis v Department of Health (Review and Regulation) [2024] VCAT 490

Dawking v Secretary (Department of Education) [2022] NSWPIC 611

For Women Scotland Ltd (Appellant) v The Scottish Ministers (Respondent) UKSC/2024/0042

Gary Newman v Minister for Health and Aged Care, Federal Court of Australia, NSD 388/2021

Johnston & Ors v Carroll (Commissioner of the Queensland Police Service) & Anor; Witthahn & Ors v Wakefield (Chief Executive of Hospital and Health Services and Director General of Queensland Health); Sutton & Ors v Carroll (Commissioner of the Queensland Police Service) [2024] QSC 2

Kassam v Hazzard; *Henry v Hazzard* [2021] NSWSC 1320

Knowles & Ors v Commonwealth of Australia & Ors, Federal Court of Australia, VID 579/2021

LibertyWorks Inc v Commonwealth, Federal Court of Australia, NSD 1312/2020

Loielo v Giles [2020] VSC 722

Re: Devin [2025] FedCFamC1F 211

Rose v Secretary of the Department of Health and Aged Care [2025] FCA 339

Secretary To the Department of Health V The Hon David Davis MLC [2025] VSCA 40

Sutton & Ors v Carroll (Commissioner of the Queensland Police Service) [2024] QSC 2

Tickle v Giggle for Girls Pty Ltd (No 2) [2024] FCA 960

U.S. v. Skrmetti U.S. Supreme Court 23-477 18 June 2025

Books and journals

Abel E K, 2007. *Tuberculosis and the Politics of Exclusion: A History of Public Health and Migration to Los Angeles*. Rutgers University Press: New Brunswick

Abel E K, 2003. From exclusion to expulsion: Mexicans and tuberculosis control in Los Angeles, 1914-1940. *Bulletin of the History of Medicine*, 77(4)

Aboriginal Affairs NSW, 2025. *Monitoring, Evaluation and Learning Package: Closing the Gap Grant Program*

Aboriginal Health and Medical Research Council of NSW, 2015. *Aboriginal Communities Improving Aboriginal Health: An Evidence Review on the Contribution of Aboriginal Controlled Health Services to Improving Aboriginal Health*

ACIL Allen, 2014. *Counting the Costs of Alcohol Policy-relevant Costs to Australia*

Actuaries Australia and Australian Institute of Health and Welfare submissions to the *Senate Inquiry into Excess Mortality 2024*

Adekunle A et al, 2020. Delaying the COVID-19 epidemic in Australia: evaluating the effectiveness of international travel bans. *Australian and New Zealand Journal of Public Health* 2020, 44(4)

Alberta COVID-19 Pandemic Data Review Task Force, 2025. *Alberta's Covid-19 Pandemic Response Final Report*

Alemayehu B & Warner K E, 2004. The lifetime distribution of health care costs. *Health Services Research* 39(3)

Alford K, 2014. *Investing in Aboriginal Community Controlled Health Makes Economic Sense.* National Aboriginal Community Controlled Health Organisation

Allais O et al, 2010. The effects of a fat tax on French households' purchases: a nutritional approach. *American Journal of Agricultural Economics* 92(1)

Allcott H, Diamond R, & Dubé J-P, 2018. The geography of poverty and nutrition: food deserts and food choices across the United States. *Working Paper No. 3631,* Graduate School of Business, Stanford University

Allen D W, 2021. Covid-19 lockdown cost/benefits: a critical assessment of the literature. *International Journal of the Economics of Business* 29(1)

Alsukaita R et al, 2020. Evaluating Saudi Arabia's 50% carbonated drink excise tax: changes in prices and volume sales. *Economics and Human Biology* 38

Altman P M, 2024. COVID-19 vaccines: a failure of the drug regulatory system, in *COVID Revisited Lessons Learned, Challenges Faced, and the Road Ahead.* Australian Medical Professionals Society

Amnesty International Australia, 2024. *Submission to the Commonwealth Government COVID-19 Response Inquiry*

Amos A, 2025. The landscape of gender affirming services in Australia. *Proceedings: The Future of Youth Gender Medicine Seminar*. NSW Parliament House

Amuedo-Dorantesa C et al, 2021. Early adoption of non-pharmaceutical interventions and COVID-19 mortality. *Economics and Human Biology* 42 (101003)

Anderberg J, 2022. *The Herd: How Sweden Chose its Own Path Through the Worst Pandemic in 100 Years.* Scribe Publications

Anderson I P S et al, 2009. Indigenous medical workforce development: current status and future directions. *Medical Journal of Australia* 190(10)

Anderson J J et al, 2017. Adiposity among 132479 UK Biobank participants; contribution of sugar intake vs other macronutrients. *International Journal of Epidemiology*, 46(2)

Annas G J, 2007. Your liberty or your life. Talking point on public health versus civil liberties. *EMBO Reports* 8(12)

Anton C J et al, 2012. Social origin, schooling and individual change in intelligence during childhood influence long-term mortality: a 68-year follow-up study. *International Journal of Epidemiology* 41

Aotearoa New Zealand Royal Commission Covid-19, 2024. *Lessons Learned: Main Report*

Appleby G, O'Sullivan M & Partlett W, 2021. *The Public Health and Wellbeing Amendment (Pandemic Management) Bill 2021* (Vic). The Centre for Public

Integrity

Armstrong J S & Green K C, 2022. *The Scientific Method: A Guide to Finding Useful Knowledge*. Cambridge University Press

Arnoldussen M et al, 2020. Re-evaluation of the Dutch approach: Are recently referred transgender youth different compared to earlier referrals? *European Child and Adolescent Psychiatry* 29

Aspin C et al, 2012. Strategic approaches to enhanced health service delivery for Aboriginal and Torres Strait Islander people with chronic illness: a qualitative study. *BMC Health Services Research* 12

Australian Bureau of Statistics, 2025. *Deaths in Australia*

Australian Bureau of Statistics, 2025. *Patient Experiences*

Australian Bureau of Statistics, 2025. *Taxation Revenue, Australia 2023-23 Financial Year*

Australian Bureau of Statistics, 2024. *Disability, Ageing and Carers, Australia: Summary of Findings*

Australian Bureau of Statistics, 2024. *Measuring Australia's Excess Deaths During the Covid-19 Pandemic until December 2023*

Australian Bureau of Statistics, 2023. *National Health Survey 2022*

Australian Bureau of Statistics, 2023. *National Study of Health and Wellbeing*

Australian Bureau of Statistics, 2019. *Apparent Consumption of Alcohol, Australia*

Australian Bureau of Statistics, 2018, *Government Benefits, Taxes and Household Income, Australia*

Australian Bureau of Statistics, 2016. *Australian Health Survey: Consumption of Added Sugars 2011-12*

Australian Bureau of Statistics, 2015. *Apparent Consumption of Alcohol, Australia, 2013-14*

Australian Bureau of Statistics, 2014. *Australian Health Survey: Nutrition First Results: Foods and Nutrients, 2011-12*

Australian Bureau of Statistics, 2010. *Year Book Australia, 2009-10*

Australian Bureau of Statistics, 2007. *Deaths, Australia, 2004*

Australian Catholic Bishops Conference, 2024. *Submission to the to the Commonwealth Government Covid-19 Response Inquiry*

Australian Charities and Not-for-profits Commission, 2015. Commissioner's interpretation statement: health promotion charities. *CIS 2015/01*

Australian Commission on Safety and Quality in Health Care, 2014. *National Statement on Health Literacy*

Australian Criminal Intelligence Commission, 2022. *Illicit Drug Data Report 2020–21*

Australian Curriculum, Assessment and Reporting Authority, 2025. *Student Attendance: Key Facts*

Australian Government the Treasury, 2013. *Fairer, Simpler and More Effective Tax Concessions for the Not-for-profit Sector*. Not-for-Profit Sector Tax Concession Working Group. Final Report

Australian Health Practitioner Regulation Agency and National Boards, 2021. *Registered Health Practitioners and Students: What You Need to Know About the COVID-19 Vaccine Rollout*. 21 March

Australian Health Promotion Association https://www.healthpromotion.org.au

Australian Indigenous Doctors' Association, 2017. *Report on the Findings of the 2016 AIDA Member Survey on Bullying, Racism and Lateral Violence in the Workplace*

Australian Institute of Health and Welfare, 2025. *Aboriginal and Torres Strait Islander Specific Primary Health Care: Results from the Online Service Reports and National Key Performance Indicators Collections*

Australian Institute for Health and Welfare, 2024. *Alcohol, Tobacco & other Drugs in Australia*

Australian Institute of Health and Welfare, 2024. *Australian Burden of Disease Study 2024*

Australian Institute of Health and Welfare, 2024. *Deaths in Australia*

Australian Institute of Health and Welfare, 2024. *National Drug Strategy Household Survey 2022–2023: Alcohol, Tobacco, ecigarette and Illicit Drug use by Population Groups: Interactive Data*

Australian Institute of Health and Welfare, 2024. *Determinants of Health for First Nations People*

Australian Institute of Health and Welfare, 2024. *General Practice, Allied Health and other Primary Care Services*

Australian Institute of Health and Welfare, 2024. *What Are Determinants of Health?*

Australian Institute of Health and Welfare, 2024. *Overweight and Obesity*

Australian Institute of Health and Welfare, 2023. *Deaths By Suicide Among Young People*

Australian Institute of Health and Welfare, 2021. *Australian Burden of Disease Study 2018*

Australian Institute of Health and Welfare, 2016. *Impact and Causes of Illness and Deaths in Australia 2011*

Australian Institute of Health and Welfare, 2016. *Skin Cancer in Australia*

Australian Institute of Health and Welfare, 2014. Healthy life expectancy in Australia: patterns and trends 1998 to 2012. *Bulletin 126*

Australian Institute of Health and Welfare, 2012. *Australia's Health 2012*

Australian Institute of Health & Welfare and National Indigenous Australians Agency, 2024. *ATSI Health Performance Framework*

Australian Medical Association, 2025. *Public Hospital Report Card*

Australian Medical Association, 2024. *Member Consultation Draft, Revised Code of Ethics*

Australian Medical Network, 2023. *Deinstitutionalisation of Mental Health*

Australian Medical Professionals' Society, 2025. *Follow the Money: WHO's Directing Global Health Policy?*

Australian Government, 2024. *COVID-19 Response Inquiry Report*

Australian Government Department of Health, 2019. *Australian Health Management Plan for Pandemic Influenza* and 2020 *Australian Health Sector Emergency Response for Novel Coronavirus (COVID-19)*

Australian Government Department of Health and Aged Care Therapeutic Goods Administration, 2023. *COVID-19 Vaccine Safety Report*

Australian Health Ministers' Advisory Council, 2016. *Cultural Respect Framework for Aboriginal and Torres Strait Islander Health 2016–2026: A National Approach to Building a Culturally Respectful Health System*

Australian Human Rights Commission, 2025. *Collateral Damage: What the Untold Stories from the COVID-19 Pandemic Expose About Human Rights in Australia*

Australian Human Rights Commission, 2025. *Health Inequities in Australia: A Scoping Review on the Impact of Racism on Indigenous and Other Negatively Racialised Communities' Health Outcomes and Healthcare Access*

Australian Prevention Partnership Centre https://preventioncentre.org.au/work/research-projects/

Australian Taxation Office, 2024. *Tobacco Tax Gap: Compare the 2022 Previous Years*

Australian Taxation Office, 2024. *Latest Estimates and Findings: How we Combat Illicit Tobacco Behaviours with Help from other Government Agencies*

Australian Taxation Office, 2024. *Excise Duty Rates for Tobacco*

Australia's Future Tax System, 2009. *Final Report*

Axfors C & Ioannidis J P A, 2022. Infection fatality rate of COVID-19 in community-dwelling elderly populations. *European Journal of Epidemiology* 37

Baba J T et al, 2014. Aboriginal medical services cure more than illness: a qualitative study of how Indigenous services address the health impacts of discrimination in Brisbane communities. *International Journal for Equity in Health* 13:56

Backholer K et al, 2021. Australia in 2030: what is our path to health for all? *Medical Journal of Australia* May 214(Supplement 8)

Bailey J et al, 2020. 'We Are working for our people': growing and strengthening the Aboriginal and Torres Strait Islander health workforce. *Career Pathways Project Report*, Melbourne: The Lowitja Institute

Banks G, 2011. Evidence and social policy: the case of gambling. *Presentation to South Australian Centre for Economic Studies, Corporate Seminar*, Adelaide

Bardosh K et al, 2024. COVID-19 Vaccine boosters for young adults: a risk-benefit assessment and ethical analysis of mandate policies at universities. *Journal of Medical Ethics* 50

Bardosh K et al, 2022. The unintended consequences of COVID-19 vaccine policy: why mandates, passports and restrictions may cause more harm than good. *BMJ Global Health* May 7(5)

Bartlett A & McCambridge J, 2021. Doing violence to evidence on violence? How the alcohol industry created doubt in order to influence policy. *Drug and Alcohol Review*. 41

Baxendale S, 2024. The impact of suppressing puberty on neuropsychological function: a review. *Acta Paediatrica* 113

Bay W, 2024. *Submission to the Commonwealth Government Covid-19 Response Inquiry*

Beaglehole R, Bonita R, Horton R, Adams O & McKee M, 2004. Public health in the new era: improving health through collective action. *Lancet*, 363

Becker M H & Joseph J G, 1988. AIDS and behavioral change to reduce risk: a review. *American Journal of Public Health* 78(4)

Beloin V, 2009. *Public Policies Guided by The Precautionary Principle.* National Collaborating Centre for Healthy Public Policy

Bennett S, Jessurun M & Orban H, 2025. *Saving The NDIS: How To Rebalance Disability Services To Get Better Results*. Grattan Institute

Berkman N D et al, 2011. Low health literacy and health outcomes: an updated systematic review. *Annals of Internal Medicine* 155(2)

Bidadanure J U, 2019. The political theory of universal basic income. *Annual Review of Political Science* 22

Biggs H, 1911. Public health is purchasable. *Monthly Bulletin of the Department of Health of the City of New York*, 1(10)

Black N, Hughes R & Jones A M, 2018. The health care costs of childhood obesity in Australia: an instrumental variables approach. *Economics & Human Biology* 31

Bleich S N et al, 2013. Systematic review of community-based childhood obesity prevention studies. *Pediatrics* 132 (1)

Bloodgood E et al, 2013. National styles of NGO regulation. *Nonprofit and Voluntary Sector Quarterly* 43(4)

Bødker M et al, 2015. The Danish fat tax: effects on consumption patterns and risk of ischaemic heart disease. *Preventive Medicine* 77

Bødker M et al, 2015. The rise and fall of the world's first fat tax. *Health Policy* 119

Borger P et al, 2020, External peer review of the RTPCR test to detect SARS-CoV-2 reveals 10 major scientific flaws at the molecular and methodological level: consequences for false positive results (Review Report - Corman-Drosten). *Eurosurveillance*

Bouchard M, 2007. On the resilience of illegal drug markets. *Global Crime* 8(4)

Bowker G & Star S L, 2000. *Sorting Things Out: Classification and Its Consequences*. MIT Press: Cambridge, MA

Bretherton I et al, 2021. The health and well-being of transgender Australians: a national community survey. *LGBT Health* 8(1)

Bridle B, 2024. Baby steps: back in my office, miracles still happen, but I still can't access my lab. *COVID Chronicles Substack*. 17 December

Buchmueller T & Meliyanni J, 2015. Obesity and health expenditures: evidence from Australia. *Economics and Human Biology* 17

Burcham P, 2025. An injured toxicologist on Covid vaccines, parts I, II and III. *Quadrant* April-June

Bureau of Infrastructure and Transport Research Economics, 2022. *Road Trauma Australia, Statistical Summary 2021*

Burnet Institute, 2023. *The Burnet Institute's Response to the Commonwealth Government COVID-19 Response Inquiry*

Byrne L et al, 2011. Parental status and childhood obesity in Australia. *International Journal of Pediatric Obesity* 6

Byrnes J et al, 2013. Can harms associated with high-intensity drinking be reduced by increasing the price of alcohol? *Drug and Alcohol Review* 32(1)

Byrnes M, 2024. Mandatory workplace vaccination: some recent COVID-19 vaccination cases. *Governance Institute of Australia Journal*

California State Board of Health, 1906. *Monthly Bulletin* 2(7)

Campbell M A et al, 2018. Contribution of Aboriginal community-controlled health services to improving Aboriginal health: an evidence review. *Australian Health Review* 42(2)

Campaign for Tobacco-Free Kids, 2008. A decade of broken promises: the 1998 state tobacco settlement ten years later. *Robert Wood Johnson Foundation*

Campos P et al, 2006. The epidemiology of overweight and obesity: public health crisis or moral panic? *International Journal of Epidemiology* 35(1)

Carrad A, 2022. Australian local government policies on creating a healthy, sustainable, and equitable food system: analysis in New South Wales and Victoria. *Australian and New Zealand Journal of Public Health* 46(3)

Carter D J, 2020. The use of coercive public health and human biosecurity law in Australia: an empirical analysis. *University of New South Wales Law Journal* 43(1)

Cass H, 2024. *Independent Review of Gender Identity Services for Children and Young People: Final Report*

Chaufan C et al, 2025. 'It isn't about health, and it sure doesn't care': a qualitative exploration of healthcare workers' lived experience of the policy of vaccination mandates in Ontario, Canada. *Journal of Public Health and Emergency* (9)16

Chaufan C, Hemsing N & Moncrieffe R, 2024. Covid-19 vaccination decisions and impacts of vaccine mandates: a cross-sectional survey of healthcare workers in British Columbia, Canada. *medRxiv* 10 December

Chemaitelly H et al, 2022. Effectiveness of COVID-19 vaccines. *Lancet* 399

Chu L et al, 2024. Submission to *Response to Commonwealth Government COVID-19 Response Inquiry*

Clancy R & McCann M (Eds) 2025. *Covid Through Our Eyes: An Australian Story of Mistakes, Mistreatment and Misinformation.* Halstead Press

Clark G, 2014. *The Son Also Rises: Surnames and the History of Social Mobility.* Princeton University Press

Clayton A, 2025. What went wrong. *Gender Clinic News | Bernard Lane* 7 May

Clayton A, 2023. Genderaffirming treatment of gender dysphoria in youth: a perfect storm environment for the placebo effect: the implications for research and clinical practice. *Archives of Sexual Behavior* 52

Coatsworth N, 2023. *Submission to the Commonwealth Government COVID-19 Response Inquiry*

Cobiac L et al, 2017. Taxes and subsidies for improving diet and population health in Australia: a cost-effectiveness modelling study. *PLoS ONE* 14(2)

Cohn, J. 2025. Censorship of essential debate in gender medicine research. *Journal of Controversial Ideas* 5(3)

Colagiuri P et al, 2025. The Fossil Fuel Non-proliferation Treaty: what it is, its importance for health, and why Australia should endorse it. *Medical Journal of Australia* 222 (6)

Colagiuri S, 2016. Is obesity a disease?: economic implications. *Obesity Australia Summit Papers*

Collins D & Lapsley H, 2008. The costs of tobacco, alcohol and illicit drug abuse to Australian society in 2004-05. Department of Health and Ageing. *Monograph Series no. 64*

Comans T et al, 2013. The cost-effectiveness and consumer acceptability of taxation strategies to reduce rates of overweight and obesity among children in Australia: study protocol. *BMC Public Health* 13(1182)

Commission on Social Determinants of Health, 2008. *Closing the Gap in a Generation*

Committee for the Economic Development of Australia, 2022. *Duty Of Care: Aged Care Sector in Crisis*

Committee for the Study of the Future of Public Health; Division of Health Care Services, 1988. *The Future of Public Health.* National Academy Press: Washington, D.C.

Commonwealth Government, 2024. *COVID-19 Response Inquiry*

Commonwealth of Australia Department of Foreign Affairs and Trade, 2025. *Global Health Reform*

Commonwealth of Australia Department of Health, 2021. *National Preventive Health Strategy, 2012-2030*

Commonwealth of Australia Department of Health, 2019. *National Alcohol Strategy 2019–2028*

Commonwealth of Australia Department of Health, Disability and Ageing, 2025. *The Interim Australian Centre for Disease Control*

Constantino V, Heslop D J & MacIntyre C R, 2020. The effectiveness of full and partial travel bans against COVID-19 spread in Australia for travellers from China during and after the epidemic peak in China. *Journal of Travel Medicine* 27(5)

Corfield C, 2024. *Submission to the COVID-19 Response Inquiry*

Craig C (Health Advisory and Recovery Team), 2023. Unsafe and Defective. *Submission to the People's Vaccine Inquiry UK*

Crampton E, 2010. Excess costs of smoking. *Offsetting Behaviour* 16 June

Crampton E, 2008. Cost-benefit analysis when the conclusion drives the method: a review of 'Report on Tobacco Taxation in New Zealand'. *The New Zealand Medical Journal* 121(1269)

Crime Statistics Agency, Victoria, 2025. *Key Figures: Year Ending March 2025*

Croucher R, 2022. Executive discretion at a time of COVID-19: promoting, protecting and fulfilling human rights in the contemporary public health context. *11th Austin Asche Oration in Law and Governance*. Australian Human Rights Commission

Cuijpers P, Smit F & Furukawa T A, 2021. Most at-risk individuals will not develop a mental disorder: the limited predictive strength of risk factors. *World Psychiatry* 20(2)

Cussen K, 2009. Handle with care: assessing the risks of the precautionary principle. *Australasian Journal of Environmental Management* 16(2)

d'Abbs P & Hewlett N, 2023. *Learning from 50 Years of Aboriginal Alcohol Programs*. Springer

Dalgleish A, 2024. The cost of ignoring science. In C H Klotz & P McCullough (Eds) *Canary In a (Post) Covid World: Money, Fear and Power*. Canary House Publishing

Dalton A, 2018. *Economic Evaluation of the Indigenous Australians' Health Programme Phase I*. Deakin Health Economics Centre for Population Health Research, Faculty of Health Deakin University

Daraganova G & Thornton L, 2013. Eating behaviour: socio-economic determinants and parental influence. *Longitudinal Study of Australian Children Annual Statistical Report 2013*

Darmon N et al, 2014. Food price policies improve diet quality while increasing socioeconomic inequalities in nutrition. *The International Journal of Behavioral Nutrition and Physical Activity* 11(1)

Davidson S, 2016. *Submission to Parliamentary Joint Committee on Law Enforcement Inquiry into Illicit Tobacco*. Australian Parliament

Dawson A & Verweij M (Eds) 2007. *Ethics, Prevention, and Public Health*. Oxford University Press: Oxford

Deary I J, Weiss A & Batty G D, 2010. Intelligence and personality as predictors of illness and death: how researchers in differential psychology and chronic disease epidemiology are collaborating to understand and address health inequalities. *Psychological Science in the Public Interest* 11(2)

Deaton A, 2013. *The Great Escape: Health, Wealth, and the Origins of Inequality*. Princeton University Press 2015 Edition

Delaney L et al, 2013. Why do some Irish drink so much? Family, historical and regional effects on students' alcohol consumption and subjective normative thresholds. *Review of Economics of the Household* 11(1)

Department of Health Victoria, 2016. *Healthy Choices: Healthy Eating Policy and Catering Guide for Workplaces*

Department of the Prime Minister and Cabinet, 2023. *Working Together to Deliver the NDIS - Independent Review into the National Disability Insurance Scheme: Final Report*

Detels R & Breslow L, 2005. Current scope and concerns in public health. In R Detels J McEwen, R Beaglehole & H Tanaka (Eds) *Oxford Textbook of Public Health 4th Ed. Vol. l. The Scope of Public Health.* Oxford University Press: Oxford

de Witt A et al, 2018. 'It's just presence,' the contributions of Aboriginal and Torres Strait Islander health professionals in cancer care in Queensland. *Frontiers in Public Health* 6(1-8)

Doble B et al, 2020. The effect of implicit and explicit taxes on the purchasing of 'high-in-calorie' products: A randomized controlled trial. *Economics and Human Biology* 37

Doherty T, Jose K & Cleland V, 2022. *Healthy Tasmania Research and Evaluation Framework.* Menzies Institute for Medical Research, University of Tasmania

Doran C M et al, 2022. Scope and quality of economic evaluations of Aboriginal and Torres Strait Islander health programs: a systematic review. *Australian and New Zealand Journal of Public Health* 46

Doshi P, 2008. The elusive definition of pandemic influenza. *Bulletin of the World Health Organization* 89(7)

Downward P & Dawson P, 2016. Is it pleasure or health from leisure that we benefit from most? An analysis of well-being alternatives and implications for policy. *Social Indicators Research* 126(1)

Duckett S, 2022. Public health management of the COVID-19 pandemic in Australia: the role of the Morrison government. *International Journal of Environmental Research and Public Health* 19

Duckett S & Swerissen H, 2016. *A Sugary Drinks Tax: Recovering the Community Costs of Obesity.* Grattan Institute

Edwards R, 2011. Commentary: soda taxes, obesity, and the shifty behavior of consumers. *Preventive Medicine* 52(6)

Elliott Z, 2023. *Binary: Debunking the Sex Spectrum Myth.* Paradox Press

Equity Economics, 2022. *Measuring the Gap in Health Expenditure: Aboriginal and Torres Strait Islander Australians.* NACCHO

Expert Advisory Panel Report to the Australian Government, 2024. *Review of General Practice Incentives*

Expósito-Campos P et al, 2023. Evolution and trends in referrals to a specialist gender identity unit in Spain over 10 years (2012-2021). *The Journal of Sexual Medicine* 20(3)

Eythorsson E et al, 2022. Rate of SARS-CoV-2 reinfection during an Omicron wave in Iceland. *JAMA Network Open* 2022(5)

Faksova K et al, 2024. COVID-19 vaccines and adverse events of special interest: a multinational Global Vaccine Data Network (GVDN) cohort study of 99 million vaccinated individuals. *Vaccine* 42(2200)

Fayaz Farkhad B & Albarracín D, 2021. Insights on the implications of COVID-19 mitigation measures for mental health. *Economics and Human Biology* 40(100963)

Fee E & Brown T M, 2005. The Public Health Act of 1848. *Bulletin of the World Health Organization*, 83(11)

Feinleib J A & Michael R T, 1998. Reported changes in sexual behavior in response to AIDS in the United States. *Preventive Medicine* 27(3)

Feldstein L R et al, 2025. Protection from COVID-19 vaccination and prior SARS-CoV-2 infection among children aged 6 Months-4 Years, United States, September 2022-April 2023. *Journal of Pediatric Infectious Diseases Society* 14

Ferguson F et al, 2020. Impact of non-pharmaceutical interventions to reduce COVID-19 mortality and healthcare demand. *Imperial College COVID-19 Response Team Report 9* 16 March

Fielding J, 2014. Foreword. In T H Tulchinsky & E A Varavikova (Eds) *The New Public* Health. Third Edition. Academic Press: Netherlands

Fischer B & Poland B, 1998. Exclusion, 'risk', and social control: reflections on community policing and public health. *Geoforum* 29(2)

Flanigan J, 2024. Political ideology and public health. *Social Philosophy and Policy* 41(2)

Fletcher J et al, 2010. Can soft drink taxes reduce population weight? *Contemporary Economic Policy* 28(1)

Fletcher J et al, 2010. The effects of soft drink taxes on child and adolescent consumption and weight outcomes. *Journal of Public Economics* 94

Forbes G, 2024. *Submission to Commonwealth Government COVID-19 Pandemic Response Inquiry*

Foster G & Sabhlok S, 2023. Response to understanding the impact of lockdowns on short-term excess mortality in Australia by Philip Clarke and Andrew Leigh. *BMJ Global Health* 29 August

Foster G with Sabhlok S, 2022. *Do Lockdowns and Border Closures Serve the Greater Good?* Connor Court

Foucault M, Bertani M, Fontana A, Ewald F & Macey D, 1997. *'Society Must Be Defended': Lectures at the Collège de France, 1975-1976*. Macmillan: London

Foulkes L & Andrews J L, 2023. Are mental health awareness efforts contributing to the rise in reported mental health problems? A call to test the prevalence inflation hypothesis. *New Ideas in Psychology* 69(10110)

Fox A, 2015. Understanding behaviour in the Australian and New Zealand night-time economies: an anthropological study. *Unpublished*

Fraiman J et al, 2022. Serious adverse events of special interest following mRNA COVID-19 vaccination in randomized trials in adults. *Vaccine* 40

Frances A, 2013. *Saving Normal: An Insider's Revolt Against Out-of-control Psychiatric Diagnosis, DSM-5, Big Pharma, and the Medicalization of Ordinary*. William Morrow

Freeman T et al, 2014. Cultural respect strategies in Australian Aboriginal primary health care services: beyond education and training of practitioners. *Australian and New Zealand Journal of Public Health* 38(4)

Fries J, 2005. The compression of morbidity. *The Milbank Quarterly* 83(4)

Fries J & Pietschnig J, 2022. An intelligent mind in a healthy body? Predicting health by cognitive ability in a large European sample. *Intelligence* 93

Gakh M, 2015. Law, the health in all policies approach, and cross-sector collaboration. *Public Health Reports* 130(1)

Gartner C et al, 2023. International progress toward a commercial tobacco endgame is an opportunity for advancing tobacco control. *Australia Australian and New Zealand Journal of Public Health* 47(2)

Geboers B et al, 2016. The association between health literacy and self-management abilities in adults aged 75 and older, and its moderators. *Quality of Life Research* 25(11)

Gilmore A B, 2023. Defining and conceptualising the commercial determinants of health. *The Lancet* 2023(401)

Girma S & Paton D, 2024. Covid-19 Vaccines as a condition of employment: impact on uptake, staffing, and mortality in elderly care homes. *Management Science* 70, 2882

Goodman M & Nash R, 2019. Examining health outcomes for people who are transgender. *Patient-Centred Outcomes Research Institute*

Gostin L O, 2000. *Public Health Law: Power, Duty, Restraint*. University of California Press

Gottfredson L S & Deary I J, 2004. Intelligence predicts health and longevity, but why? *Current Directions in Psychological Science* 13(1)

Gottfredson M R & Hirschi T, 1990. *A General Theory of Crime*. Stanford University Press

Goymann W, Brumm H & Kappeler P, 2022. Biological sex is binary, even though there is a rainbow of sex roles. *BioEssays*, 45(2)

Gracner T, Boone C & Gertler P J, 2024. Exposure to sugar rationing in the first 1000 days of life protected against chronic disease. *Science* 386(6725)

Great Barrington Declaration, 2020. https://gbdeclaration.org

Greenhalgh E M et al (Eds) 2024. *Tobacco in Australia: Facts and Issues*. Cancer Council Victoria

Greenland S, 1988. Probability versus Popper: an elaboration of the insufficiency of current Popperian approaches for epidemiologic analysis. In K. Rothman (Ed) *Causal Inference*. Epidemiology Resources Inc.

Grossman M, 2023. *Lost in Trans Nation: A Child Psychiatrist's Guide out of the Madness*. Skyhorse Publishing

Grove N J & Zwi A B, 2006. Our health and theirs: forced migration, othering, and public health. *Social Science & Medicine*, 62

Guastella A J, 2024. Executive function in children with neurodevelopmental conditions: a systematic review and meta-analysis. *Nature Human Behaviour* (8) December

Günther M, Rockenfeller R and Walach H, 2025. A calibration of nucleic acid (PCR) by antibody (IgG) tests in Germany: the course of SARS-CoV-2 infections estimated. *Frontiers in Epidemiology* 5(1592629)

Gur-Arie R et al, 2023. The ethics of COVID-19 vaccine mandates for healthcare workers: public health and clinical perspectives. *Bioethics*

Gupta S, The lost lessons of lockdown. *UnHerd* 22 November 2025

Gwynne K & Lincoln M, 2017. Developing the rural health workforce to improve Australian Aboriginal and Torres Strait Islander health outcomes: a systematic review. *Australian Health Review* 41(2)

Hakeem A, 2023. *Detrans: When Transition is Not the Solution*. Independent

Halsbury's, 2013. *Laws of Australia*. LexisNexis Butterworths 75

Hanks A et al, 2014. Chocolate milk consequences: a pilot study evaluating the consequences of banning chocolate milk in school cafeterias. *PLoS ONE* 9(4)

Hanks A et al, 2013. From Coke to Coors: a field study of a fat tax and its unintended consequences. *Journal of Nutrition Education and Behaviour* 45(4)

Hanna J, 1998. The vaccination status of Aboriginal and Torres Strait Island children in Far North Queensland. *Australian and New Zealand Journal of Public Health* 22(6)

Harfield S G et al, 2018. Characteristics of indigenous primary health care service delivery models: A systematic scoping review. *Globalization and*

Health 14(1)

Hawkes C et al, 2015. Smart food policies for obesity prevention. *The Lancet* 385(9985)

Hayman N, 1999. The poor health status of Aboriginal and Torres Strait Islander peoples. Can more indigenous doctors make a difference? *New Doctor* Summer

Haynes K & Stone C, 2004. Predictors of incomplete immunisation in Victorian children. *Australian and New Zealand Journal of Public Health*, 28(1)

Heckelman J C & Wilson B, 2013. Institutions, lobbying, and economic performance. *Economics and Politics* 25(3)

Heenan M, Ralph M & Shantosh J, 2024. Why public health acts could be our best chance to stem the tide of non-communicable diseases. *Australian and New Zealand Journal of Public Health*

Herby J, Jonung L & Hanke S H, 2022. A literature review and meta-analysis of the effects of lockdowns on COVID-19 mortality. *Studies in Applied Economics* 200(January)

Hickie I B et al, 2025. Novel youth mental health services in Australia: what differences are being reported about the clinical needs of those who attend and the outcomes achieved? *Australian & New Zealand Journal of Psychiatry* 59(2)

Hickman, C et al, 2021. Climate anxiety in children and young people and their beliefs about government responses to climate change: a global survey. *The Lancet Planetary Health* 5(12)

Hirono K T & Smith K E, 2018. Australia's $40 per pack cigarette tax plans: the need to consider equity. *Tobacco Control* 27(2)

House of Commons, 1842. *Report on the Sanitary Condition of the Labouring Population of Great Britain*. Parliament of Great Britain: London

House of Commons, 1840. *Report from the Select Committee on the Health of Towns*. Parliament of Great Britain: London

Hughes M, 2024. The WPATH files pseudoscientific surgical and hormonal experiments on children, adolescents, and vulnerable adults. *Environmental Progress* 4 March

Hull B et al, 2004. Evaluation of immunisation coverage for Aboriginal and Torres Strait Islander children using the Australian Childhood Immunisation Register. *Australian and New Zealand Journal of Public Health* 28(1)

Hunt G, 2024. *Submission to Commonwealth Government Covid-19 Response Inquiry*

Inacio M C et al, 2024. Excess mortality in residents of aged care facilities during COVID-19 in Australia, 2019–2022. *International Journal of*

Epidemiology 53(1)

International Council of Nurses, 2021. *The ICN Code of Ethics for Nurses*

Ioannidis J P A, Bhattacharya J et al, 2020. COVID-19 antibody seroprevalence in Santa Clara County, California. *medRxiv* April

Ioannoua P et al, 2021. Transmission of SARS-CoV-2 variant B.1.1.7 among vaccinated health care workers. *Infectious Diseases* 53(11)

Iveson, M H et al, 2018. Intelligence and all-cause mortality in the 6-Day Sample of the Scottish Mental Survey 1947 and their siblings: testing the contribution of family background, *International Journal of Epidemiology* 47(1)

James L P et al, 2021. The use and misuse of mathematical modeling for infectious disease policymaking: lessons for the COVID-19 pandemic. *Medical Decision Making* 41(4)

Jarrett S, 2013. *Liberating Aboriginal People from Violence*. Connor Court

Jefferson T et al, 2020. Physical interventions to interrupt or reduce the spread of respiratory viruses. *Cochrane Database Systematic Reviews* 11

Jennings W et al, 2021. Rapid review of five years of Aboriginal and Torres Strait Islander health research in Australia: persisting under-representation of urban populations. *Australian and New Zealand Journal of Public Health* 45

Jensen J D & Smed S, 2013. The Danish tax on saturated fat: short run effects on consumption, substitution patterns and consumer prices of fats. *Food Policy* 42

Johns G, 2015. *No Contraception, No Dole: Tackling Intergenerational Welfare*. Connor Court

Joint Standing Committee on the National Disability Insurance Scheme, 2024. *General Issues: Annual Report No. 2 of the 47th Parliament*

Jones J et al, 2020. *Rainbow Tick Standards: A Framework for LGBTIQ Cultural Safety*. Third Edition

Jones T et al, 2018. *Preventing Harm, Promoting Justice: Responding to LGBT Conversion Therapy in Australia*. Melbourne: Gay and Lesbian Health Victoria, Australian Research Centre in Sex, Health and Society and the Human Rights Law Centre

Jongen C et al, 2019. Working well: strategies to strengthen the workforce of the indigenous primary healthcare sector. *BMC Health Services Research* 19(910)

Jorm A F, 2018. Australia's 'Better Access' scheme: has it had an impact on population mental health? *Australian & New Zealand Journal of Psychiatry* 52(11)

Junger N & Hirsch O, 2024. Ethics of nudging in the COVID-19 crisis and the necessary return to the principles of shared decision making: a critical review. *Cureus* 2024(16)

Kaltiala R et al, 2020. Time trends in referrals to child and adolescent gender identity services: a study in four Nordic countries and in the UK. *Nordic Journal of Psychiatry* 74(1)

Kao K et al, 2020. The health and financial impacts of a sugary drink tax across different income groups in Canada. *Economics and Human Biology* 38

Kapeke K et al, 2024. Young voices, healthy futures: the rationale for lowering the voting age to 16. *Medical Journal of Australia* 221(10)

Kavanaugh M et al, 2025. Considering the nutritional benefits and health implications of red meat in the era of meatless initiatives. *Frontiers in Nutrition* 12(1525011)

Kelly T, 2024. Beyond blame: dissecting the systemic roots of societal disease exposed by the covid era. *The Hope Accord*

Kenny D, 2025. Psychotherapy for gender dysphoria in adolescents: a comprehensive and ethical approach. *Proceedings: The Future of Youth Gender Medicine Seminar*. NSW Parliament House

Kenny D, 2024. *Gender Ideology, Social Contagion, and the Making of a Transgender Generation*. Cambridge Scholars Press

Kevat D, 2021. Medico-legal considerations of mandatory COVID-19 vaccination for high risk workers. *Medical Journal of Australia* 215(1)

Kildea S, 2018. Birthing on Country (in Our Community): a case study of engaging stakeholders and developing a best-practice Indigenous maternity service in an urban setting. *Australian Health Review* 42

Kim, H J et al, 2025. Broad-spectrum adverse events of special interests based on immune response following COVID-19 vaccination: a large-scale population-based cohort study. *Journal of Clinical Medicine* 14

Kirkbride J B et al, 2024. The social determinants of mental health and disorder: evidence, prevention and recommendations. *World Psychiatry* 23(1), 58

Koener B et al, 2025. Managing gender dysphoria in minors: what insights does evidence-based medicine offer in 2024? *Disease Biology, Genetics, and Socioecology* 1(1)

Komlos J & Brabec M, 2011. The trend of BMI values of U.S. adults by deciles, birth cohorts 1882–1986 stratified by gender and ethnicity. *Economics & Human Biology* 9(3)

Kranjac A & Wagmiller R, 2016. Decomposing trends in adult body mass index, obesity, and morbid obesity, 1971-2012. *Social Science and Medicine* 167

Laba T-L et al, 2018. Medication non-adherence in a cohort of chronically ill

Australians: a case of missed opportunities. *Australian Journal of Medical Practice* 47(8)

Lacy-Nichols J et al, 2022. The public health playbook: ideas for challenging the corporate playbook. *Lancet Global Health* 10(7)

Lacy-Nichols J, Johnson M & Cullerton K, 2023. Commercial lobbying and political contributions: an Australian scoping review. *Australian and New Zealand Journal of Public Health* 47(4)

Lai G C et al, 2018. Factors affecting the retention of Indigenous Australians in the health workforce: a systematic review. *International Journal of Environmental Research and Public Health* 15(5)

Lally M, 2022. A cost-benefit analysis of COVID-19 lockdowns in Australia. *Monash Bioethics Review* 40

Lane B, 2025. Stop this sterilising of children. *Gender Clinic News*. 26 October

Laslett A-M et al, 2025. *Alcohol's Harm to Others in Australia: Patterns, Costs, Disparities and Precipitants*. Melbourne: Centre for Alcohol Policy Research, La Trobe University

Latimer E, Ray-Chaudhuri S & Waters T, 2025. *The Role of Changing Health in Rising Health-related Benefit Claims*. Institute of Fiscal Studies

LaVeist T A, Nuru-Jeter A & Jones K E, 2003. The association of doctor-patient race concordance with health services utilization. *Journal of Public Health Policy* 24(3-4)

Laws P et al, 2006. Smoking and pregnancy. *Australian Institute of Health and Welfare, National Perinatal Statistics Unit* No. 33

Lewis J E et al, 2025. Examining gender-specific mental health risks after gender-affirming surgery: a national database study. *The Journal of Sexual Medicine* 22(4)

Liberman, J. 2024. Litigation brought by Australian consumer and regulatory groups against the tobacco industry. In E M Greenhalgh et al (Eds) *Tobacco in Australia: Facts and Issues*. Cancer Council Victoria

Liester M et al, 2025. A narrative review of the COVID-19 infodemic and censorship in healthcare. *Secrecy and Society* 3(2)

Life Without Barriers, 2022. *Elevate Reconciliation Action Plan 2022-2025*

Lindberg R et al, 2024. Revising a right to food road map: perspectives of Australian key informants. *Australian and New Zealand Journal of Public Health* 48(5)

Littman L, 2019. Correction: parent reports of adolescents and young adults perceived to show signs of a rapid onset of gender dysphoria. *PLoS ONE* 14(3)

Lomborg B, 2023. *Best Things First.* Copenhagen Consensus Center

Looi J C L et al, 2024. The corrosion of adult mental healthcare in Australia: can we meet the needs of those who need the most? *Australasian Psychiatry* 32(4)

Lowitja Institute, 2024. *2024 Aboriginal and Torres Strait Islander Health Roundtable: Outcomes Report*

Luciano M et al, 2018. Personality, intelligence and genes. In M Kivimäki et al (Eds) *The Routledge International Handbook of Psychosocial Epidemiology*

Ludvigsson J F, 2023. How Sweden approached the COVID-19 pandemic: summary and commentary on the National Commission Inquiry. *Acta Paediatrica* 112(1)

Macedo S & Lee F, 2025. *In Covid's Wake: How Our Politics Failed Us*. Kindle Edition

MacKean C et al, 2024. *State of the Nation's Food Industry Report.* The Food Foundation

MacMahon T F & Pugh B (Eds) 1970. *Epidemiology: Principles and Methods.* Little Brown & Co: Boston

Magnusson R, 2016. Is obesity a disease?: legal implications. *Obesity Australia Summit Papers*

Maher P, 1999. A review of 'traditional' Aboriginal health beliefs. *Australian Journal of Rural Health* 7(4)

Malhotra A, 2022. Curing the pandemic of misinformation on COVID-19 mRNA vaccines through real evidence-based medicine - Part 1. *Journal of Insulin Resistance* 5(1)

Malhotra A, 2022. Curing the pandemic of misinformation on COVID-19 mRNA vaccines through real evidence-based medicine - Part 2. *Journal of Insulin Resistance* 5(1)

Malik V S et al, 2013. Global obesity: trends, risk factors and policy implications. *National Review of Endocrinology* 9(1)

Marmot M. 2016. Fair Australia: social justice and the health gap. *2016 Boyer Lectures*. Australian Broadcasting Commission

Martin J & Bright D, 2024. Australia's restrictive vaping and tobacco policies are fuelling a lucrative and dangerous black market. *The Conversation* 12 March

Marvanova M et al, 2011. Health literacy and medication understanding among hospitalized adults. *Journal of Hospital Medicine* 6(9)

Masters R et al, 2017. Return on investment of public health interventions: a systematic review. *Journal of Epidemiology Community Health* 71

Maxwell Parkin D & Bray F, 2005. Descriptive studies. In W Ahrens & I Pigeot

(Eds) *Handbook of Epidemiology*. Springer: London

Mazzocchi M & Traill W B, 2011. Calories, obesity and health in OECD countries. *Applied Economics* 43(26)

McCaw, J. 2024. *Submission to the Commonwealth Government Covid-19 Response Inquiry*

McCormack S W, 2010. Taking the good with the bad: recognizing the negative externalities created by charities and their implications for the charitable deduction. *Arizona Law Review* 52

McGonagle D G, 2022. Health-care workers recovered from natural SARS-CoV-2 infection should be exempt from mandatory vaccination edicts. *Lancet Rheumatol* (4)

McGorry P D et al, 2024. The Lancet Psychiatry Commission on youth mental health. *The Lancet Psychiatry* 11(9)

McGrath et al, 2007. The case for Aboriginal health workers in palliative care. *Australian Health Review* 31(3)

McKinsey Global Institute, 2014. Overcoming obesity: an initial economic analysis. *Discussion Paper*

Mclean H & Huf B, 2020. Emergency powers, public health and COVID-19. *Research Paper No. 2, August*. Research & Inquiries Unit Parliamentary Library & Information Service, Victorian Parliament

Mendoza-Jiménez M J, van Exel J & Brouwer W, 2024. On spillovers in economic evaluations: definition, mapping review and research agenda. *European Journal of Health Economics* 25(7)

Miao Z et al, 2013. Accounting for product substitution in the analysis of food taxes targeting obesity. *Health Economics* 22

Michon K, 2015. Tobacco litigation: history and recent developments. *NOLO* 30 December

Miles H et al, 2022. Describing and characterising on-demand delivery of unhealthy commodities in New Zealand. *Australian and New Zealand Journal of Public Health* 46(4)

Miller T A, 2016. Health literacy and adherence to medical treatment in chronic and acute illness: a meta-analysis. *Patient Education and Counseling* 99(7)

Mitchell S E et al, 2012. Health literacy and 30-day post discharge hospital utilization. *Journal of Health Communication* 17(3)

Mithen V et al, 2021. Aboriginal patient and interpreter perspectives on the delivery of culturally safe hospital-based care. *Health Promotion Journal of Australia* 32(S1)

Moens G, 2025. An abominable law. *Quadrant* 26 April

Moloney S, 2025. You can't say that! The Medical Board of Australia and other governors – whither freedom of speech and political communication for doctors, lawyers and the public? *Address to the Medico Legal Society of Victoria*. Melbourne Club 6 September

Morris P, 2025. Rebalancing diagnosis and clinical treatment: the contribution of NAPP to clinical discourse on youth gender medicine. *Proceedings: The Future of Youth Gender Medicine Seminar*. NSW Parliament House

Morrison J, 2014. *Social Licence: How To Keep Your Organisation Legitimate*. London: Palgrave McMillan

Morrison S, 2024. *Submission to the Commonwealth Government COVID-19 Response Inquiry*

Mouliou D S & Gourgoulianis K I, 2021. False-positive and false-negative COVID-19 cases: respiratory prevention and management strategies, vaccination, and further perspectives. *Expert Review of Respiratory Medicine* 15(8)

Mundy L K et al, 2023. Adolescents at risk of mental health problems in the COVID-19 pandemic: a prospective population-based study of the effects of government mandates and school closures. *Australian Journal of Social Issues* 58(1)

Murray R B et al, 2005. Sustaining remote-area programs: retinal camera use by Aboriginal health workers and nurses in a Kimberley partnership. *Medical Journal of Australia* 182(10)

Myers M et al, 2023. An ethical analysis of the arguments both for and against COVID-19 vaccine mandates for healthcare workers. *Journal of Emergency Medicine* 64(2)

Nakhimovsky S et al, 2016. Taxes on sugar-sweetened beverages to reduce overweight and obesity in middle-income countries: a systematic review. *PLoS ONE* 11(9)

Nasrullah M et al, 2017. Factors associated with condom use among sexually active U.S. adults, national survey of family growth, 2006–2010 and 2011–2013. *Journal of Sexual Medicine* 14(4)

National Aboriginal Community Controlled Health Organisation, 2025. *Key Facts February 2025*

National Disability Insurance Agency, 2024. *Annual Report 2023–24*

National Disability Insurance Scheme, 2024. *Quarterly Report*. December

National Disability Insurance Scheme, 2024. *Report to Disability Ministers Quarter 2 2024-25, Supplement*

National Disability Insurance Scheme, undated. *A Framework for Information, Linkages and Capacity Building*

National Disability Insurance Scheme Review, 2023. *Our Final Report: A Guide for People with Disability and Their Families*

National Drug and Alcohol Research Centre UNSW, 2025. Kava. *NDARC Fact Sheet*

National Suicide Prevention Office, 2025. *National Suicide Prevention Strategy 2025–2035*

New South Wales Auditor-General, 2013. *Cost of Alcohol Abuse to the NSW Government.* Auditor-General's Report Performance Audit

New South Wales Government, 2018. Forecasting future outcomes. *2018 Insights Report*

Norstrom T & Pape H, 2010. Alcohol, suppressed anger and violence. *Addiction* 105(9)

Nyberg T et al, 2022. Comparative analysis of the risks of hospitalisation and death associated with Sars-Cov-2 Omicron and Delta variants in England: a cohort study. *The Lancet* 399(10332)

Nyquist C B et al, 2025. Treatment trajectories among children and adolescents referred to the Norwegian National Center for Gender Incongruence. *Acta Paediatrica* 114

Obesity Australia, 2015. *Rethink Obesity: A Media Guide on How to Report on Obesity*, Sydney

Obesity Australia, 2013. *Action Agenda.* Sydney

O'Brien P & Waters E, 2021. COVID-19: public health emergency powers and accountability mechanisms in Australia. *Journal of Law and Medicine* 28(2)

O'Connor M, Adair T, Australian Medical Professionals Association, and Australians for Science and Freedom, 2024. Submissions to *Senate Standing Committees on Community Affairs Inquiry into Excess Mortality 2024*

O'Dea B et al, 2024. Breaking the cycle: effect of a multi-agency maternity service redesign on reducing the over-representation of Aboriginal and Torres Strait Islander newborns in out-of-home care: a prospective, non-randomised, intervention study in urban Australia. *Child Abuse & Neglect* 149(106664)

Olson K R et al, 2022. Gender identity 5 years after social transition. *Pediatrics* 150(2)

Ong J et al, 2012. Contraception matters: indicators of poor usage of contraception in sexually active women attending family planning clinics in Victoria, Australia. *BMC Public Health* 23(12)

Ong K et al, 2012. Differences in primary health care delivery to Australia's indigenous population: a template for use in economic evaluations. *BMC Health Services Research* 12(1)

Ooi J Y et al, 2021, A trial of a six-month sugar-sweetened beverage intervention in secondary schools from a socio-economically disadvantaged region in Australia. *Australian and New Zealand Journal of Public Health* 45(6)

Ophir Y et al, 2025. A step-by-step evaluation of the claim that COVID-19 vaccines saved millions of lives. *ResearchGate preprint*

Oster E, 2012. HIV and sexual behavior change: why not Africa? *Journal of Health Economics* 31(1)

Owen R, 1817. *Observations on the effect of the manufacturing system: with hints for the improvement of those parts of it which are most injurious to health and morals: dedicated most respectfully to the British legislature.* Second Edition. Multiple publishers: London

Parkinson P, 2025. Legal issues in treatment of minors. *Proceedings: The Future of Youth Gender Medicine Seminar.* NSW Parliament House

Parliament of Victoria, 2022. Transcript. *Pandemic Declaration Accountability and Oversight Committee Review of Pandemic Orders.* Melbourne, 31 January

Parliament of Victoria Public Accounts and Estimates Committee, 2024. *Vaping and Tobacco Controls*

Parry P, 2025. How did we get to where we are today? *Proceedings: The Future of Youth Gender Medicine Seminar.* NSW Parliament House

Pawson R, 2023. Do lockdowns work? Evidence from the UK. In P Eliadis, I Naidoo, & R Rist (Eds) *Policy Evaluation in the Era of COVID-19.* Taylor and Francis

Pearson O et al, 2020. Aboriginal community-controlled health organisations address health equity through action on the social determinants of health of Aboriginal and Torres Strait Islander peoples in Australia. *BMC Public Health* 20

Perkins A, 2016. *The Welfare Trait: How State Benefits Affect Personality.* Palgrave Macmillan

Pettigrew S et al, 2023. The inexorable rise of automated food deliveries and potential anticipatory policy actions. *Australian and New Zealand Journal of Public Health* 47(4)

Pezzullo A M, 2023. Age-stratified infection fatality rate of COVID-19 in the non-elderly population. *Environmental Research* 216(114655)

Pinker S, 2011. *The Better Angels of Our Nature: A History of Violence and Humanity* Penguin

Pinker S, 2003. *The Blank Slate: The Modern Denial of Human Nature.* Penguin 2019 Edition

Plomin R, 2018. *Blueprint: How DNA Makes Us Who We Are.* Penguin Random

House

Poirier B et al, 2025. The causes of the causes: Aboriginal and Torres Strait Islander oral health and the neoliberalisation of Australia's dental health system. *Humanities and Social Sciences Communications* 12

Price Waterhouse Coopers, 2015. *Weighing the Cost of Obesity: A Case for Action*

Productivity Commission, 2024. *Fairly Equal? Economic Mobility in Australia.* Research paper, Canberra

Productivity Commission, 2024. *Review of the National Agreement on Closing the Gap Study report: Supporting Paper Volume 2*

Productivity Commission, 2017. *NDIS Costs*

Productivity Commission, 2011. *Disability Care and Support*

Public Health Association of Australia, 2018. Top 10 public health successes over the last 20 years. *PHAA Monograph Series No. 2*

Queensland Health, 2023. *Chief Health Officer Public Health Directions and Revoked Public Health Directions*

Raciti M & Gibson C, 2025. A call to Indigenise occupational wellbeing. *Medical Journal of Australia* 222 (11)16 June

Radobuljac M D, 2024. ESCAP statement on the care for children and adolescents with gender dysphoria: an urgent need for safeguarding clinical, scientific, and ethical standards. *European Child & Adolescent Psychiatry* 33

Rajan R & Topp S M, 2022. Accountability mechanisms of inquiries and investigations into Australian governments' responses to the COVID-19 pandemic. *Australian and New Zealand Journal of Public Health* 46(4)

Rank C & Menzies R, 2007. How reliable are Australian childhood immunisation register coverage estimates for indigenous children? An assessment of data quality and coverage. *Communicable Diseases Intelligence* 31(3)

Redfern Legal Centre, 2024. *Submission to the Commonwealth Government Covid-19 Response Inquiry*

Revenue South Australia, *Wagering Tax Announcement.* 7 July 2016

Rickles D, 2011. Public health. In F. Gifford (Ed) *Handbook of the Philosophy of Science.* Volume 16. Elsevier: Netherlands

Ridd P, 2024. Trump's revolution is coming for the health technocrats. *The Australian* 5 December

Roberts C M et al, 2022. Continuation of gender-affirming hormones among transgender adolescents and adults. *The Journal of Clinical Endocrinology & Metabolism* 107(9)

Robson S, 2025. Drinking risks are real – women should know them. *The*

Australian 5 January

Room R & Mäkelä K, 2000. Typologies of the cultural position of drinking. *Journal of the Study of Alcohol* 61(3)

Rose G, 1992. *The Strategy of Preventive Medicine*. Oxford University Press: Oxford

Roseby R et al, 2019. Not just a policy; this is for real. An affirmative action policy to encourage Aboriginal and Torres Strait Islander peoples to seek employment in the health workforce. *Internal Medicine Journal* 49(7)

Rosen G, 1958. Industrialism and the sanitary movement (1830-1875). In G. Rosen, *A History of Public Health*. MD Publications: New York

Royal Australian College of General Practitioners, 2025. *Reaffirming our Commitment to the Uluru Statement from the Heart*. 13 June

Royal Commission into Violence, Abuse, Neglect and Exploitation of People with a Disability, 2023. *Final Report*

Russell L, 2009. Preventing chronic disease: an important investment, but don't count on cost savings. *Health Affairs* 28(1)

Sabhlok S, 2024. Non-pharmaceutical interventions should be approved by the drugs regulator – Parts 1 and 2. *The Times of India* December 24

Sánchez-Izquierdo M et al, 2023. Intelligence and life expectancy in late adulthood: a meta-analysis. *Intelligence* 98

Sarma S et al, 2014. The effect of physical activity on adult obesity: evidence from the Canadian NPHS panel. *Economics & Human Biology* 14

Scally G, 2014. Public health profession. *Encyclopedia of Health Economics* 3

Schonberger L B et al, 1979. Guillain-Barre syndrome following vaccination in the national influenza immunization program, United States, 1976–1977. *American Journal of Epidemiology* 110(2)

Scrimgeour M & Scrimgeour D, 2007. Health care access for Aboriginal and Torres Strait Islander people living in urban areas, and related research issues: a review of the literature. *Cooperative Research Centre for Aboriginal Health*, Darwin

Schwartz S, 2025. Cancer warning labels on wine? Put a cork in it. *The Australian* 4 January

Seddon N, 2007. *Who Cares? How State Funding and Political Activism Change Charity*. Civitas: Institute for the Study of Civil Society London

Sharp C A, 2023. *Submission to the Commonwealth Government COVID-19 Response Inquiry*

Shepherd S et al, 2020. Closing the (incarceration) gap: assessing the socio-economic and clinical indicators of indigenous males by lifetime incarceration status. *BMC Public Health* 20(1)

Sherry C, 2023. All about the land: the (mis)application of public health orders to strata schemes during the delta variant COVID-19 outbreak in Sydney, Australia. *Sydney Law Review* 45(2)

Shopping Centre Council of Australia, 2024. *Submission to the Commonwealth Government Covid-19 Response Inquiry*

Shrier A, 2021. *Irreversible Damage: Teenage Girls and the Transgender Craze*. Swift Press

Silva S J R, 2022. Viral load in COVID-19 patients: implications for prognosis and vaccine efficacy in the context of emerging SARS-CoV-2 variants. *Frontiers in Medicine* 8

Smith K, 2024. *Devastated: How Gender Ideology is Tearing Australian Families Apart*. Gender Awareness Australia Limited

Snowdon C, 2015. Death and taxes: why living longer costs money. Institute for Economic Affairs, *Discussion Paper* 67

Sorli A S, 2025. The discrepancy between the number of saved lives with COVID-19 vaccination and statistics of our world data. *Journal of Clinical Trials* S32(001)

South Australia Report of the Auditor General, 2023. *Gambling Harm Minimisation*

Sowell T, 2019. *Discrimination and Disparities*. Basic Books

Spencer J & Clarke P, 2025. AusPATH: activism influencing health policy. *Australasian Psychiatry* 33(2)

Spencer J, D'Angelo R & Clarke P, 2025. The Profession that failed. *Gender Clinic News* 29 August

Staszak J-F, 2020. Other/Otherness. In A Kobayashi (Ed) *International Encyclopedia of Human Geography* Second Edition. Elsevier: New York

St Vincent's Health Australia, 2016. *Restoring the Balance: A New Approach to Alcohol in Australia*. Melbourne: St. Vincent's Health Australia

Stein M, 2025. The Ozempic effect: how one drug reshaped health, hype and regulation in Australia. *Hall & Wilcox*

Stoked-Walker C, 2022. What do we know about COVID vaccines and preventing transmission? *British Medical Journal* 376

Strecker J, 2023. Pandemic survivors and the silent victims of excess mortality. *The Spectator* 6 January

Suicide Prevention Australia, 2025. *National Policy Platform*

Suraweera A, 2022. *Palmer v Western Australia*: pandemic border closures and section 92 of the Australian Constitution. *Sydney Law Review* 13 44(2)

Sutton B, 2024. Pandemic lessons learned and future public health strategies. *Microbiology Australia* 45(1)

Sutton P, 2006. Custom not in common: cultural relativism and customary law. *Macquarie Law Bulletin* 6

Swinburn B A et al, 2019. The global syndemic of obesity, undernutrition, and climate change: the Lancet Commission report. *Lancet* 393(10173)

Sy W, 2023. Early indication of long-term impact of COVID injections. *Medical & Clinical Research* 8(10)

Sydenstricker E, 1928. The statistician's place in public health work. *Journal of the American Statistical Association* 23(162)

Tasmanian Government Department of Health, 2023. *Healthy Tasmania Five-Year Strategic Plan 2022–2026 Report for Years 1 and 2*

Taylor J et al, 2023. Council of Academic Public Health Institutions Australasia, public health education for a sustainable future 'Call to Action', 2021. *Australian and New Zealand Journal of Public Health* 47(2)

Taylor K P et al, 2009. Exploring the impact of an Aboriginal health worker on hospitalised Aboriginal experiences: lessons from cardiology. *Australian Health Review* 33(4)

Telfer M M et al, 2020. *Australian Standards of Care and Treatment Guidelines for Trans and Gender Diverse Children and Adolescents*. Melbourne: Royal Children's Hospital version 1.3

Temple N, 2012. Why prevention can increase health-care spending. *European Journal of Public Health* 22(5)

Therapeutic Goods Administration, *$8 million of illicit vapes located in collaboration between TGA and Victoria Police*. 30 October 2024

Thomas K & Mcintyre A, 2025. Controlled by confidence: the unchecked power of AHPRA and the state. *The Spectator* 12 August

Thompson L & Kumar A, 2011. Responses to health promotion campaigns: resistance, denial and othering. *Critical Public Health* 21(1)

Tollit M A et al, 2021. The clinical profile of patients attending a large Australian pediatric gender service: a 10-year review. *International Journal of Transgender Health* 24(1)

Trewin D & Madden R, 2005. *The Health and Welfare of Australia's Aboriginal and Torres Strait Islander Peoples*. Australian Bureau of Statistics

Twenge J M, 2025. *Generations: The Real Differences Between Gen Z, Millennials, Gen X, Boomers, and Silents—and What They Mean for America's Future*. Atria Paperback

UK COVID Inquiry, 2025. *A Report by The Rt Hon The Baroness Hallett*

DBE, Chair of the UK Covid-19 Inquiry on the Core Decision-Making and Political Governance

United Nations, 2025. *Social Determinants Of Health: Key Facts*

United Nations, 2019. *Non-pharmaceutical Public Health Measures for Mitigating the Risk and Impact of Epidemic and Pandemic Influenza*

Unsafe and Defective, 2024. *Submission to the People's Vaccine Inquiry UK*

U.S. Department of Health and Human Services, 2025. *Treatment for Pediatric Gender Dysphoria: Review of Evidence and Best Practices*

U.S. House of Representatives, 2024. *Final Report of the Select Subcommittee on the Coronavirus Pandemic Committee on Oversight and Accountability*

van Baal et al, 2008. Lifetime medical costs of obesity: prevention no cure for increasing health expenditure. *PLOS Medicine*

Vandenbussche E, 2022. Detransition-related needs and support: a cross-sectional online survey. *Journal of Homosexuality* 69(9)

van der Loos M et al, 2022. Continuation of gender-affirming hormones in transgender people starting puberty suppression in adolescence: a cohort study in the Netherlands. *The Lancet Child & Adolescent Health* 6(12)

Van Scoy L J et al, 2022. 'Us-Versus-Them': othering in COVID-19 public health behavior compliance. *PLoS ONE* 17(1)

Veerman L et al, 2016. The impact of a tax on sugar-sweetened beverages on health and health care costs: a modelling study. *PLoS ONE* 11(4)

Victorian Equal Opportunity and Human Rights Commission, 2020. Human rights and Victoria's *COVID-19 Omnibus (Emergency Measures) Act* May 2020

Victorian Gambling and Casino Control Commission, *Gambling Data*

Victorian Ombudsman, 2020. *Investigation into the Detention and Treatment of Public Housing Residents Arising from a COVID-19 'Hard Lockdown' in July 2020*

Victorian State Government Department of Treasury and Finance, 2024. *Community Support Fund financial overview 2023-24*

von Unger H, Scott P & Odukoya D, 2019. Constructing im/migrants and ethnic minority groups as 'carriers of disease': power effects of categorization practices in tuberculosis health reporting in the UK and Germany. *Ethnicities* 19(3)

Vos T, Carter R & Barendregt J, 2010. *Assessing Cost-effectiveness in Prevention ACE: Prevention Final Report*. Brisbane: University of Queensland

Walter M, 2017. Doing Indigenous family. In M Walter, K Martin & G Bodkin-Andrews (Eds) *Indigenous Children Growing Up Strong: A Longitudinal*

Study of Aboriginal and Torres Strait Islander Families. Palgrave Macmillan

Warrier V et al, 2020. Elevated rates of autism, other neurodevelopmental and psychiatric diagnoses, and autistic traits in transgender and gender-diverse individuals. *Nature Communications* 11

Webb S, 1995. *Palaeopathology of Aboriginal Australians: Health and Disease Across a Hunter-gatherer Continent*. Cambridge University Press

Webster E et al, 2022. Building cultural responsiveness in a mainstream health organisation with '8 Aboriginal Ways of Learning': a participatory action research study. *Australian and New Zealand Journal of Public Health* 46

Weeramanthri T S et al, 2020. *Climate Health WA Inquiry: Final Report*. Department of Health, Government of Western Australia

West R, Usher K, & Foster K, 2010. Increased numbers of Australian Indigenous nurses would make a significant contribution to 'closing the gap' in Indigenous health: what is getting in the way? *Contemporary Nurse* 36(1–2)

West S, et al 2026. Weight regain after cessation of medication for weight management: systematic review and meta-analysis. *BMJ* 392:e085304

Wexler M, 2025. The shifting tide: part 1. *Democrats for an Informed Approach to Gender*. Substack

White H R, 1997. Longitudinal perspective on alcohol use and aggression during adolescence. *Recent Developments in Alcohol* 13

Whitehall J, 2025. A review of the physiology and side effects of puberty blockers and cross sex hormones, *Proceedings: The Future of Youth Gender Medicine Seminar*. NSW Parliament House

Whyte J, 2013. *Quack Policy Abusing Science in the Cause of Paternalism*. The Institute of Economic Affairs

Williams R, 1999. Cultural safety: what does it mean for our work practice? *Australian and New Zealand Journal of Public Health* 23(2)

Winsberg E & Harvard S, 2024. *Scientific Models and Decision Making, Elements in the Philosophy of Science*. Cambridge University Press

Winslow C E A, 1923. *The Evolution and Significance of the Modern Public Health Campaign*. Yale University Press: New Haven

Winter G, 2022. Nutrition and the surgical patient. *The Bulletin of the Royal College of Surgeons of England* 104(1)

Wolf G, 2023. How to manage a pandemic?: decision-making under the Public Health and Wellbeing Amendment (Pandemic Management) Act 2021 (Vic). *Journal of Law and Medicine* May

World Health Organization, 2025. Intergovernmental Negotiating Body to draft and negotiate a WHO convention, agreement or other international instrument on pandemic prevention, preparedness and response *Report by the Director-General 14 May*

World Health Organization, 2022. *WHO Calls on Countries to Tax Sugar-sweetened Beverages to Save Lives*

World Health Organization, 2020. *Coronavirus Disease (COVID-19) Serology, Antibodies and Immunity* 9 June 2020, 13 November 2020, 31 December 2020

World Health Organization, 2020. Advice on the Use of Masks in the Context of COVID-19. *Interim Guidance* 5 June

World Health Organization, 2020. *Report of the WHO-China Joint Mission on Coronavirus Disease 2019 (COVID-19)* 16-24 February

World Health Organization, 2019. *Global Influenza Program Non-Pharmaceutical Public Health Measures for Mitigating the Risk and Impact of Epidemic and Pandemic Influenza*

Wraw C et al, 2015. Intelligence in youth and health at age 50. *Intelligence* 53

Wucher M et al, 2024. *COVID-19 Spike Protein Pathogenicity Research Library*

Yoo J H, 2025. On the controversies surrounding the *Lab-Leak* theory of COVID-19. *Journal of Korean Medical Science* 40(16)

Zhang S et al, 2022. Why does COVID-19 continue to spread despite mass vaccination? *Frontiers in Public Health* Jul 25(10)

Zhu W, Bazzi S A & Bazzi A R, 2019. Behavioral changes following HIV seroconversion during the historical expansion of HIV treatment in the United States. *AIDS* 33(1)

Ziesing S et al, 2023. Is it time to increase the cost of tobacco licences after 10 years of stagnation? *Australian and New Zealand Journal of Public Health* 47(5)

www.ingramcontent.com/pod-product-compliance
Lightning Source LLC
LaVergne TN
LVHW052037200926
848481LV00005B/1708